STEM CELLS - LABORATORY AND CLINICAL RESEARCH

HEMATOPOIETIC STEM CELLS

NEW RESEARCH

STEM CELLS - LABORATORY AND CLINICAL RESEARCH

Additional books in this series can be found on Nova's website under the Series tab.

Additional E-books in this series can be found on Nova's website under the E-book tab.

STEM CELLS AND REGENERATIVE MEDICINE

Additional books in this series can be found on Nova's website under the Series tab.

Additional E-books in this series can be found on Nova's website under the E-book tab.

STEM CELLS - LABORATORY AND CLINICAL RESEARCH

HEMATOPOIETIC STEM CELLS

NEW RESEARCH

WESLEY G. MONTGOMERY
AND
HEATHER I. BURTON
EDITORS

New York

For permission to use material from this book please contact us:
Telephone 631-231-7269; Fax 631-231-8175
Web Site: http://www.novapublishers.com

Library of Congress Cataloging-in-Publication Data

Library of Congress Control Number: 2012942452

ISBN: 978-1-62257-468-1

Published by Nova Science Publishers, Inc. † New York

CONTENTS

Preface		**vii**
Chapter 1	Pulmonary Complications Following Hematopoietic Stem Cell Transplantation *Jihane Zaza Dit Yafawi, Emad S. Shehada and Ayman O. Soubani*	**1**
Chapter 2	Hematopoietic Stem Cells: Potential New Applications for Translational Medicine *Hady Felfly and Gabriel G. Haddad*	**51**
Chapter 3	Psychological Health and Adjustment of Families of Children Who Undergo Hematopoietic Stem Cell Transplantation *Marta Tremolada, Sabrina Bonichini and Marta Pillon*	**97**
Chapter 4	New Insights into the Immunogenetics of Unrelated Hematopoietic Stem Cell Transplantation for Thalassemia *G. Caocci, R. Littera, S. Orrù, C. Carcassi and G. La Nasa*	**117**
Chapter 5	Hematopoietic Stem Cell Therapy for Inflammatory Bowel Diseases *W. K. van Deen, G. M. Crooks and D. W. Hommes*	**135**
Chapter 6	Concise Review: Extramedullary Hematopoiesis Leading to the Production of a Novel Antigen-Presenting Cell Type in Murine Spleen *Rebecca A. Hinton and Helen C. O'Neill*	**151**
Index		**165**

PREFACE

Hematopoietic Stem Cell Transplantation (HSCT) is an established treatment for a variety of malignant and nonmalignant conditions. In autologous HSCT, the stem cells are collected from the patient then infused back after high dose chemotherapy. On the other hand, in allogeneic HSCT, the stem cells are donated from another individual (who may be related or unrelated and unmatched or matched). In this book, the authors present new research in the study of hematopoietic stem cells including pulmonary complications following HSCT; psychological health and adjustment of families of children who undergo HSCT; the immunogenetics of unrelated HSCT for thalassemia; HSCT for inflammatory bowel diseases; and extramedullary hematopoiesis leading to the production of a novel antigen-presenting cell type in the murine spleen.

Chapter 1 - Hematopoietic Stem Cell Transplantation (HSCT) is an established treatment for a variety of malignant and nonmalignant conditions. In autologous HSCT, the stem cells are collected from the patient then infused back after high dose chemotherapy. On the other hand, in allogeneic HSCT, the stem cells are donated from another individual (who may be related or unrelated and matched or unmatched). Despite significant advances, HSCT remains limited by significant complications related to conditioning regimen and graft versus host disease (GVHD) and its management. Pulmonary complications, infectious and noninfectious, are major cause of morbidity and mortality following HSCT. There are significant advances in the diagnosis, prophylaxis and treatment of infectious complications. However there are still challenges related to a variety of pulmonary infections such fungal and viral infections. The recent progress in management of infectious complications increased the significance of noninfectious pulmonary conditions. Acute lung injury due to diffuse alveolar hemorrhage or idiopathic pneumonia syndrome are the main acute complications, however bronchiolitis obliterans remains the most challenging late pulmonary complication facing clinicians who are taking care of HSCT recipients. This chapter provides a clinical update of the incidence, risk factors, pathogenesis, clinical characteristics and management of the main infectious and noninfectious pulmonary complications following HSCT.

Chapter 2 - Hematopoietic stem cells (HSC) are multipotent cells that produce the various lineages of blood and HSC transplantations (HSCT) are widely used to reconstitute damaged bone marrow (BM). Over time, HSCT has evolved for the treatment of non-blood diseases as well, brain in particular. However, HSCT required total myeloablation through irradiation and/or chemotherapy for the treatment of BM-related diseases, and HSCs are difficult to safely deliver in large amounts into the brain. In blood disorders, for a minimal myelosuppression to be sufficient and allow donor cells to engraft, it is necessary to determine the minimal percentage of normal BM cells needed to achieve phenotypic correction. Recent studies on animal models of β-thalassemia and sickle cell disease (SCD), through Competitive Repopulation Assay (CRA) following lethal irradiation of recipients, demonstrated that an average of 25% normal BM cells allows the production of enough normal red blood cells to significantly correct the β-thalassemia and SCD phenotypes, at the levels of BM, blood, histology, and survival, with normal donor cells contributing to 50-60% of peripheral red blood cells. Further assays using mild myelosuppression showed that long term sustained phenotypic correction can be obtained for both diseases through a novel transplantation strategy based on modulating four parameters: dose of irradiation/ myelosuppression, number of transplanted cells, timing of cell injections, and number of cell doses. Through a minimal dose of irradiation of 1Gy (100 Rads) or 2Gy, two injections of BM cells within the first 24h after myelosuppression resulted in engraftment in 100% of mice and a sustained therapeutic mixed chimerism in β-thalassemia, while three to four injections were needed to achieve a similar outcome in SCD. Following the success of these trials, we modified this novel HSCT strategy and applied it to determine whether we can protect mice from lethal stroke induced through the Middle Cerebral Artery Occlusion (MCAO). Ischemia/reperfusion resulted in a major infarct that propagated over time to encompass ~70% of the affected hemisphere. When two doses of HSCs were injected at 2h and 24h after the reperfusion, 40% of mice survived, visible neurological defects disappeared, and the infarct size was reduced by two to four fold. Histological examination of brains in surviving mice revealed very few donor cells in the recipient brains, decreased total neurons count and increased glial cell numbers. These data suggest that the neuro-protection was not dependent on cell-supplementation, but rather the protection is manifested likely through growth factor secretion. Combined, these studies create a novel HSCT approach that has proved efficient for the treatment of various disorders. A "window of opportunity" exists for each disease where the donor cells should be administered, and multiple injections of donor HSCs can rescue diseases that would otherwise not be treatable. We hypothesize that the initial injection primes the affected tissue, and subsequent ones help in repair. This new strategy has opened the way for a new era of HSCT for the potential treatments and possibly cures of many diseases.

Chapter 3 - *Background:* Having a child undergoing Hematopoietic Stem Cell Transplantation (HSCT) is a stressful and upsetting experience for parents.

Especially mothers have a key role in children's everyday adaptation to the transplantation experience and for this reason their psychological health has received comparatively large attention in the literature in different phases of medical treatment (pre-HSCT, during the isolation, post HSCT). The presence of a child undergoing HSCT in the family may place also siblings at risk for psychological difficulties.

Aims: This chapter reviews the research published in the last 20 years on the psycho-social health and adaptation of parents and siblings of children who have undergone HSCT.

Method: Articles were found using four electronic databases (PubMed, PsycINFO, Web of Science and SCOPUS) employing various search strategies: the search terms used included MeSH, headings, text words, or keywords relevant to the following terms: "QoL," "adaptation," "psychology," "HSCT", "parents" and "siblings". The search was limited to English-language literature published in the last 20 years and to those articles including families of patients who received any type of HSCT as children.

Results: A corpus of 38 empirical studies was selected and will be presented here. From this selection three main topics emerged: psychological health and adaptation of parents of children undergoing HSCT (N=24); psychosocial adjustment of siblings of HSCT patients (N=8); psychosocial interventions for families of children undergoing HSCT (N=8, 2 of which also included in the second topic).

The information emerged from the review of the literature will be discussed with special attention to methodological issues and directions for future research will be proposed.

Chapter 4 - Beta-thalassemia major, also known as Cooley's anemia, is designated by the World Health Organization (WHO) as one of the world's most common inherited genetic blood disorders. Although regular transfusions of red blood cells can correct the anemia and effectively suppress the ineffective erythropoiesis, patients will eventually develop some of the typical clinical complications of iron overload such as cardiac dysfunction, liver disease and impairment of the endocrine system. Allogeneic hematopoietic stem cell transplantation (HSCT) is currently the only treatment potentially capable of liberating patients from the weight of chronic lifelong transfusion therapy. The first successful bone marrow transplantation (BMT) for beta thalassemia major was performed in Seattle, Washington in 1981. Since then, enormous progress has been made, and estimates for overall survival (OS) and thalassemia-free survival (TFS) now range from 70%-95% and 65%-90%, respectively, depending upon the patient's age and clinical conditions before HSCT. The parallel availability of an international network of voluntary stem cell donor registries has significantly increased the odds of being able to find a suitable human leukocyte antigen (HLA) matched donor for patients lacking a compatible family donor. Graft versus host disease (GVHD) remains a prominent cause of death and morbidity following HSCT. The complex mechanisms that mediate induction of donor-specific tolerance and facilitate engraftment have tempted many investigators. Scientific studies conducted in recent years have uncovered a correlation between certain immunogenetic variables and the occurrence of GVHD which is bound to lead to considerable improvement in donor selection criteria. This review addresses some of the most intriguing new findings within this field.

Chapter 5 - Inflammatory bowel diseases (IBD) are chronic debilitating inflammatory disorders of potentially any part of the gastrointestinal tract, leading to various intestinal but also extra-intestinal symptoms. It is thought that dysregulation of the normally controlled immune response to commensal bacteria in genetically susceptible patients drives the disease. Although medical therapy for IBD has improved due to an extensive repertoire of immunosuppressive drugs and the introduction of anti tumor necrosis factor-α (TNFα) compounds, the clinical course of the disease cannot be adequately controlled in a substantial group of patients. More than half of the patients require one or more surgical resections during the course of the disease. Therefore, there is an unmet need for more effective therapeutic strategies.

Evidence that hematopoietic stem cell transplantation (HSCT) would be an effective treatment for autoimmune diseases firstly came from several animal models and from incidental case reports on HSCT recipients with coexistent autoimmune disease. Already more than 15 years ago a case report on the positive effect of HSCT on active IBD was published, followed by many others showing improvement of the clinical course of disease after HSCT indicated for other diseases. In the last couple of years, various cases have been reported of successful remission induction of patients with (therapy refractory) Crohn's disease (CD) by means of an autologous HSCT. The most extensive experience on autologous

HSCT applied specifically for CD has been reported by the group of Oyama. All treated patients went into remission with a Crohn's Disease Activity Index (CDAI) score of <150. There was no inpatient mortality and neutropenic fever was the most important complication. Recently published long-term follow follow-up data showed a clinical relapse-free survival of 57% at 3 years and 19% at 5 years. The percentage of patients in remission (CDAI<150), steroid free, or medication free at any post-transplant evaluation interval over 5 years post-transplant was 70%, 80% and 60%, respectively.

Although the observed benefit is remarkable, the exact mechanism behind this 'resetting' of the immune system needs to be elucidated. Although the prolonged T cell depletion will probably add to the therapeutic benefit, the thymus most likely plays a dominant role in resetting the T cell repertoire in IBD patients. This chapter will review the evidence for HSCT for IBD and discuss potential mechanisms of HSCT important for clinical benefit.

Chapter 6 - The concept of extramedullary hematopoiesis for production of organ-specific antigen presenting cells has importance in immunity in terms of the compartmentalisation of the immune response in different tissue sites. A new and distinct dendritic-like antigen presenting cell subtype is described which is dependent on the spleen microenvironment for development. Cells arise by a unique developmental pathway distinct from other dendritic cells (DC). In particular, a self-renewing progenitor of these cells has been identified in spleen upstream of the earliest DC progenitor currently identified in bone marrow. This progenitor depends on the splenic microenvironment for maintenance and proliferation, adding further support for spleen as a site for hematopoiesis.

In: Hematopoietic Stem Cells: New Research ISBN 978-1-62257-468-1
Editors: Wesley G. Montgomery and Heather I. Burton

Chapter 1

PULMONARY COMPLICATIONS FOLLOWING HEMATOPOIETIC STEM CELL TRANSPLANTATION

Jihane Zaza Dit Yafawi, Emad S. Shehada and Ayman O. Soubani*

Division of Pulmonary, Critical Care and Sleep Medicine
Karmanos Cancer Center and Wayne State University School of Medicine, Detroit, MI, US

ABSTRACT

Hematopoietic Stem Cell Transplantation (HSCT) is an established treatment for a variety of malignant and nonmalignant conditions. In autologous HSCT, the stem cells are collected from the patient then infused back after high dose chemotherapy. On the other hand, in allogeneic HSCT, the stem cells are donated from another individual (who may be related or unrelated and matched or unmatched). Despite significant advances, HSCT remains limited by significant complications related to conditioning regimen and graft versus host disease (GVHD) and its management. Pulmonary complications, infectious and noninfectious, are major cause of morbidity and mortality following HSCT. There are significant advances in the diagnosis, prophylaxis and treatment of infectious complications. However there are still challenges related to a variety of pulmonary infections such fungal and viral infections. The recent progress in management of infectious complications increased the significance of noninfectious pulmonary conditions. Acute lung injury due to diffuse alveolar hemorrhage or idiopathic pneumonia syndrome are the main acute complications, however bronchiolitis obliterans remains the most challenging late pulmonary complication facing clinicians who are taking care of HSCT recipients. This chapter provides a clinical update of the incidence, risk factors, pathogenesis, clinical characteristics and management of the main infectious and noninfectious pulmonary complications following HSCT.

---

* Correspondence to Ayman O. Soubani, MD. Professor of Medicine, Wayne State University School of Medicine, Chief, Pulmonary and Critical Care Service, Karmanos Cancer Center, Medical Director, Medical ICU, Harper University Hospital, 3990 John R- 3 Hudson, Detroit, MI 48201. Tel: 313-745-8471; Fax: 313-993-0562; asoubani@med.wayne.edu.

INTRODUCTION

Hematopoietic stem cell transplantation (HSCT) is a treatment option for several malignant and nonmalignant disorders [1]. In autologous HSCT, the stem cells are collected from the patient then infused back after high dose chemotherapy. In allogeneic HSCT, the stem cells are donated from another individual (who may be related or unrelated and matched or unmatched). The hematopoietic stem cells may be obtained from bone marrow or peripheral blood, or harvested from umbilical cord blood. Allogeneic HSCT is further classified according to the intensity of the conditioning regimen. In myeloablative regimen, supralethal doses of chemotherapy with or without irradiation are given, leading to significant toxicity and immunosuppression._More recently, nonmyeloablative regimens have been used to extend transplant to older patients and those with co-morbidities.

Despite the advances in HSCT, the procedure remains limited by the high rate of severe complications that are generally related to toxicity of conditioning regimen, immunosuppression, and graft-vs.-host disease (GVHD). Pulmonary complications following HSCT both infectious and noninfectious develop in up to 60% of patients and are a significant cause of morbidity and mortality (Table 1) [2]. These complications tend to follow a characteristic sequence, and are more common following allogeneic HSCT especially in the setting of GVHD (Figure 1) [2].

Table 1. Spectrum and frequency of respiratory infectious and noninfectious complication following HSCT [2]

Disease	Autologous	Allogeneic
Infectious		
- Bacteria	++	++
- Mycobacteria	+/-	+
- Nocardia	+/-	+
- Aspergillus	+	++
- Non-aspergillus fungal	+/-	+
- P jiroveci	+/-	+
- CMV	+	++
- Community respiratory viruses	+/-	+
Non-infectious		
- Pulmonary edema	++	++
- Engraftment syndrome	++	+
- Diffuse alveolar hemorrhage	+	++
- Idiopathic pneumonia syndrome	+	++
- Delayed pulmonary toxicity syndrome	++	+
- Bronchiolitis obliterans organizing pneumonia	+	+
- Bronchiolitis obliterans	+/-	++

++ = high incidence (>10%), + = low incidence (<10%), +/- = very rare (<1%).

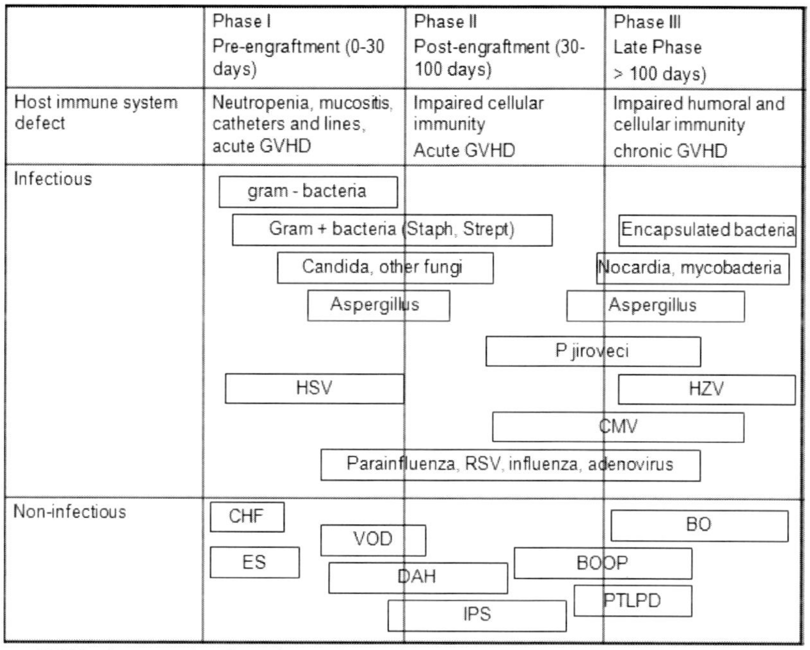

Abbreviations: HSV= herpes simplex virus, HZV= herpes zoster virus, CMV= cytomegalovirus, RSV= respiratory syncytial virus, CHF= congestive heart failure, BO= bronchiolitis obliterans, VOD= veno-occlusive disease, ES= engraftment syndrome, DAH= diffuse alveolar hemorrhage, BOOP= bronchiolitis obliterans organizing pneumonia, IPS= idiopathic pneumonia syndrome, PTLPD= post transplant lymphoproliferative disorder.

Figure 1. The time line of the main pulmonary complications following HSCT [2, 3, 4, 5].

Table 2. Factors that predispose to respiratory infections following HSCT [2]

Pre-transplantation
- older age
- pre-transplant immune status
- underlying pulmonary disease
- CMV status of the donor and recipient
- residence in endemic areas

Transplantation
- allogeneic
- type and intensity of conditioning regimen
- total body irradiation
- delayed engraftment

Post-transplantation
- mucositis
- severity and duration of neutropenia
- acute GVHD and its treatment
- chronic GVHD and its treatment
- T-cell depleting strategies
- hospital environment (construction, type of air filtration, transmission of infection by healthcare providers)

Infectious Pulmonary Complications Following HSCT

Despite the advances in prophylaxis and treatment of respiratory infections, they remain a cause of death in more than 40% of HSCT recipients [2]. Table 2 summarizes the general factors that predispose to respiratory infections following HSCT.

Bacterial Pneumonia

Bacterial pneumonia accounts for 15% of all respiratory infections in HSCT recipients with mortality rate around 22% [6, 7, 8].

Risk factors include pre-transplantation immune status, type of conditioning regimen, degree and duration of neutropenia [9]. Allogeneic HSCT and the presence of GVHD significantly increase the risk of bacterial pneumonia due to slower reconstitution of the immune system, impairment of the reticuloendothelial system, and opsonization9.

HSCT recipients are at highest risk for bacterial pneumonia in the pre-engraftment phase within the first 30 days following transplantation. Factors that increase the risk of bacterial pneumonia in this phase are neutropenia, mucositis as well as indwelling catheters that predispose to bacteremia and septic embolization to the lungs [10].

Patients may present with neutropenic fever with no localizing symptoms and signs due to blunted inflammatory response [11]. Radiological signs may be scarce. The chest radiograph usually shows focal consolidation, however may be normal. The infiltrates may progress quickly to multifocal or diffuse changes compatible with ARDS. HRCT of the chest may show pulmonary infiltrates in up to 50% of patients with negative chest radiograph and is recommended in febrile neutropenic patients [12, 13].

Identification of the causative microorganism may be difficult especially during the pre-engraftment period due to colonization of respiratory airways or contamination of respiratory specimens by upper airways organisms. The main organisms identified in the pre-engraftment phase are gram negative bacteria such as pseudomonas, klebseilla, and enterobacter [10, 14, 15, 16]. There is an increasing incidence of gram positive bacteria such as S. Aureus, E. Faecium, and α- hemolytic streptococcus which may be associated with septic shock and ARDS. Anaerobic organisms may be causative agents in the case of aspiration. Broad spectrum antibiotics with activity against pseudomonas and gram positive cocci should be started immediately in all patients suspected to have bacterial pneumonia during this phase [13].

Bacterial pneumonia is less common in the post-engraftment period. Allogeneic HSCT with acute GVHD increase the risk [11, 18]. The clinical and radiological picture is usually classical for bacterial pneumonia. Invasive pseudomonas infection and legionella pneumonia have been reported during this period. Risk factors for poor outcome following invasive pseudomonas include the presence of co-pathogens and high dose corticosteroid therapy [17].

After the first 100 days, the risk of bacterial pneumonia is generally low except in patients with chronic GHVD, commonly due to encapsulated organisms such as S. Pneumoniae and H. Influenza. Gram negative organisms may be the etiology in up to 25% of patients 6, 9, 10, 19]. Pneumococcal vaccine breakthrough has also been reported [20]. The infection occurs a mean of 433 +/- 669 days post-transplantation. It is more common in patients with lymphoma and those on high dose corticosteroid therapy. The one year survival of these patients is around 70% [19].

Table 3. Suggested prophylactic options against respiratory infections following HSCT [23]

Infection	First choice	Alternate choice	Comments
Bacteria (general) Pneumococcus H. Influenza	- IVIG - pneumococcal vaccine at 12, 24months - Hib vaccine at 12, 14, 24 months	- Penicillin VK - Fluoroquinolone - TMP-SMZ	IVIG only if IgG level < 400 mg/dl
Mycobacteria	Isoniazid 300mg/day		9 month therapy Add pyridoxine 25-50mg daily
Aspergillus	Posaconazole 200mg three times daily	- Voriconazole - Itraconazole - Echinocandins	
Candida	Fluconazole 400mg/day orally or IV	- Echinocandins	Until engraftment and during neutropenia
P. Jiroveci	TMP/SMX I double strength tablet/day or 3 times/wk	- Dapsone - Aerosolized pentamidine	From engraftment for 6 months and during immunosuppressive therapy for GVHD
CMV	Gancyclovir 5mg/kg/dose bid for 7-14 days, followed by 5 mg/kg/day for 5 day/wk	- Foscarnet - Valgancyclovir	Until day 100 or for a minimum of 3 wks. Monitor CMV antigen for duration of treatment
RSV	RSV IVIG 750 mg/kg/month	Aerosolized ribavirin	Based on pediatric HSCT during the high season months
Influenza	Lifelong annual seasonal Influenza vaccine before HSCT, and restarting 6 months after HSCT	- Rimantadine - Amantadine	
Herpes	Acyclovir 200mg orally 3 times/day or 250mg/m2/dose bid intravenously	Valacyclovir	Until engraftment or day 30
HZV	HZ IG 625 U IM		

Empiric broad spectrum antibiotics should be started immediately when bacterial pneumonia is suspected following HSCT. The American Thoracic Society guidelines for the treatment of healthcare associated pneumonia in patients with risk factors such as HSCT or neutropenia recommend a regimen that includes antipseudomonal cephalosporin or carbapenem, or B-lactam plus antipseudomonal fluoroquinolone, or aminoglycoside plus linezolid or vancomycin if methicillin resistant S. Aureus is suspected. In patients who develop bacterial pneumonia late following HSCT, coverage of encapsulated organisms with a fluoroquinolone is recommended. The antibiotic regimen should be narrowed if the etiologic agent is identified [21, 22].

Prophylactic measures against bacterial pneumonia include intravenous immunoglobulins in allogeneic HSCT recipients with low IgG level [23] (Table 3). Antibiotics with activity against encapsulated organisms are recommended during the treatment of chronic GVHD, however it should be noted that the routine use of prophylactic fluoroquinolones in the early post-transplant phase may be associated with increased infections due to coagulase negative staphylococci and gram negative rods resistant to fluoroquinolones [24].

Nocardia Pneumonia

Nocardia infection in HSCT recipients is rare with an incidence ranging between 0.3-1.7% [25, 26], almost always affecting allogeneic HSCT recipients on treatment for severe GVHD. The infection occurs a median of 210 days following transplantation. The main predisposing factors are neutropenia, active acute or chronic GVHD and lack of prophylaxis with trimethoprim- Sulfamethoxezole (TMP-SMZ). Most infections are caused by N. Astroides. Pulmonary involvement occurs in 56% of patients and the most common radiological findings are nodules with or without infiltrates. The diagnosis of nocardia pneumonia is usually made by BAL, although occasionally the organism is detected by culture of sputum or tracheal secretions. The diagnosis can be confirmed by CT guided aspirate of a pulmonary nodule or open lung biopsy. In about third of patients there is co-infection with other organisms such as CMV and Aspergillus.

Treatment of nocardia infection is by prolonged administration of TMP-SMZ. Second line agents include amikacin, minocycline, cephalosporin or imipenem. Response to treatment is generally good, and long term survival in patients with nocardiosis is not significantly different from controls [26]. Prophylaxis against P. Jiroveci using low dose TMP-SMZ has an added benefit of reducing the incidence of nocardia infection in HSCT recipients.

Mycobacterial Infection

Mycobacterium tuberculosis is reported in 0.4-5.5% of HSCT recipients [27-32], and is a concern in endemic areas or in patients who lived in an endemic area prior to HSCT. The prevalence of TB in autologous HSCT is similar to the general population but increases 3 folds in allogeneic HSCT recipients [28].

TB occurs in only 2% of infections developing during neutropenia, 23% during the first 100 days post-transplantation, and 75% after the first 100days [32]. The median time for TB infection is 324 days [28]. The main risk factors are allogeneic transplantation, total body irradiation, chronic GVHD, corticosteroid therapy and residence in endemic areas [28-32]. The clinical and radiological picture of TB infection in HSCT recipients is similar to non-transplant patients; however atypical presentations including rapidly progressive disease can be seen [33].

Treatment is similar to non-transplant patients; however rifampin should be avoided because of potential interaction with commonly used medications in these patients such as fluconazole and calcineurin inhibitors [13, 34]. Some studies suggest a full one year of treatment [32]. It is important to mention in this context that treatment of latent TB is indicated in patients with Tuberculin skin test showing 5 mm or more induration and in patients with significant exposure to patients with active TB infection even with a negative tuberculin skin test [13].

Nontuberculous mycobacterial infections (such as M. Avium complex, M. Kansasii, M. Chelonae) are rare in HSCT recipients, occurring in less than 1% of all patients with about half the infections in patients with GVHD [35]. The median time to diagnosis of nontuberculous mycobacteria is 4 months. The infection usually resolves with medical therapy and the attributed mortality is 7.5% [35].

It is known that nontuberculous mycobacteria colonize the airways of patients with chronic lung disease which may create a challenge in determining the significance of isolating them from lower respiratory tract samples of HSCT recipients. The diagnostic criteria of pulmonary nontuberculous mycobacteria infection were detailed in published guidelines and should include signs and symptoms compatible with the diagnosis and isolation of nontuberculous mycobacteria from respiratory tract specimen or other body tissues [36,37]. In the case of Mycobacterium Avium Intracellulare, first line agents include clarithromycin, azithormycin, ethambutol, rifampin, and rifabutin for 18 months and 12 months negative culture.

Invasive Pulmonary Apergillosis

Invasive pulmonary aspergillosis (IPA) is a major problem following HSCT due to neutropenia and defects in T-helper cell function. There is a steady rise in the documented cases of IPA post-transplantation. The risk for IPA is much higher following allogeneic HSCT when compared to autologous HSCT (incidence is 2.3-15% and 0.5-4% respectively) [38-42]. After autologous HSCT, IPA is mainly seen during the neutropenic phase. In allogeneic HSCT, the highest risk is in patients with severe GVHD (grade III-IV). The probability of IPA is approximately 5% at 2 months, 9% at 6 months, and 10% at 1 year following allogeneic HSCT. By the third year after transplantation, further increase in probability of IPA is minimal [40]. In these patients, the timeline for IPA infection follows a bimodal distribution, with a peak in the first month following HSCT, which is associated with neutropenia and the second peak is during the treatment for GVHD (median 78-112 days post-transplantation) [39, 41, 43]. The first peak is currently less significant due to the routine use of stem cell instead of bone marrow for transplantation, the use of non-myeloablative regimens, the use of colony stimulating factors during neutropenia, and the widespread use of antifungal agents [39, 44]. On the other hand, the incidence of IPA during the treatment of GVHD has become more significant especially with higher incidence of GVHD associated with unrelated allogeneic transplantation and non-myeloablative HSCT. Cord blood HSCT is also associated with increased risk of IPA which usually happens in the first 100 days post-transplantation (median 20 days) [45].

Other risk factors for IPA include the use of Alemutuzumab, an anti-DC52 monoclonal antibody used to deplete peripheral B and T lymphocytes [39, 40, 42], treatment of GVHD with intensive immunosuppressive therapy including corticosteroids, cyclosporine A, and anti-TNF- α agents and CMV infection [39-41, 46-49].

Patients present with symptoms that are usually non-specific and consistent with bronchopneumonia with fever unresponsive to antibiotics, cough, sputum production, and dyspnea. Patients may also present with pleuritic chest pain (due to vascular invasion leading to small pulmonary infarcts) and hemoptysis which is usually mild but could be massive. IPA is one of the most common causes of hemoptysis in neutropenic patients and has been reported to be associated with cavitation that occurs with neutrophil recovery [54]. Aspergillus infection may disseminate and spread hematogenously to other organs most commonly the brain (leading to seizures, ring-enhancing lesions, cerebral infarctions, intracranial hemorrhage, meningitis, and epidural abscess), and less frequently the skin, kidneys, pleura, heart, esophagus, and liver [50-53, 55].

The diagnosis of IPA is challenging. Early diagnosis in HSCT recipients remains difficult and high index of suspicion is necessary in patients with risk factors for invasive disease. Histopathological diagnosis by examining lung tissue obtained by thoracoscopic or open lung biopsy remains the "gold standard" for the diagnosis of IPA56. The presence of septate acute branching hyphae invading the lung tissue samples along with a positive culture for Aspergillus from the same site are diagnostic of IPA. The histopathological findings associated with IPA have been recently shown to differ according to the underlying host. In patients with allogeneic HSCT and GVHD there is intense inflammation with neutrophilic infiltration, minimal coagulation necrosis, and low fungal burden; while in neutropenic patients, IPA is characterized by scant inflammation, extensive coagulation necrosis associated with hyphal angioinvasion, and high fungal burden. Dissemination to other organs is equally high in both groups [57].

The chest radiograph has small role in early stages of the disease because the incidence of non-specific changes is high. Usual findings include rounded densities, pleural-based infiltrates that are suggestive of pulmonary infarctions, and cavitations. Pleural effusions are uncommon [58, 59]. Chest CT, especially when combined with high resolution images (HRCT), is a much more helpful tool in the diagnosis of IPA. The routine use of chest HRCT early in the course of IPA leads to earlier diagnosis and improved outcome of these patients [60, 61, 62]. The typical chest CT findings include ill defined consolidation (48%), nodules with halo sign (44%), centrilobular nodules (44%), ground glass attenuation (22%), and pleural effusion (26%) [65, 66]. The halo sign is mainly seen in neutropenic patients early in the course of infection (usually in the first week), and appears as a zone of low attenuation due to hemorrhage surrounding the pulmonary nodule. The air crescent sign, which represents crescent-shaped lucency in the region of the original nodule secondary to necrosis is another late radiological sign [59, 63]. Both, the halo and the air crescent signs are neither sensitive nor pathognomonic of IPA [64].

In HSCT recipients, isolating Aspergillus species from sputum is highly predictive of invasive disease with a positive predictive value of 80-90% [67-69]. However, negative sputum samples don't rule out IPA [69, 70]. Blood cultures are rarely positive [71].

Bronchoscopy with BAL is generally helpful in the diagnosis of IPA, especially in patients with diffuse lung involvement. The sensitivity and specificity of a positive result of BAL are around 50% and 97% respectively. This yield of BAL in the diagnosis of IPA is not consistent, and there are reports of much lower diagnostic yield [67, 68, 72-76]. Transbronchial biopsies usually do not add much to the diagnosis and are associated with increased risk of bleeding, so they are usually not performed [67].

The most recent advances in the diagnosis of IPA are related to detecting Aspergillus antigens in body fluids. Galactomannan (GM) is a polysaccharide cell-wall component that is released by Aspergillus during growth. A double sandwich ELISA for the detection of serum GM was approved by the Food and Drug Administration for the diagnosis of IPA, with a threshold of 0.5 ng/ml with 71% sensitivity and 89% specificity [86-90]. Serum GM can be detected several days before the presence of clinical signs, an abnormal chest radiograph, or positive culture. Thus, GM detection may allow earlier confirmation of the diagnosis and serial determination of serum GM values may be useful in assessing the evolution of infection during treatment [83, 84].

Serum GM assay is more useful in patients who have hematological malignancy or who have undergone allogeneic HSCT than in solid-organ transplant recipients or nonneutropenic patients. Furthermore, BAL Galactomannan assay can add to the sensitivity of serum GM and to other diagnostic methods [85, 91-94]. In patients with hematologic malignancies and patients following HSCT, the sensitivity and specificity of BAL GM in diagnosing proven or probable IPA are 73% and 89% respectively when using a cutoff of ≥0.5 and 67% and 95% respectively when using a cutoff of ≥0.85 [85].

Polymerase chain reaction (PCR) is another way to diagnose IPA by the detection of Aspergillus DNA in BAL fluid and serum. A positive Aspergillus PCR in BAL fluid has an estimated sensitivity of 67%-100% and specificity between 55% and 95% [95]. PCR sensitivity and specificity have also been reported at 100% and 65%-92% respectively in serum samples [95-98]. However this test is often associated with false positive results because it doesn't discriminate between colonization and infection. Detection of serum (1→3)-β-D-glucan, a fungal cell wall constituent has recently received Food and Drug Administration approval. Determination of plasma (1→3)-β-D-glucan has been reported to be a highly sensitive and specific test for invasive deep mycosis, including candidiasis, fusariosis, and aspergillosis, and could be useful in immunocompromised patients [99]. However, the utility of this assay in allogeneic HSCT recipients at high risk for IPA is not yet defined. The EORTC/ MSG has proposed several criteria for the diagnosis of invasive fungal infections [100]. These criteria consist of host factors, microbiologic, minor and major clinical criteria (Table 4). These criteria are meant to serve as a guide for clinical and epidemiological research, and need not be present in every patient to treat for IPA.

The treatment of IPA is difficult and mortality rate is still high despite the introduction of several new antifungal agents. Therapy should be considered as soon as there is a clinical suspicion of IPA, and while a workup is underway. For many years, amphotericin B has been the first line of therapy for IPA. The recommended dose is 1 to 1.5 mg/kg/day. Amphotericin B is known to cause serious side effects including nephrotoxicity, electrolyte disturbances, and hypersensitivity. For these reasons, newer lipid-based preparations of amphotericin B (e.g. liposomal amphotericin B and lipid complex amphotericin B) have been introduced. Voriconazole is a new broad-spectrum triazole which is approved as the initial treatment of invasive aspergillosis, and is currently considered the treatment of choice [101-104]. It is available in both intravenous and oral formulations. The recommended dose is 6 mg/kg twice daily intravenously on day one followed by 4 mg/kg/day. After seven days, switching to 200mg orally twice daily may be considered. Voriconazole has a milder side effect profile, and is much better tolerated than amphotericin B. The most frequent adverse effect is visual disturbances described as blurred vision, photophobia, and altered color perception. Liver function test abnormalities and skin reactions are less common side effects [101].

Table 4. The Diagnostic Criteria for IPA [100]

Diagnosis	Criteria
Proven IPA	Histopathologic or cytopathologic examination of lung tissue showing hyphae from needle aspiration or biopsy specimen with evidence of associated tissue damage; *OR* Positive culture result for Aspergillus from a sample obtained by sterile procedure from the lung and clinically or radiologically abnormal site consistent with infection
Probable IPA	Host risk factor; *AND* Microbiological criteria (positive Aspergillus microscopy or culture from the sputum or BAL, or positive GM assay); *AND* Clinical criteria consistent with the infection (1 major or 2 minor)*
Possible IPA	Host risk factor; *AND* Microbiological criteria (positive Aspergillus microscopy or culture from the sputum or BAL, or positive GM assay); *OR* Clinical criteria consistent with the infection (1 major or 2 minor)*

* Major clinical criteria are: new characteristic infiltrates on CT imaging (halo sign, air-crescent sign, or cavity within area of consolidation). Minor Clinical criteria are: Symptoms of LRTI (cough, chest pain, hemoptysis, or dyspnea); physical finding of pleural rub; any new infiltrate not fulfilling major criterion; pleural effusion.

Posaconazole is another broad-spectrum triazole that is effective and safe as salvage therapy in patients with invasive aspergillosis refractory to standard antifungal therapy [82, 105, 106].

Echinocandin derivatives such as caspofungin, micafungin, and anidulafungin are effective agents in the treatment of IPA refractory to standard treatment and can be used as second line agents or as in combination therapy [107-114].

Surgical resection has a limited role in the management of patients with IPA; however it should be considered in cases of massive hemoptysis, or pulmonary lesions close to the great blood vessels or pericardium, or for resection of residual localized pulmonary lesions in patients with continuing immunosuppression [61, 115-120].

Immunomodulatory therapy such as colony stimulating factors (i.e. granulocyte-colony stimulating factors, granulocyte macrophage-colony stimulating therapy) or interferon-γ could be used to decrease the degree of immunosuppression, as an adjunct to antifungal therapy for the treatment of IPA [121-127]. There is a concern about the use of interferon-γ in allogeneic HSCT recipients, since it may worsen GVHD, however a recent trial showed that GVHD may actually improve during this therapy [128, 129]. Granulocyte transfusion is another potential supportive therapy for patients with prolonged neutropenia and life-threatening infections refractory to conventional therapy130. Additionally, it is important in patients with IPA, whenever possible, to decrease the dose of systemic corticosteroids and immunosuppressive agents.

The management of IPA is difficult, so prophylaxis is an important approach for those patients at increased risk. Avoiding hospitalization of patients in construction areas and the use of high-efficiency particulate air (HEPA) filtration with or without laminar air flow ventilation have proven to be efficient [131]. Itraconazole Is effective in preventing fungal infections in neutropenic patients and posaconazole is effective in the prophylaxis against IPA in patients with severe GVHD and other hematological malignancies [132-134].

While A.fumigatus is the most common cause of IPA, there are increasing reports of IPA in cancer patients due to other species such as A.niger, A.terreus and A.flavus [77-81]. Some of these species (such as A.terreus and A.nidulans) are resistant to amphotericin B [78, 81]. A.terreus is the second most common species isolated with frequency of 23%. The risk factors and outcome for A.terreus infection are similar to those for A.fumigatus infection, however the former is significantly more likely to be nosocomial in origin, and more likely to be resistant to amphotericin B [80]. The new triazole antifungal agents such as voriconazole and posaconazole have significantly better efficacy against A.terreus [78, 79, 82].

Other Fungal Infections

HSCT predisposes to other invasive fungal infections that primarily involve the lungs but may disseminate to other organs. These infections are mainly seen in patients with neutropenia, allogeneic HSCT, and GVHD [42, 135-139].

Hyaline hyphomycetes such as fusarium and scedosporium are the main non-aspergillus molds reported following HSCT. These organisms resemble Aspergillus histologically with septate hyphae that invade blood vessels [42, 140, 141]. Culture is the only means to distinguish these organisms from Aspergillus. The lungs are the primary site of infection, however these organisms have the tendency to disseminate [42]. Fungemia due to fusarium is reported in 20-70% of patients [142]. These infections usually occur early (in the first 2 months) following allogeneic HSCT. Scedosporium has been isolated from the air in hospitals [141]. In the lungs, these organisms usually present with thin wall cavities or nodules with or without air-crescent sign that are refractory to antibiotics and antifungal therapy143. The diagnosis is usually confirmed by culture of BAL fluid or lung tissue obtained by open lung biopsy and occasionally by fungal blood cultures.

These fungal agents are resistant to amphotericin B, however respond to voriconazole in 40-60% of cases [139]. S.prolificans is resistant to all available antifungal agents including the newer azoles [144, 145]. Mortality associated with these fungal infections remains very high, in the range of 70-100% [142, 146].

Zygomycetes such as Rhizopus and mucor are characterized by sparsely septate, broad hyphae with irregular branching. They have the tendency to invade blood vessels with thrombosis and tissue necrosis. They usually involve the sino-pulmonary tree and dissemination to other organs is rare. The incidence of zygomycetes infections in HSCT recipients is rare (0.5-1.9%) [42, 137, 138]. The best approach to treatment is the combination of high dose amphtericin B and surgical debridement. These organisms may be resistant to voriconazole but may have a good response to posaconazole [147, 148]. Mortality is 75-80% [42, 137, 138].

Endemic mycoses such as histoplasmosis, blastomycosis, and coccidiomycosis are rare after HSCT [149]. These infections tend to have geographical distribution, and are usually caused by endogenous reactivation or a latent infection. The infection usually presents with progressive pulmonary disease that disseminate to other organs. Treatment is high dose amphotericin B [140]. After controlling the infection, an azole such as itraconazole (or fluconazole in the case of coccidiomycosis) can be used as a continuing treatment [139].

Invasive candida infection develops in 11-16% of HSCT recipients and pulmonary involvement is usually secondary to disseminated candidiasis or candidemia. Autopsy studies suggest that 50% of infected patients have pulmonary involvement [150]. The universal prophylaxis with fluconazole has significantly decreased the incidence of candida infections and primary candida pneumonia is extremely rare. There is a shift in the candida species from C. albicans to more resistant species such as C. glabarata and C. krusei.

Pneumocystis pneumonia is caused by P. jiroveci. Infection is caused by inhalation of aerosolized organisms [151]. The incidence of pneumocystis pneumonia following HSCT was historically 5-15%, usually in the second to the sixth month following HSCT2. However the routine prophylaxis with TMX/SMZ during this period has significantly decreased the incidence to negligible values. Breakthrough infection in patients on TMP/SMZ prophylaxis is extremely rare, however is possible in patients on other prophylactic agents such as low dose atevaquone, or aerosolized pentamidine [152-154]. The incidence of P. jiroveci infection is about 2.5% in patients undergoing allogeneic HSCT. The majority of cases occur late (median 14.5 months) in patients with low CD4+ T cell count and in patients on immunosuppressive therapy for chronic GVHD who are not receiving prophylaxis against P. jiroveci [155].

Patients usually present with progressive dyspnea, nonproductive cough, fever and hypoxemia. Radiologically, there are perihilar interstitial or alveolar infiltrates. Ground glass opacification may be the prominent finding on HRCT of the chest. LDH may be elevated. The diagnosis is usually made by bronchoscopy with BAL, however the sensitivity of this procedure is lower than that reported in patients with AIDS due to the lower burden of the organism2. Treatment of choice is TMP/SMZ with or without systemic corticosteroids. Alternative agents are less effective and include intravenous pentamidine, dapsone and trimethoprim, atevaqoune, or clindamycin and primaqine [13]. Mortality is around 34%, and the only predictor of poor outcome is the use of mechanical ventilation [156]. Prophylaxis against P. jiroveci pneumonia is initiated by starting TMP/SMZ following engraftment for 120 days, however if the patient has chronic GVHD, prophylactic treatment is recommended as long as they are on treatment for chronic GVHD.

Cytomegalovirus

CMV infection is defined as isolation of the CMV virus or its proteins or nucleic acid from body fluids or tissue specimens. CMV viremia is isolation of CMV from blood by culture. CMV antigenemia is detection of CMV pp65 in circulating leukocytes or CMV nucleic acid by PCR techniques. CMV disease is the presence of signs and symptoms related to CMV infection, and may manifest as hepatitis, gastroenteritis, encephalitis, or a systemic syndrome. CMV pneumonitis is one of the most frequent and severe manifestations of CMV disease in HSCT recipient. It is defined as pulmonary signs and symptoms combined with detection of CMV in pulmonary samples (sputum, BAL, or lung tissue). It is important to note that some patients may shed CMV in sputum or BAL fluid in the absence of invasive disease. It is also important to note that CMV affects the immune system and promotes other infections. Co-infection with other organisms such as P. jiroveci, Aspergillus, or other viruses occurs in up to one third of cases [157].

Traditionally, CMV pneumonia was a relatively frequent infection in HSCT recipients. It was diagnosed in 20-35%, and 60-80% of diffuse pneumonitis following HSCT [23, 158, 159]. CMV pneumonia usually presented in the first 2 months post-transplantation (median 44 days), and was associated with high mortality ranging between 80-100% [158]. However, antiviral prophylaxis for high risk patients and preemptive therapy has changed the epidemiology of CMV pneumonia in HSCT recipients. Currently, in allogeneic HSCT recipients, the incidence of CMV pneumonia is 10-30%, while in autologous recipients, it is extremely rare (1-9%) [160-163]. The onset of CMV pneumonia in allogeneic HSCT is now delayed to after the first 100 days (median 169 days), especially in patients with non-myeloablative HSCT and during the treatment of chronic GVHD [164, 165].

CMV pneumonia is mainly seen after allogeneic HSCT, and seropositive recipients are at highest risk [166]. Additional risk factors include older age, total body irradiation, myeloablative chemotherapy, the presence and acuity of acute GVHD, and the use of T-cell depletion strategies [158, 167, 168].

In autologous HSCT, the main risk factors for CMV pneumonia are the presence of CMV infection prior to transplantation and CD-34 enriched stem cells, probably due to lower number of T cells and delayed immunologic reconstitution [169].

CMV pneumonia presents clinically with rapid onset of fever, nonproductive cough, dyspnea, and hypoxemia. Pleurisy may be present. The respiratory symptoms usually progress to acute respiratory failure within 2 weeks. Radiologically, the most common findings are an interstitial pattern with tiny pulmonary nodules and patchy areas of consolidation. Rarely CMV pneumonia may present with focal diseases [170, 171]. HRCT of the chest is more sensitive in detecting the findings related to CMV pneumonia including diffuse or patchy ground glass opacification, thickened interlobular septa and tree in bud nodular changes. Pleural effusion may be present in 25% of patients [171].

The hallmark histopathological finding of CMV pneumonia is intracytoplasmic inclusion bodies within areas of inflammation on lung biopsy. Areas of mononuclear interstitial pneumonitis with or without alveolar epithelial desquamation and hyaline membrane formation can also be found. These findings can be rarely demonstrated by bronchoscopic biopsy; open lung biopsy by video-assisted thoracoscopy is usually necessary.

Cytological examination of the BAL fluid to detect the inclusion bodies within the lower respiratory tract epithelial cells is highly specific (98%) for CMV pneumonia, but has lower sensitivity (90%) [172]. On the other hand, rapid culture of the BAL fluid using shell viral technique is highly sensitive (99%) in detecting the virus, but lacks the specificity (67-83%), since it cannot differentiate between viral shedding and invasive disease [172, 173].

The value of detecting CMV antigens in the diagnosis of CMV pneumonia is controversial. CMV pp65 antigen assay is based on staining blood neutrophil for the pp65 antigen. The test requires an adequate number of neutrophils (>1000 cells/mm3), so it is not useful in the presence of neutropenia [174]. Detecting the viral CMV DNA by PCR could be done on whole blood, plasma, leukocytes, BAL, urine, and CSF. Detection of CMV DNA in the BAL is suggestive of CMV pneumonia, however false positive results are frequent [175].

Detecting blood CMV antigens correlates well with CMV pneumonia and may precede clinical features of pneumonia by up to 3 weeks [176, 177]. It is, however, possible for CMV pneumonia to develop without antigenemia [178]. These tests are also useful in monitoring response to antiviral therapy. Persistence of CMV antigenemia after 2 weeks of therapy should raise suspicion of antiviral resistance.

Gancyclovir as a single agent or in combination with CMV immunoglobulins may be effective in the treatment of CMV pneumonia and is currently the standard of care in the management of this condition following HSCT [160, 163]. With this approach, mortality has decreased to 0-47% provided treatment is started prior to the onset of acute respiratory failure. Survival of patients with respiratory failure at the time of initiation of therapy remains infrequent.

Valgancyclovir is an oral agent that has 60% bioavailability, and a daily dose of 900mg is equivalent to 5 mg/kg/day of intravenous gancyclovir [157]. CMV IgG is prepared from pooled adult human plasma that contains CMV antibodies. It is not useful as the sole treatment for CMV pneumonia [160]. Second line agents include foscarnet and cidofivir. The combination of gancyclovir and foscarnet may provide synergy [180].

Prevention of CMV infection is the best approach to avoid disease. Use of CMV negative stem cells and seronegative or leukocyte-filtered blood products for CMV seronegative recipients decreases the risk of infection to 2- 4% [181, 182]. Antiviral prophylaxis and viral monitoring with pre-emptive therapy (when more than 10,000 DNA copies/ml are detected in serum) are at present the two main antiviral strategies used in the prevention of CMV infection and disease. Gancyclovir prophylaxis administered in seropositive patients or in seronegative subjects receiving graft from a seropositive donor, from 5 days before engraftment to 100 days after transplant reduces the risk of CMV infection and invasive disease, as well as mortality [183]. However, this approach did not change the overall survival owing to increased sepsis associated with gancyclovir-induced neutropenia, and shift in the onset of the CMV disease later in the course following HSCT when the prophylactic treatment is discontinued [184]. Other investigational interventions include infusion of donor derived CMV specific cytotoxic T lymphocyte infusion and CMV vaccine [185].

Community Respiratory Viruses

There are four main community respiratory viral agents that lead to infection following HSCT: respiratory syncytial virus (RSV), parainfluenza, influenza and adenovirus [190]. These viruses are often co-pathogens with other bacteria or fungi. Overall, the incidence of these viral infections following HSCT ranges between 11-65% [186-189]. Risk factors include allogeneic HSCT, leukemia, age older than 65 yr, and presence of severe neutropenia or lymphopenia. The overall mortality is 15%. The only independent predictor of fatal outcome is absolute lymphopenia in patients with influenza pneumonia [189].

Community respiratory viral infections lead to lower respiratory tract infections and increase the risk of bronchiolitis obliterans following allogeneic HSCT.

The diagnosis of lower respiratory tract community respiratory viral infection is usually suspected in patients with preceding upper respiratory tract infection. HRCT of the chest usually shows patchy or extensive ground glass opacities or a mixture of patterns including ground glass attenuation, thickening of the bronchial walls, and multiple small nodules that may have centrilobular or random distribution. Consolidation and pleural effusions are less common [191]. The diagnosis is usually made using the combination of direct fluorescent antibody (DFA) and indirect fluorescent antibody (IFA) testing, and viral cultures of clinical specimens which are best obtained by nasopharyngeal wash or swabs [192-194]. BAL may also be helpful when lower respiratory tract infection is suspected with a sensitivity around 70% [188].

Given the high mortality associated with community respiratory viral lower respiratory tract infections in HSCT recipients, preventive measures play an important role in avoiding infection in these patients. Simple measures such as hand washing are very effective against infection (except for influenza which is transmitted by aerosolized droplets). Other measures include isolating patients suspected to have community respiratory viral infection, even before the infection is confirmed, restricting symptomatic healthcare providers from contact with HSCT recipients and limiting visitors to HSCT recipients during the winter months [13, 196].

Respiratory Syncytial Virus (RSV)

RSV) is the most common community respiratory virus infection in HSCT recipients. It has seasonal variation with the highest incidence in late autumn and winter. Children are more affected than adults, and outbreaks of RSV infections have been described in HSCT units [197-199]. The incidence is around 3.5-6.3% following allogeneic HSCT and 0.4-1.5% following autologous HSCT [200,201].

RSV infection usually starts with upper respiratory tract symptoms including cough, rhinorrhea, and sinus congestion. Wheezing may develop in 30% of cases. Fever may not be present even with lower respiratory tract infection [202]. The most serious complication of RSV infection in this patient population is the development of lower respiratory tract infection which happens in 30-50% of patients and is associated with high mortality (19%) [189, 203]. It is usually characterized by progressive dyspnea and hypoxemia. Lack of RSV directed antiviral therapy and older age are associated with increased risk of progression to pneumonia [189]. The radiological findings of RSV pneumonia include multiple small nodules, tree in bud pattern, diffuse ground glass infiltrates, and bronchial thickening [204].

The role of pharmacological therapy in RSV infection following HSCT remains controversial. Ribavirin (intravenously, orally or aerosolized) with or without RSV specific intravenous immunoglobulins may be beneficial [205, 206, 208]. Care should be taken during Ribavirin aerosolization since exposure to the medication may cause headache, skin rash, and conjunctivitis. Furthermore, ribavirin has teratogenic effects and pregnant women should not enter the patient's room during treatment [206]. Other therapeutic modalities, such as high titer monoclonal antibody against RSV are under investigation [207]. Starting antiviral therapy once the patient develops acute respiratory failure requiring mechanical ventilation is usually not effective, with high mortality that reaches 90% [205].

Parainfluenza Virus

Parainfluenza virus accounts for 5-50% of community respiratory viral infections, with equal incidence following autologous and allogeneic HSCT [190, 209, 210]. Parainfluenza has 4 serotypes, and serotypes 1 and 3 are reportedly the most common causes of infection in

HSCT recipients. Parainfluenza infection is variable throughout the year, with outbreaks reported in winter, and sometimes in spring and summer.

It usually presents with cough. Rhinorrhea and fever are uncommon. Lower respiratory tract infection is the most serious complication of parainfluenza infection, and is reported in 18-100% of patients, with mortality ranging between 15-73%. Up to 50% of patients with parainfluenza lower respiratory tract infection have co-infection with bacteria or fungi [195,210].

Treatment of parainfluenza infection is supportive. Ribavirin therapy is controversial [206, 210, 211]. It is recommended to consider aerosolized ribavirin in the treatment of parainfluenza lower respiratory tract infection, although experience to date provides little evidence of efficacy [206].

Influenza Virus

Influenza virus infection has been described in HSCT recipients as a community or nosocomial infection. It usually develops in the winter months, and the clinical picture is similar to normal hosts, presenting with fever, rhinorrhea, coryza, mayalgia, and headache. The frequency of influenza infection is similar in autologous and allogeneic HSCT recipients. Lower respiratory tract infections are rare, and co-infection with bacteria has been reported. The overall mortality with influenza lower respiratory tract infection following HSCT is low, however the prognosis is worse if the patient develops the infection early post-transplantation [212]. Lower respiratory tract influenza infection is more frequent in those who develop infection early post-transplantation (median 36 days vs. 61 days), and those with lymphopenia [189, 212].

The treatment of influenza infection is supportive. Antiviral agents such as amantadine, rimantadine, oseltamir, zanamivir may be considered in HSCT patients with severe infection [213]. Early treatment with oseltamivir may decrease the progression to lower respiratory tract infection and decrease viral shedding [212]. Vaccination against influenza is effective, however live attenuated preparations should be avoided in these patients. Additionally, HSCT recipients may respond poorly to vaccination in the first 2 years following transplantation [206].

Adenovirus

Adenovirus infection accounts for 0-21% of community respiratory viral infections following HSCT, and is more common in children [203, 214]. Most cases are due to reactivation of latent infection. Patients with allogeneic HSCT may have delayed adenovirus specific T-cell immune recovery, which correlates with increased risk of adenovirus associated morbidity and mortality [215].

Adenovirus infection may be asymptomatic, or may lead to pneumonia or to disseminated disease with gastroenteritis, hepatitis, and hemorrhagic cystitis, with or without respiratory involvement. Approximately 20% of HSCT recipients with adenovirus infection develop pneumonia [216]. Histologically, the diagnosis is suggested by the presence of the characteristic smudge cells [216].

Mortality ranges between 38-100%. Prognosis depends on the degree of dissemination [193, 194, 201]. Given this high mortality, early and aggressive treatment is warranted. There are limited antiviral agents with activity against adenovirus. Cidofivir has been shown to improve outcome in small studies [217]. Ribavirin and gancyclovir have no significant activity against adenovirus.

Other Virus Infection

Rhinovirus is an important cause of common cold. Its significance in HSCT recipients is not well known. In prospective studies on HSCT recipients, 25% of patients with viral infections were documented to have rhinovirus, and in 3-17% of these patients the infection progressed to the lower respiratory tract with mortality up to 33% [181, 218]. There is no specific treatment for rhinovirus infection.

Herpes viruses have been reported as a cause of lower respiratory tract infection following HSCT. Herpes simplex virus-1 reactivates in 80% of HSCT recipients and occasionally may be associated with pneumonia. Universal prophylaxis with acyclovir and gancyclovir has significantly reduced the incidence of herpes simplex virus serious infections [161]. Herpes zoster virus may also lead to lower respiratory tract infection following HSCT, and is usually preceded by the characteristic skin rash. Human herpes virus (HHV-6) has been suggested to have a role in the pathogenesis of idiopathic pneumonia syndrome following HSCT [219]. It may act as a co-pathogen with CMV or act as an isolated cause of pneumonia. Although HHV-6 can be isolated from peripheral blood or other specimen tested following HSCT, it is associated with interstitial/alveolar pneumonia in only 2% of patients. HHV-6 reactivation is significantly associated with GVHD, Epstein Barr viral co-infection, and unrelated donor transplantation [220].

NON-INFECTIOUS PULMONARY COMPLICATIONS OF HSCT

Engraftment Syndrome

Engraftment syndrome usually develops within 96 hrs of engraftment and occurs more frequently after autologous HSCT, with an incidence of 7–11% [221, 222, 223]. The etiology of this syndrome is poorly understood. Release of proinflammatory cytokines during engraftment is postulated to play a principal role. The incidence and severity of engraftment syndrome increase with the use of granulocyte colony-stimulating factor (G-CSF) that regulates the production of cytokines (TNF-α, IL-1B, and IL-8), which increase alveolar permeability and neutrophil influx [224].

Specific criteria have been suggested for the diagnosis of engraftment syndrome following HSCT. These include major criteria: temperature $\geq$ 38.3 C with no identifiable infectious etiology, erythrodermatous rash involving more than 25% of body surface area and not attributable to a medication, and noncardiogenic pulmonary edema manifested by diffuse pulmonary infiltrates consistent with the diagnosis and hypoxia. Minor criteria include: hepatic dysfunction, renal insufficiency, weight gain $\geq$ 2.5% of baseline body weight, and transient encephalopathy unexplainable by other causes. Three major or two major and one or more minor criteria are needed for the diagnosis of engraftment syndrome following HSCT [225].

The prognosis of engraftment syndrome is generally favorable. Mild cases are managed by supportive measures while strong consideration should be given to discontinue G-CSF.

More severe cases, especially those with pulmonary involvement have dramatic response to systemic corticosteroids with improvement within one day of treatment. Patients who require mechanical ventilation have the worse prognosis [222, 225-227].

Diffuse Alveolar Hemorrhage

Diffuse alveolar hemorrhage (DAH) complicates 2 to 14% of HSCT. The hallmark of the syndrome is the finding of progressively bloodier return from BAL in the absence of an identifiable respiratory tract infection. The incidence among autologous and allogeneic recipients appears to be equivalent [228, 229]. Risk factors for DAH following HSCT include age greater than 40 years, total body irradiation, transplantation for solid tumors, and the presence of high fevers, severe mucositis, leukocyte recovery, and renal insufficiency [230]. There is no relation between DAH and type of preparatory regimen, whether it is reduced intensity or myeloablative [231].

The pathogenesis of DAH in HSCT recipients remains obscure. It is possible that DAH is part of a spectrum of acute lung injury induced by conditioning chemotherapy, radiation, or occult infection. The fact that many cases occur at the time of engraftment suggests that neutrophil influx into the lung may accentuate the injury and in some way precipitate alveolar hemorrhage [228, 230, 232].

DAH is most commonly observed within the first month after HSCT (a median of 23 days) often during the preengraftment phase, but later onset is encountered in up to 42% of cases [228]. Patients present with dyspnea, nonproductive cough, fever, diffuse pulmonary infiltrates, and rarely hemoptysis. Radiological findings are usually diffuse interstitial, alveolar or ground glass changes that are more prominent in the perihilar areas and lower lobes. The radiological findings may appear up to 3 days prior to clinical diagnosis of DAH. The diagnosis is usually made by BAL that reveals progressively bloodier lavage fluid return from at least three separate subsegmental bronchi. However, it is possible to have DAH with nonbloody BAL fluid, especially if the procedure is done few days after the onset of symptoms [232]. The presence of greater than 20% hemosiderin-laden macrophages in BAL fluid is an alternative diagnostic criterion, but it may take 48–72 hours for this finding to appear [228,229].

The following diagnostic criteria have been suggested:

1) Evidence of widespread alveolar injury manifested by multilobar pulmonary infiltrates, symptoms and signs of pneumonia, and abnormal physiology with widened A-a gradient
2) BAL showing progressively bloodier return from three separate subsegmental bronchi, or more than 20% hemosiderin-laden macrophages on examination of the BAL fluid, or if a surgical lung biopsy is performed, more than 30% of the alveolar surface of the examined lung tissue is covered by blood and
3) Absence of infection compatible with the diagnosis [228].

There are no prospective randomized trials to address the management of DAH following HSCT. High-dose corticosteroids (500–1,000 mg per day of methylprednisolone for 3–4 days followed by taper over 2-4 weeks) may improve the survival rate [233-235]. The addition of an antifibrinolytic agent such as aminocaproic acid may be beneficial [236].

With supportive therapy alone, mortality rate in patients with DAH is 74–100% and is usually due to sepsis or multiorgan failure rather than respiratory failure [228, 230, 233]. Autologous HSCT, onset within the first 30 days of transplantation and lack of mechanical ventilation are associated with favorable outcome [229]. Long term survivors of DAH following HSCT have normal lung function [235].

Idiopathic Pneumonia Syndrome

Idiopathic pneumonia syndrome (IPS) is another important cause of non-infectious diffuse lung injury following HSCT. A National Institutes of Health workshop defined IPS as "diffuse lung injury occurring after marrow transplant for which an infectious etiology is not identified" [237]. This workshop put forward the following diagnostic criteria for IPS:

1) Evidence of widespread alveolar injury as manifested by multilobar infiltrates, symptoms and signs of pneumonia, and increased A-a gradient and/or restrictive lung disease based on pulmonary function tests.
2) Absence of lower respiratory tract infection after appropriate evaluation that includes BAL that is negative for bacterial and non-bacterial pathogens, lack of improvement with broad spectrum antibiotics, and a second confirmatory test within 2-14 days.
3) If lung biopsy is performed it usually reveals one of two patterns: diffuse alveolar damage or interstitial pneumonitis [237].

The incidence of IPS ranges from 2 to 17 %. It usually happens in the first 120 days post-HSCT and the median time of onset is 21 to 49 days after transplantation. IPS is more common following allogeneic HSCT [238,239].

Risk factors include older age, lower pre-transplantation performance status, **transplantation** for a malignancy other than leukemia, high-intensity conditioning regimens, total body irradiation, high-grade acute GVHD, and methotrexate-based GVHD prophylaxis [239-241].

Patients with IPS present with dyspnea, fever, nonproductive cough, increasing oxygen requirements, and diffuse radiographic infiltrates. The clinical course of IPS is typically rapid, with up to two-thirds of patients progressing within several days to respiratory failure requiring mechanical ventilation [238]. Mortality rate is 74% and is primarily related to progressive respiratory failure [239]. Factors that predict mortality include the need for mechanical ventilation and higher serum creatinine level at the onset of IPS [239, 240].

Beyond supportive care, there is no proven treatment for IPS. High-dose corticosteroid therapy does not appear to be of benefit [238, 240]. Etanercept, a soluble TNF-α–binding protein, is shown to improve pulmonary function within the first week of therapy when used with or without steroids [242, 243].

Table 5 summarizes the similarities and differences between the 3 main noninfectious causes (engraftment syndrome, DAH, and IPS) of diffuse lung injury following HSCT.

Table 5. comparison of the characteristics of the main non-infectious causes of acute lung injury following HSCT

Feature	Engraftment syndrome	DAH	IPS
Incidence	Autologous > allogeneic	Autologous = allogeneic	Allogeneic > autologous
Onset	Early/ acute	Early/ acute	Late/ subacute
Relation to stem cell engraftment	within 96 hr of engraftment	Relation to engraftment is less definite	No relation
Characteristic clinical feature	Systemic manifestations	Bloody BAL	Progressive respiratory failure
Pathology	Diffuse alveolar damage. G-CSF plays a role	Diffuse alveolar damage with release of several cytokines	Diffuse alveolar damage. TNF- α plays a role.
Response to corticosteroids	Excellent response	Moderate response	Poor response
Prognosis	Favorable prognosis	Less favorable prognosis. Usually die with multi-organ failure and sepsis	Poor prognosis usually die with respiratory failure

Bronchiolitis Obliterans

Bronchiolitis obliterans (BO) is the most important late non-infectious pulmonary complication following allogeneic HSCT, usually presents after the first 100 days following transplantation [244, 253, 267-271, 276, 278, 279]. Although there are reports of BO as early as 30 days following HSCT, 80% of cases present between 6 and 12 months post-transplantation [260, 272].

This condition is characterized by the new onset of air flow obstruction (AFO) following HSCT. Due to the lack of a standardized definition, the incidence of BO varies widely in the literature ranging from 0 to 48% [239, 244, 245]. BO is more common following peripheral blood stem cell transplantation compared with bone marrow transplantation and is more common following conventional myeloablative HSCT compared with non-myeloablative HSCT [246]. BO is uncommon following autologous HSCT or umbilical cord blood stem cell transplantation [247-250].

The presence of chronic GVHD is the most important association with BO although it may develop in a small percentage of patients who do not have manifestations of GVHD [251, 252]. The risk is higher in those with progressive chronic GVHD (which evolves without hiatus from active acute GVHD) as compared to those with quiescent chronic GVHD (that develops after an interval of response to treatment of acute GVHD) or de novo chronic GVHD (in patients who never had acute GVHD) [244, 253]. Acute GVHD alone does not appear to significantly increase the risk of BO [244, 253-255].

Other risk factors for BO include: older age of the recipient (>20 yrs); the presence of AFO (forced expiratory volume in one second (FEV1)/forced vital capacity (FVC) < 0.7) prior to HSCT, and respiratory viral infections in the first 100 days following HSCT [244, 253]. Biochemical factors (such as low pre-transplant serum surfactant D protein level) and genetic factors (such as NOD2/CARD15 polymorphism) may predispose HSCT recipients to BO [256, 257].

The pathogenesis of BO following HSCT is not well defined. The most important mechanism is probably an alloreactive immune process in which the donors T-lymphocytes target the epithelial cells of the bronchioles, leading to the inflammatory reaction characterized by an increase in cytokines, such as IL-1, IL-6, IL-8, IL-18 and TNF-α [263-266]. This mechanism is evident from the exclusive occurrence of BO following allogeneic HSCT, and the strong association between BO and chronic GVHD. Some authors suggest that BO is a manifestation of chronic GVHD [262]. These immune mechanisms are thought to trigger inflammatory reactions that lead to BO.

BO may also be the result of a lung injury precipitated by the conditioning regimen, this is supported by the higher incidence of BO in busulfan-based conditioning regimen and the apparent lower incidence in non-myeloablative HSCT compared to conventional regimen [246 ,258, 259]. BO may also have an infectious etiology [277]. Low serum immunoglobulins, secondary to slow reconstitution of B-cells following transplantation, is associated with abnormal local defense mechanisms in the lungs, predisposing them to infections that lead to BO[254, 260, 261].

The presentation of BO is usually insidious and may be preceded by upper respiratory tract symptoms[268]. The main symptoms are dry cough (60–100%) and dyspnea (50–70%) [252, 260, 268, 273]. Wheezing and sinusitis are frequent. Fever is rare unless there is a concomitant infectious process. Approximately 20% of patients are asymptomatic and the diagnosis is suspected based on pulmonary function test findings [268]. In the advanced stages of BO, the patients are physically limited due to severe obstructive airway disease and may require home oxygen therapy. Some patients may develop features of bronchiectasis with recurrent respiratory tract infections and colonization of the airways by Pseudomonas spp., Staphylococcus aureus and, occasionally, Aspergillus species.

The clinical course of BO is variable. The majority of patients have a slow progressive AFO, with episodes of acute exacerbation of AFO. In the minority of patients, the AFO progresses rapidly and patients develop respiratory failure within a few months. However, some patients may have stabilization or even improvement in the AFO [274,275].

In the early stages of BO, the chest radiograph is normal. As BO becomes more advanced, signs of hyperinflation and later changes consistent with bronchiectasis with dilated and thickened bronchi and areas of scarring are seen. Pneumothorax, pneumomediastinum, and pneumopericardium may develop in advanced cases, and are usually associated with significant morbidity and mortality [251, 280, 281]. HRCT of the chest is much more sensitive in detecting signs of BO and is the radiological procedure of choice in evaluating these patients [282, 283]. While the study may still be normal in the early stages of BO, it usually shows signs of hyperinflation with areas of decreased attenuation. Bronchiectasis is seen in advanced cases. The most common radiological sign of BO on HRCT of the chest is the presence of air trapping during the expiratory phase of imaging. These views show areas of hypoattenuation that correspond to obstructed airways interspaced with areas of ground glass appearance corresponding to the pulmonary lobules with patent airways. This ''mosaic'' appearance is highly suggestive of BO, and has sensitivity and specificity ranging between 74–91% and 67–94%, respectively [284,285]. In addition, HRCT of the chest is helpful in excluding co-existing conditions such as infections, bronchiolitis obliterans organizing pneumonia (BOOP), or idiopathic pneumonia syndrome that are usually associated with parenchymal infiltrates [275]. In summary, it is recommended that a HRCT of the chest with inspiratory and expiratory views be performed on all patients under evaluation for BO following HSCT.

Spirometry is the main study used to diagnose and follow-up patients with BO following HSCT. It usually shows evidence of new AFO with reduction in forced expiratory volume in the first second (FEV1) and FEV1 to forced vital capacity (FVC) ratio (FEV1/FVC). However, there is a lack of consensus on the spirometric criteria for the diagnosis of BO following HSCT. Recently, the National Institutes of Health sponsored a consensus development project for clinical trials on chronic GVHD [286]. The workshop considered BO as the only diagnostic manifestation of chronic GVHD in the lung. Table 6 proposes diagnostic criteria of BO following HSCT [287].

Table 6. Suggested Diagnostic Criteria of BO Following HSCT [287]

1.	Allogeneic HSCT
2.	Chronic GVHD
3.	Insidious onset of dyspnea, cough and wheezing usually after 100 days following transplantation
4.	Normal chest radiograph
5.	HRCT of the chest (with inspiratory and expiratory views) showing areas of air trapping on expiratory views (mosaic pattern), hyperinflation, micronodular changes, or bronchial dilatation, with no parenchymal involvement.
6.	PFT showing new onset of airflow obstruction (FEV1/FVC <0.7 and FEV1 <75% of predicted), not responsive to bronchodilators
7.	Exclusion of an infectious process by appropriate radiological, serological and microbiological studies (obtained by sinus aspirate, upper respiratory tract viral screen, sputum culture or BAL).

Bronchoscopy has a limited role in the diagnosis of BO following HSCT. BAL is mainly carried out to rule out an infectious process in HSCT recipients who present with respiratory symptoms suggestive of BO. The main infections to be considered in this setting, and in which BAL may be useful are viral infections such as CMV, RSV, influenza, parainfluenza, or HSV. In addition, fungal infections and Pneumocystis jiroveci need to be considered if the patient is on systemic corticosteroids and/or immunosuppressive therapy [288].

Transbronchial biopsy is generally not recommended for the diagnosis of BO following HSCT because the disease is patchy and peripheral, and the biopsy samples are usually too small to show bronchiolar pathology. If histological confirmation of BO is necessary, the best approach is a surgical lung biopsy obtained by video-assisted thoracoscopy.

In general, the management of BO is difficult as the pathogenesis is incompletely understood and treatment does not result in reversible improvement of lung function. Goals of therapy are directed towards stabilization at best. In general, the management of BO is similar to that of chronic GVHD and consists of high dose systemic corticosteroids and reinstitution or augmentation of immunosuppressive therapy. Systemic corticosteroids are suggested in the form of prednisone at 1–1.5 mg/ kg daily (up to 100 mg/day) for 2–6 weeks. If there is clinical and physiological stabilization, the dose is tapered every 2 weeks over 3–12 months [252, 267, 268, 270, 289-293]. The immunosuppressive agents used are similar to those used in the treatment of chronic GVHD, namely cyclosporine A or tacrolimus [252, 270, 271, 275, 289]. This treatment regimen is recommended for 3 – 12 months although some studies suggest that further improvement is unlikely after 9 months of treatment [289, 293]. Intravenous immunoglobulins have been given to patients with BO, with no proven benefit [294]. Based on the experience using macrolides in the treatment of diffuse panbronchiolitis, cystic fibrosis and treatment of BO following lung transplantation, this class of medications is increasingly considered in the management of BO following HSCT [295-298]. Macrolides down-regulate pro-inflammatory cytokines, such as TNF-α and may decrease the inflammatory reaction that leads to BO [299]. The suggested medication is azithromycin at a dose of 250 mg three times a week for 12 weeks [300]. High-dose inhaled corticosteroids such as fluticasone propionate may be effective in treatment of BO and may improve symptoms of airway obstruction and stabilize FEV1 3-6 months after treatment [300-303]. There are limited studies on the combination of inhaled corticosteroids and long acting B2 agonist in these patients [267, 268, 272].

Extracorporeal photodynamic (ECP) therapy is an immunotherapeutic modality that has been used in the treatment of chronic GVHD and BO. This therapy involves extracorporeal exposure of peripheral blood mononuclear cells to photoactivated 8-methoxypsoralen, by exposure to ultraviolet A light, followed by re-infusion of the treated cells [304]. The photoactivated 8-methoxypsoralen binds to DNA leading to initiation of apoptosis with a selective effect on autoreactive T cells [305]. The role of ECP in the management of BO following HSCT has not been well studied and benefits are limited to case reports or small trials [306-308].

Other suggested treatments for BO following HSCT include anti- TNF-α monoclonal antibodies (such as infliximab), Imatinib mesylate, alefacept, dacluzimab, and rituximab [309-312].

Supportive treatment is essential in the management of patients with BO following HSCT. Infectious processes should be excluded prior to starting immunosuppressive therapy. Once treatment is started, patients should be maintained on appropriate prophylactic measures against P. jiroveci. Prophylaxis against fungi and CMV should be considered in high-risk patients. In addition, appropriate vaccinations including those against influenza and pneumococcus are recommended. Prompt treatment of pulmonary infections is essential, since these tend to worsen the course and outcome of BO. Patients with advanced BO may require long-term oxygen therapy and may benefit from outpatient pulmonary rehabilitation. There are a few reports of lung transplantation in patients with advanced BO with encouraging results [313]. Table 7 summarizes a management approach to patients with BO following HSCT [287].

Table 7. Suggested Approach to the Management of BO Following HSCT [287]

1. Confirm the diagnosis of BO- *See Table 6*
2. Systemic corticosteroids (Prednisone 1-1.5 mg/kg/day). Taper gradually over 6-12 months
3. Immunosuppressive therapy (such as cyclosporine A or tacrolimus)
4. Maintenance macrolide treatment
5. Inhaled bronchodilators
6. Prophylactic therapy against *P. jiroveci*, fungi and CMV
7. Anti-reflux measures
8. *Consider* Inhaled corticosteroids
9. *Consider* Extracorporeal Photodynamic Therapy
10. *consider* intravenous immunoglobulins
11. In advanced cases:
    - long term oxygen therapy
    - outpatient pulmonary rehabilitation
    - *consider* lung transplantation

BO following HSCT is a progressive disease that leads, in the majority of patients, to irreversible AFO. The decline in lung function is usually slow over several months to years. During this course there may be exacerbations that are associated with temporary worsening of the lung function. Some patients may have a rapidly progressive AFO that leads to respiratory failure. Aggressive therapy results in improvement of lung function in only 8-20% of patients, while in most patients, treatment is aimed to stabilize and prevent further drops in FEV1 [246, 259, 289, 314]. The mortality of BO following HSCT is usually due to pneumonia. It is 9% at 3 years, 12% at 5 years, and 18% at 10 years [253]. The mortality doubles in those with associated chronic GVHD [253]. Factors that are associated with increased mortality include rapid deterioration of FEV1 (more than 10% annually), age >60years, progressive chronic GVHD, underlying disease relapse, and history of respiratory viral infection [245, 253, 260]. In addition, the prognosis of BO is worse in patients who don't respond to the primary treatment regimen [239]. The prognosis of BO appears not to be influenced by the presence of AFO prior to transplantation, the source of stem cells, degree of matching, CMV serologic status, or type of GVHD prophylaxis [253].

Bronchiolitis Obliterans Organizing Pneumonia (BOOP)

BOOP is a specific inflammatory condition that develops following HSCT. The term bronchiolitis obliterans organizing pneumonia (BOOP) following HSCT is commonly confused with bronchiolitis obliterans (BO). However these are two different entities with characteristic clinical, radiological and pathological findings. Table 8 summarizes the characteristics of BO and BOOP following HSCT [276].

BOOP has been described following autologous and allogeneic HSCT, although more frequently following the latter. The incidence following allogeneic HSCT ranges between 0.9-10.3% [293, 315]. Predictors of the development of BOOP are: primary diagnosis of leukemia, radiation-containing preparative regimens and the presence of acute and chronic

GVHD. The strong association between BOOP and acute and chronic GVHD suggests that the donor T-cell mediated immune response against the recipient lung tissue may play a role in the pathogenesis of BOOP in these patients. Strategies to deplete T-cells may prevent BOOP in allogeneic HSCT recipients [263]. BOOP following autologous HSCT is rare and may be related to infections or medications.

Table 8. comparison between bronchiolitis obliterans and bronchiolitis obliterans organizing pneumonia [276]

Features	Bronchiolitis obliterans	BOOP
Incidence	0-48%	<2%
HSCT	Allogeneic	Allogeneic and autologous
Onset following HSCT	Late (around 1 year)	Usually in the first 100 days
Clinical presentation	Insidious; dyspnea, cough, wheezing	Acute; dyspnea, cough, fever
Radiological findings	Normal; hyperinflation, air trapping, bronchiectasis	Patchy consolidation (usually peripheral), ground glass attenuation, nodular opacities
Pulmonary function test	Obstructive; normal diffusing capacity	Restrictive; reduction in diffusing capacity
BAL	Predominantly neutrophils	Predominantly lymphocytes
Diagnosis	Clinical, radiological and physiological criteria	Usually requires tissue, best by surgical lung biopsy
Histolopathology	Granular plugs obliterating the bronchioles with inflammation and scarring; sparing of the alveoli and alveolar ducts	Granular plugs of bronchioles, extending to alveoli; interstitial inflammation and fibrosis
Treatment	Corticosteroids and immunosuppressive therapy	Corticosteroids
Outcome	Poor response to therapy; progressive disease with high mortality	Good response to therapy; potentially reversible

BOOP usually develops earlier than BO following HSCT. The onset of BOOP ranges from 5-2800 days with a median of 108 days [315]. The clinical presentation is usually acute or subacute with 2 weeks of fever, nonproductive cough, and dyspnea. Radiologically, findings include patchy (multifocal, diffuse or focal) consolidations that tend to be peripheral and/or peribronchovascular, ground glass opacities or nodular lesions [315]. Pulmonary function tests typically show mild to moderate restrictive pattern and characteristically low diffusing capacity and usually no airflow obstruction. Bronchoscopy is very useful in patients with BOOP to exclude other conditions such as infections. BAL fluid reveals lymphocytosis with low CD4/CD8 ratio [316]. Histological confirmation is usually necessary, and can be made by transbronchial biopsies, however most patients require surgical lung biopsy by video-assisted thoracoscopy. Pathologically, BOOP is characterized by patchy distribution of plugs of granulation tissue that fill the lumens of the distal airways extending to the alveolar ducts and spaces associated with chronic interstitial inflammation. Contrary to BO, patients with BOOP following HSCT have more favorable response to systemic corticosteroid therapy with initial dose of prednisone 1mg/kg daily then tapered over 3-6 months [315]. In 78% of patients, BOOP either resolves or remains stable. Patients who progress on corticosteroids therapy usually die of respiratory failure. The mortality of BOOP following HSCT is around 19% [317].

Other Non-Infectious Pulmonary Complications

Pulmonary Veno-Occlusive Disease

Pulmonary veno-occlusive disease is a rare complication after both autologous and allogeneic HSCT which is characterized by intimal proliferation and fibrosis of the pulmonary venules and small veins, leading to progressive vascular obstruction and increased pulmonary capillary and arterial pressures [318, 319]. It may be the result of an infectious or toxic injury to the endothelium (such as injury by chemotherapeutic agents like BCNU, mitomycin C and bleomycin). Patients typically present several months after transplantation with progressive dyspnea on exertion and fatigue. The triad of pulmonary arterial hypertension, radiographic signs of pulmonary edema, and a normal pulmonary artery occlusion pressure strongly suggests the diagnosis, but may not be present concurrently in all patients [320]. Surgical lung biopsy is the only way to confirm the diagnosis [320].

Arterial vasodilatation in the setting of fixed pulmonary venous resistance can markedly increase transcapillary hydrostatic pressure and precipitate or worsen pulmonary edema. Treatment of pulmonary veno-occlusive disease with vasodilators is therefore potentially dangerous and must be initiated under close observation. Response to high-dose corticosteroid therapy has been anecdotally reported [319]. Prognosis is generally poor.

Post-Transplant Lymphoproliferative Disorder

Post-transplant lymphoproliferative disorder is an infrequent but serious complication following allogeneic HSCT with a typical onset within the first 6 months. It represents an uncontrolled expansion of donor-derived, EBV-infected B lymphocytes as the result of weakened cytotoxic T cell immunity. Major risk factors include the use of unrelated or HLA-mismatched related donors, T cell-depleted donor stem cells, and anti-thymocyte globulin or monoclonal anti-T cell antibodies for the prevention or treatment of GVHD [321]. Although the overall incidence of post-transplant lymphoproliferative disorder is only 1%, the incidence increases to 8% for those with two risk factors and to 22% for those with three risk factors [321].

This disease is characterized by involvement of lymph nodes, liver, and spleen. Pulmonary involvement occurs in about 20% of cases [322]. Definitive diagnosis requires biopsy but quantitative EBV DNA monitoring by PCR is emerging as a noninvasive diagnostic technique [323]. Treatment includes the administration of anti-B cell monoclonal antibodies combined with a reduction in the dose of immunosuppressive agents [322,324]. Survival among HSCT recipients with post-transplant lymphoproliferative disorder is considerably lower than that of solid organ transplant recipients and is particularly poor for those who had received HSCT for hematologic malignancies [322].

Pulmonary Cytolytic Thrombi

Pulmonary cytolytic thrombi is a rare noninfectious pulmonary complication following HSCT characterized by pulmonary thrombi associated with infiltration by monocytes from donor and recipient origin in the small and medium pulmonary vessels. This disorder is reported exclusively following allogeneic HSCT in patients with other features of acute or chronic GVHD [325]. It has been primarily reported in pediatric population, with onset between 8 and 343 days (median 72 days) following HSCT [326, 327]. The pathogenesis is not known, however it may be a manifestation of GVHD. Patients present with fever, cough, chest pain and dyspnea. Chest CT reveals multiple peripheral opacities consistent with pulmonary infarcts. Treatment consists of intensification of immunosuppressive therapy usually associated with clinical improvement in 1-2 weeks and radiological resolution over weeks or months [328].

Sarcoidosis

Development of sarcoidosis post-HSCT has been reported with possible transmission of sarcoidosis from the donor stem cells to the allogeneic HSCT recipients, although some patients may develop it with no known history of sarcoidosis in the donor. Sarcoidosis occurs following stem cell engraftment a mean of 25 months (range 3-120 months) post-HSCT [329-331]. This reaction may be due to an abnormal immunological host response to common antigenic triggers. It is postulated that post-HSCT lung environment may promote the development of non-caseating graunlomas by high levels of chemokines such as MCP-1,CCRI, CCR2 and IL-8 [321]. Symptomatic patients with sarcoidosis following HSCT respond well to corticosteroids and prognosis is good [321].

Pulmonary Fibrosis

There are patients who develop nonspecific pulmonary fibrosis that does not fit into any of the other non-infectious pulmonary complications following HSCT. These patients are primarily long term survivors following allogeneic HSCT. They usually have dyspnea on exertion with cough, and develop frequent exacerbations consistent with acute bronchitis or pneumonia. The patients commonly have evidence of chronic GVHD, however it is usually quiescent. Pulmonary function tests usually reveal restrictive pattern with reduction in diffusing capacity. Radiologically, there are fibrotic changes that tend to involve the lower lobes associated with areas of bronchiectasis. The exact etiology of this presentation is not clear, however it could be a late manifestation of pulmonary drug toxicity or a late stage of BOOP or IPS, or it may be due to chronic GVHD with scleroderma like changes, or due to recurrent aspiration associated with esophageal involvement by GVHD. These patients are usually managed supportively, and may require oxygen therapy and antibiotics when there are acute exacerbations.

Asthma

Asthma and other allergic conditions such as allergic rhinitis may develop in allogeneic HSCT recipients from donors with atopy, possibly due to the transfer of marrow-derived immune cells from allergic donors [332]. New onset of asthma following HSCT should be differentiated from BO, which is much more common in this patient population.

Pulmonary Alveolar Proteinosis

It is characterized by the accumulation of periodic acid-Schiff stain- positive amorphous material in the pulmonary alveolar space due to decreased clearance of the surfactant proteins. Recent evidence suggests that GM-CSF plays a role in the development of pulmonary alveolar proteinosis [333]. There are few reports of acquired pulmonary alveolar proteinosis following HSCT during the period of leukopenia after myeloablative conditioning [3334, 335]. These patients develop acute respiratory failure with diffuse alveolar pulmonary infiltrates. Prognosis is generally poor [335]. The role of interventions such as frequent BAL and administration of aerosolized recombinant GM-CSF to reverse the pulmonary disease in these patients is not known.

REFERENCES

[1] www.ibmtr.org. Accessed september 2007.

[2] Soubani AO, Miller KB, Hassoun PM. Pulmonary complications of bone marrow transplantation. *Chest* 1996;109(4):1066-77.

[3] Paulin T, Ringden O, Lonnqvist B. Faster immunological recovery after bone marrow transplantation in patients without cytomegalovirus infection. *Transplantation* 1985;39(4):377-84.

[4] Witherspoon RP, Storb R, Ochs HD, et al. Recovery of antibody production in human allogeneic marrow graft recipients: influence of time posttransplantation, the presence or absence of chronic graft-versus-host disease, and antithymocyte globulin treatment. *Blood* 1981;58(2):360-8.

[5] Aucouturier P, Barra A, Intrator L, et al. Long lasting IgG subclass and antibacterial polysaccharide antibody deficiency after allogeneic bone marrow transplantation. Blood 1987;70(3):779-85.

[6] Kotloff RM, Ahya VN, Crawford SW. Pulmonary complications of solid organ and hematopoietic stem cell transplantation. *Am J Respir Crit Care Med* 2004;170(1):22-48.

[7] Sloane JP, Depledge MH, Powles RL, Morgenstern GR, Trickey BS, Dady PJ. Histopathology of the lung after bone marrow transplantation. *J Clin Pathol* 1983;36(5):546-54.

[8] Lossos IS, Breuer R, Or R, et al. Bacterial pneumonia in recipients of bone marrow transplantation. A five-year prospective study. *Transplantation* 1995;60(7):672-8.

[9] Wingard JR. Opportunistic infections after blood and marrow transplantation. Transpl Infect Dis 1999;1(1):3-20.

[10] Poutsiaka DD, Price LL, Ucuzian A, Chan GW, Miller KB, Snydman DR. Blood stream infection after hematopoietic stem cell transplantation is associated with increased mortality. *Bone Marrow Transplant* 2007;40(1):63-70.

[11] Rolston KV. The spectrum of pulmonary infections in cancer patients. *Curr Opin Oncol* 2001;13(4):218-23.

[12] Heussel CP, Kauczor HU, Heussel G, Fischer B, Mildenberger P, Thelen M. Early detection of pneumonia in febrile neutropenic patients: use of thin-section CT. *AJR Am J Roentgenol* 1997;169(5):1347-53.

[13] Guidelines for preventing opportunistic infections among hematopoietic stem cell transplant recipients. *MMWR Recomm Rep* 2000;49(RR-10):1-125, CE1-7.
[14] Hofmeister CC, Czerlanis C, Forsythe S, Stiff PJ. Retrospective utility of bronchoscopy after hematopoietic stem cell transplant. *Bone Marrow Transplant* 2006;38(10):693-8.
[15] Laws HJ, Kobbe G, Dilloo D, et al. Surveillance of nosocomial infections in paediatric recipients of bone marrow or peripheral blood stem cell transplantation during neutropenia, compared with adult recipients. *J Hosp Infect* 2006;62(1):80-8.
[16] Narreddy S, Mellon-Reppen S, Abidi MH, et al. Non-bacterial infections in allogeneic non-myeloablative stem cell transplant recipients. *Transpl Infect Dis* 2007;9(1):3-10.
[17] Hakki M, Limaye AP, Kim HW, Kirby KA, Corey L, Boeckh M. Invasive Pseudomonas aeruginosa infections: high rate of recurrence and mortality after hematopoietic cell transplantation. *Bone Marrow Transplant* 2007;39(11):687-93.
[18] Oren I, Zuckerman T, Avivi I, Finkelstein R, Yigla M, Rowe JM. Nosocomial outbreak of Legionella pneumophila serogroup 3 pneumonia in a new bone marrow transplant unit: evaluation, treatment and control. *Bone Marrow Transplant* 2002;30(3):175-9.
[19] Chen CS, Boeckh M, Seidel K, et al. Incidence, risk factors, and mortality from pneumonia developing late after hematopoietic stem cell transplantation. *Bone Marrow Transplan*t 2003;32(5):515-22.
[20] Youssef S, Rodriguez G, Rolston KV, Champlin RE, Raad, II, Safdar A. Streptococcus pneumoniae infections in 47 hematopoietic stem cell transplantation recipients: clinical characteristics of infections and vaccine-breakthrough infections, 1989-2005. *Medicine* (Baltimore) 2007;86(2):69-77.
[21] Niederman MS, Mandell LA, Anzueto A, et al. Guidelines for the management of adults with community-acquired pneumonia. Diagnosis, assessment of severity, antimicrobial therapy, and prevention. *Am J Respir Crit Care Med* 2001;163(7):1730-54.
[22] Guidelines for the management of adults with hospital-acquired, ventilator-associated, and healthcare-associated pneumonia. *Am J Respir Crit Care Med* 2005;171(4):388-416.
[23] Sullivan KM, Dykewicz CA, Longworth DL, et al. Preventing opportunistic infections after hematopoietic stem cell transplantation: the Centers for Disease Control and Prevention, Infectious Diseases Society of America, and American Society for Blood and Marrow Transplantation Practice Guidelines and beyond. *Hematology Am Soc Hematol Educ Program* 2001:392-421.
[24] Bonadio M, Morelli G, Mori S, Riccioni R, Papineschi F, Petrini M. Fluoroquinolone resistance in hematopoietic stem cell transplant recipients with infectious complications. *Biomed Pharmacother* 2005;59(9):511-6.
[25] Daly AS, McGeer A, Lipton JH. Systemic nocardiosis following allogeneic bone marrow transplantation. *Transpl Infect Dis* 2003;5(1):16-20.
[26] van Burik JA, Hackman RC, Nadeem SQ, et al. Nocardiosis after bone marrow transplantation: a retrospective study. *Clin Infect Dis* 1997;24(6):1154-60.
[27] Roy V, Weisdorf D. Mycobacterial infections following bone marrow transplantation: a 20 year retrospective review. *Bone Marrow Transplant* 1997;19(5):467-70.
[28] de la Camara R, Martino R, Granados E, et al. Tuberculosis after hematopoietic stem cell transplantation: incidence, clinical characteristics and outcome. Spanish Group on

Infectious Complications in Hematopoietic Transplantation. *Bone Marrow Transplant* 2000;26(3):291-8.

[29] Cordonnier C, Martino R, Trabasso P, et al. Mycobacterial infection: a difficult and late diagnosis in stem cell transplant recipients. *Clin Infect Dis* 2004;38(9):1229-36.

[30] Ip MS, Yuen KY, Woo PC, et al. Risk factors for pulmonary tuberculosis in bone marrow transplant recipients. *Am J Respir Crit Care Med* 1998;158(4):1173-7.

[31] Ku SC, Tang JL, Hsueh PR, Luh KT, Yu CJ, Yang PC. Pulmonary tuberculosis in allogeneic hematopoietic stem cell transplantation. *Bone Marrow Transplant* 2001;27(12):1293-7.

[32] Yuen KY, Woo PC. Tuberculosis in blood and marrow transplant recipients. Hematol Oncol 2002;20(2):51-62.

[33] Keung YK, Nugent K, Jumper C, Cobos E. Mycobacterium tuberculosis infection masquerading as diffuse alveolar hemorrhage after autologous stem cell transplant. *Bone Marrow Transplant* 1999;23(7):737-8.

[34] Mycobacterium tuberculosis. *Am J Transplant* 2004;4 Suppl 10:37-41.

[35] Doucette K, Fishman JA. Nontuberculous mycobacterial infection in hematopoietic stem cell and solid organ transplant recipients. *Clin Infect Dis* 2004;38(10):1428-39.

[36] Nontuberculous mycobacteria. *Am J Transplant* 2004;4 Suppl 10:42-6.

[37] Griffith DE, Aksamit T, Brown-Elliott BA, et al. An official ATS/IDSA statement: diagnosis, treatment, and prevention of nontuberculous mycobacterial diseases. *Am J Respir Crit Care Med* 2007;175(4):367-416.

[38] Morgan J, Wannemuehler KA, Marr KA, et al. Incidence of invasive aspergillosis following hematopoietic stem cell and solid organ transplantation: interim results of a prospective multicenter surveillance program. *Med Mycol* 2005;43 Suppl 1:S49-58.

[39] Wald A, Leisenring W, van Burik JA, Bowden RA. Epidemiology of Aspergillus infections in a large cohort of patients undergoing bone marrow transplantation. *J Infect Dis* 1997;175(6):1459-66.

[40] Marr KA, Carter RA, Boeckh M, Martin P, Corey L. Invasive aspergillosis in allogeneic stem cell transplant recipients: changes in epidemiology and risk factors. *Blood* 2002;100(13):4358-66.

[41] Fukuda T, Boeckh M, Carter RA, et al. Risks and outcomes of invasive fungal infections in recipients of allogeneic hematopoietic stem cell transplants after nonmyeloablative conditioning. *Blood* 2003;102(3):827-33.

[42] Marr KA, Carter RA, Crippa F, Wald A, Corey L. Epidemiology and outcome of mould infections in hematopoietic stem cell transplant recipients. *Clin Infect Dis* 2002;34(7):909-17.

[43] Baddley JW, Stroud TP, Salzman D, Pappas PG. Invasive mold infections in allogeneic bone marrow transplant recipients. *Clin Infect Dis* 2001;32(9):1319-24.

[44] Junghanss C, Marr KA, Carter RA, et al. Incidence and outcome of bacterial and fungal infections following nonmyeloablative compared with myeloablative allogeneic hematopoietic stem cell transplantation: a matched control study. *Biol Blood Marrow Transplant* 2002;8(9):512-20.

[45] Miyakoshi S, Kusumi E, Matsumura T, et al. Invasive fungal infection following reduced-intensity cord blood transplantation for adult patients with hematologic diseases. *Biol Blood Marrow Transplant* 2007;13(7):771-7.

[46] Warris A, Bjorneklett A, Gaustad P. Invasive pulmonary aspergillosis associated with infliximab therapy. N Engl J Med 2001;344(14):1099-100.

[47] Cordonnier C, Ribaud P, Herbrecht R, et al. Prognostic factors for death due to invasive aspergillosis after hematopoietic stem cell transplantation: a 1-year retrospective study of consecutive patients at French transplantation centers. *Clin Infect Dis* 2006;42(7):955-63.

[48] Ribaud P, Chastang C, Latge JP, et al. Survival and prognostic factors of invasive aspergillosis after allogeneic bone marrow transplantation. *Clin Infect Dis* 1999;28(2):322-30.

[49] Nichols WG, Corey L, Gooley T, Davis C, Boeckh M. High risk of death due to bacterial and fungal infection among cytomegalovirus (CMV)-seronegative recipients of stem cell transplants from seropositive donors: evidence for indirect effects of primary CMV infection. *J Infect Di*s 2002;185(3):273-82.

[50] Iwen PC, Rupp ME, Langnas AN, Reed EC, Hinrichs SH. Invasive pulmonary aspergillosis due to Aspergillus terreus: 12-year experience and review of the literature. *Clin Infect Dis* 1998;26(5):1092-7.

[51] Young RC, Bennett JE, Vogel CL, Carbone PP, DeVita VT. Aspergillosis. The spectrum of the disease in 98 patients. *Medicine* (Baltimore) 1970;49(2):147-73.

[52] Prystowsky SD, Vogelstein B, Ettinger DS, et al. Invasive aspergillosis. *N Engl J Med* 1976;295(12):655-8.

[53] Allo MD, Miller J, Townsend T, Tan C. Primary cutaneous aspergillosis associated with Hickman intravenous catheters. *N Engl J Med* 1987;317(18):1105-8.

[54] Albelda SM, Talbot GH, Gerson SL, Miller WT, Cassileth PA. Pulmonary cavitation and massive hemoptysis in invasive pulmonary aspergillosis. Influence of bone marrow recovery in patients with acute leukemia. *Am Rev Respir* Dis 1985;131(1):115-20.

[55] Denning DW. Invasive aspergillosis. *Clin Infect Dis* 1998;26(4):781-803; quiz 4-5.

[56] Ruhnke M, Bohme A, Buchheidt D, et al. Diagnosis of invasive fungal infections in hematology and oncology--guidelines of the Infectious Diseases Working Party (AGIHO) of the German Society of Hematology and Oncology (DGHO). *Ann Hematol* 2003;82 Suppl 2:S141-8.

[57] Chamilos G, Luna M, Lewis RE, et al. Invasive fungal infections in patients with hematologic malignancies in a tertiary care cancer center: an autopsy study over a 15-year period (1989-2003). *Haematologica* 2006;91(7):986-9.

[58] Libshitz HI, Pagani JJ. Aspergillosis and mucormycosis: two types of opportunistic fungal pneumonia. *Radiology* 1981;140(2):301-6.

[59] Kuhlman JE, Fishman EK, Siegelman SS. Invasive pulmonary aspergillosis in acute leukemia: characteristic findings on CT, the CT halo sign, and the role of CT in early diagnosis. *Radiology* 1985;157(3):611-4.

[60] Caillot D, Casasnovas O, Bernard A, et al. Improved management of invasive pulmonary aspergillosis in neutropenic patients using early thoracic computed tomographic scan and surgery. *J Clin Oncol* 1997;15(1):139-47.

[61] Caillot D, Mannone L, Cuisenier B, Couaillier JF. Role of early diagnosis and aggressive surgery in the management of invasive pulmonary aspergillosis in neutropenic patients. Clin Microbiol Infect 2001;7 Suppl 2:54-61.

[62] Kuhlman JE, Fishman EK, Burch PA, Karp JE, Zerhouni EA, Siegelman SS. Invasive pulmonary aspergillosis in acute leukemia. The contribution of CT to early diagnosis and aggressive management. *Chest* 1987;92(1):95-9.

[63] Curtis AM, Smith GJ, Ravin CE. Air crescent sign of invasive aspergillosis. *Radiology* 1979;133(1):17-21.

[64] Gaeta M, Blandino A, Scribano E, Minutoli F, Volta S, Pandolfo I. Computed tomography halo sign in pulmonary nodules: frequency and diagnostic value. *J Thorac Imaging* 1999;14(2):109-13.

[65] Greene R. The radiological spectrum of pulmonary aspergillosis. *Med Mycol* 2005;43 Suppl 1:S147-54.

[66] Kojima R, Tateishi U, Kami M, et al. Chest computed tomography of late invasive aspergillosis after allogeneic hematopoietic stem cell transplantation. *Biol Blood Marrow Transplant* 2005;11(7):506-11.

[67] Soubani AO, Qureshi MA. Invasive pulmonary aspergillosis following bone marrow transplantation: risk factors and diagnostic aspect. *Haematologia* (Budap) 2002;32(4):427-37.

[68] Horvath JA, Dummer S. The use of respiratory-tract cultures in the diagnosis of invasive pulmonary aspergillosis. *Am J Med* 1996;100(2):171-8.

[69] Yu VL, Muder RR, Poorsattar A. Significance of isolation of Aspergillus from the respiratory tract in diagnosis of invasive pulmonary aspergillosis. Results from a three-year prospective study. *Am J Med* 1986;81(2):249-54.

[70] Tang CM, Cohen J. Diagnosing fungal infections in immunocompromised hosts. *J Clin Pathol* 1992;45(1):1-5.

[71] Duthie R, Denning DW. Aspergillus fungemia: report of two cases and review. *Clin Infect Dis* 1995;20(3):598-605.

[72] Albelda SM, Talbot GH, Gerson SL, Miller WT, Cassileth PA. Role of fiberoptic bronchoscopy in the diagnosis of invasive pulmonary aspergillosis in patients with acute leukemia. *Am J Med* 1984;76(6):1027-34.

[73] Kahn FW, Jones JM, England DM. The role of bronchoalveolar lavage in the diagnosis of invasive pulmonary aspergillosis. *Am J Clin Pathol* 1986;86(4):518-23.

[74] Levy H, Horak DA, Tegtmeier BR, Yokota SB, Forman SJ. The value of bronchoalveolar lavage and bronchial washings in the diagnosis of invasive pulmonary aspergillosis. *Respir Med* 1992;86(3):243-8.

[75] Reichenberger F, Habicht J, Matt P, et al. Diagnostic yield of bronchoscopy in histologically proven invasive pulmonary aspergillosis. *Bone Marrow Transplant* 1999;24(11):1195-9.

[76] Maschmeyer G, Beinert T, Buchheidt D, et al. Diagnosis and antimicrobial therapy of pulmonary infiltrates in febrile neutropenic patients--guidelines of the Infectious Diseases Working Party (AGIHO) of the German Society of Hematology and Oncology (DGHO). *Ann Hematol* 2003;82 Suppl 2:S118-26.

[77] Walsh TJ, Groll AH. Overview: non-fumigatus species of Aspergillus: perspectives on emerging pathogens in immunocompromised hosts. *Curr Opin Investig Drugs* 2001;2(10):1366-7.

[78] Lass-Florl C, Griff K, Mayr A, et al. Epidemiology and outcome of infections due to Aspergillus terreus: 10-year single centre experience. *Br J Haematol* 2005;131(2):201-7.

[79] Steinbach WJ, Benjamin DK, Jr., Kontoyiannis DP, et al. Infections due to Aspergillus terreus: a multicenter retrospective analysis of 83 cases. *Clin Infect Dis* 2004;39(2):192-8.
[80] Hachem RY, Kontoyiannis DP, Boktour MR, et al. Aspergillus terreus: an emerging amphotericin B-resistant opportunistic mold in patients with hematologic malignancies. Cancer 2004;101(7):1594-600.
[81] Kontoyiannis DP, Lewis RE, May GS, Osherov N, Rinaldi MG. Aspergillus nidulans is frequently resistant to amphotericin B. *Mycoses* 2002;45(9-10):406-7.
[82] Walsh TJ, Raad I, Patterson TF, et al. Treatment of invasive aspergillosis with posaconazole in patients who are refractory to or intolerant of conventional therapy: an externally controlled trial. *Clin Infect Dis* 2007;44(1):2-12.
[83] Boutboul F, Alberti C, Leblanc T, et al. Invasive aspergillosis in allogeneic stem cell transplant recipients: increasing antigenemia is associated with progressive disease. *Clin Infect Dis* 2002;34(7):939-43.
[84] Marr KA, Balajee SA, McLaughlin L, Tabouret M, Bentsen C, Walsh TJ. Detection of galactomannan antigenemia by enzyme immunoassay for the diagnosis of invasive aspergillosis: variables that affect performance. *J Infect Dis* 2004;190(3):641-9.
[85. Nguyen MH, Leather H, Clancy CJ, Cline C, Jantz MA, Kulkarni V, Wheat LJ, Wingard JR. Galactomannan testing in bronchoalveolar lavage fluid facilitates the diagnosis of invasive pulmonary aspergillosis in patients with hematologic malignancies and stem cell transplant recipients. *Biol Blood* Marrow Transplant.
[2011 Jul;17(7):1043-50. Epub 2010 Nov 16. PubMed PMID: 21087680.
[86] Pfeiffer CD, Fine JP, Safdar N. Diagnosis of invasive aspergillosis using a galactomannan assay: a meta-analysis. *Clin Infect Dis* 2006;42(10):1417-727.
[87] Herbrecht R, Letscher-Bru V, Oprea C, et al. Aspergillus galactomannan detection in the diagnosis of invasive aspergillosis in cancer patients. *J Clin Oncol* 2002;20(7):1898-906.
[88] Singh N, Obman A, Husain S, Aspinall S, Mietzner S, Stout JE. Reactivity of platelia Aspergillus galactomannan antigen with piperacillin-tazobactam: clinical implications based on achievable concentrations in serum. *Antimicrob Agents Chemother* 2004;48(6):1989-92.
[89] Marr KA, Laverdiere M, Gugel A, Leisenring W. Antifungal therapy decreases sensitivity of the Aspergillus galactomannan enzyme immunoassay. *Clin Infect Dis* 2005;40(12):1762-9.
[90] Ansorg R, van den Boom R, Rath PM. Detection of Aspergillus galactomannan antigen in foods and antibiotics. *Mycoses* 1997;40(9-10):353-7.
[91] Busca A, Locatelli F, Barbui A, et al. Usefulness of sequential Aspergillus galactomannan antigen detection combined with early radiologic evaluation for diagnosis of invasive pulmonary aspergillosis in patients undergoing allogeneic stem cell transplantation. *Transplant Proc* 2006;38(5):1610-3.
[92] Musher B, Fredricks D, Leisenring W, Balajee SA, Smith C, Marr KA. Aspergillus galactomannan enzyme immunoassay and quantitative PCR for diagnosis of invasive aspergillosis with bronchoalveolar lavage fluid. *J Clin Microbiol* 2004;42(12):5517-22.
[93] Klont RR, Mennink-Kersten MA, Verweij PE. Utility of Aspergillus antigen detection in specimens other than serum specimens. *Clin Infect Dis* 2004;39(10):1467-74.

[94] Salonen J, Lehtonen OP, Terasjarvi MR, Nikoskelainen J. Aspergillus antigen in serum, urine and bronchoalveolar lavage specimens of neutropenic patients in relation to clinical outcome. *Scand J Infect Dis* 2000;32(5):485-90.

[95] Hizel K, Kokturk N, Kalkanci A, Ozturk C, Kustimur S, Tufan M. Polymerase chain reaction in the diagnosis of invasive aspergillosis. *Mycoses* 2004;47(7):338-42.

[96] Buchheidt D, Baust C, Skladny H, et al. Detection of Aspergillus species in blood and bronchoalveolar lavage samples from immunocompromised patients by means of 2-step polymerase chain reaction: clinical results. *Clin Infect Dis* 2001;33(4):428-35.

[97] Loeffler J, Kloepfer K, Hebart H, et al. Polymerase chain reaction detection of aspergillus DNA in experimental models of invasive aspergillosis. *J Infect Dis* 2002;185(8):1203-6.

[98] Halliday C, Hoile R, Sorrell T, et al. Role of prospective screening of blood for invasive aspergillosis by polymerase chain reaction in febrile neutropenic recipients of haematopoietic stem cell transplants and patients with acute leukaemia. *Br J Haematol* 2006;132(4):478-86.

[99] Obayashi T, Yoshida M, Mori T, et al. Plasma (1-->3)-beta-D-glucan measurement in diagnosis of invasive deep mycosis and fungal febrile episodes. *Lancet* 1995;345(8941):17-20.

[100] Ascioglu S, Rex JH, de Pauw B, et al. Defining opportunistic invasive fungal infections in immunocompromised patients with cancer and hematopoietic stem cell transplants: an international consensus. *Clin Infect Dis* 2002;34(1):7-14.

[101] Johnson LB, Kauffman CA. Voriconazole: a new triazole antifungal agent. *Clin Infect Dis* 2003;36(5):630-7.

[102] Sambatakou H, Dupont B, Lode H, Denning DW. Voriconazole treatment for subacute invasive and chronic pulmonary aspergillosis. *Am J Med* 2006;119(6):527 e17-24.

[103] Ghannoum MA, Kuhn DM. Voriconazole -- better chances for patients with invasive mycoses. *Eur J Med Res* 2002;7(5):242-56.

[104] Herbrecht R, Denning DW, Patterson TF, et al. Voriconazole versus amphotericin B for primary therapy of invasive aspergillosis. *N Engl J Med* 2002;347(6):408-15.

[105] Segal BH, Barnhart LA, Anderson VL, Walsh TJ, Malech HL, Holland SM. Posaconazole as salvage therapy in patients with chronic granulomatous disease and invasive filamentous fungal infection. *Clin Infect Dis* 2005;40(11):1684-8.

[106] Pitisuttithum P, Negroni R, Graybill JR, et al. Activity of posaconazole in the treatment of central nervous system fungal infections. *J Antimicrob Chemother* 2005;56(4):745-55.

[107] Spanakis EK, Aperis G, Mylonakis E. New agents for the treatment of fungal infections: clinical efficacy and gaps in coverage. *Clin Infect Dis* 2006;43(8):1060-8.

[108] Cohen-Wolkowiez M, Benjamin DK, Jr., Steinbach WJ, Smith PB. Anidulafungin: a new echinocandin for the treatment of fungal infections. Drugs Today (Barc) 2006;42(8):533-44.

[109] Aliff TB, Maslak PG, Jurcic JG, et al. Refractory Aspergillus pneumonia in patients with acute leukemia: successful therapy with combination caspofungin and liposomal amphotericin. *Cancer* 2003;97(4):1025-32.

[110] Kontoyiannis DP, Hachem R, Lewis RE, et al. Efficacy and toxicity of caspofungin in combination with liposomal amphotericin B as primary or salvage treatment of invasive aspergillosis in patients with hematologic malignancies. *Cancer* 2003;98(2):292-9.

[111] Graybill JR, Bocanegra R, Gonzalez GM, Najvar LK. Combination antifungal therapy of murine aspergillosis: liposomal amphotericin B and micafungin. *J Antimicrob Chemother* 2003;52(4):656-62.

[112] Marr KA, Boeckh M, Carter RA, Kim HW, Corey L. Combination antifungal therapy for invasive aspergillosis. *Clin Infect Dis* 2004;39(6):797-802.

[113] Perea S, Gonzalez G, Fothergill AW, Kirkpatrick WR, Rinaldi MG, Patterson TF. In vitro interaction of caspofungin acetate with voriconazole against clinical isolates of Aspergillus spp. *Antimicrob Agents Chemother* 2002;46(9):3039-41.

[114] Denning DW, Marr KA, Lau WM, et al. Micafungin (FK463), alone or in combination with other systemic antifungal agents, for the treatment of acute invasive aspergillosis. J Infect 2006;53(5):337-49.

[115] Moreau P, Zahar JR, Milpied N, et al. Localized invasive pulmonary aspergillosis in patients with neutropenia. Effectiveness of surgical resection. *Cancer* 1993;72(11):3223-6.

[116] Reichenberger F, Habicht J, Kaim A, et al. Lung resection for invasive pulmonary aspergillosis in neutropenic patients with hematologic diseases. *Am J Respir Crit Care Med* 1998;158(3):885-90.

[117] Habicht JM, Reichenberger F, Gratwohl A, Zerkowski HR, Tamm M. Surgical aspects of resection for suspected invasive pulmonary fungal infection in neutropenic patients. *Ann Thorac Surg* 1999;68(2):321-5.

[118] Pidhorecky I, Urschel J, Anderson T. Resection of invasive pulmonary aspergillosis in immunocompromised patients. *Ann Surg Oncol* 2000;7(4):312-7.

[119] Matt P, Bernet F, Habicht J, et al. Predicting outcome after lung resection for invasive pulmonary aspergillosis in patients with neutropenia. *Chest* 2004;126(6):1783-8.

[120] Baron O, Guillaume B, Moreau P, et al. Aggressive surgical management in localized pulmonary mycotic and nonmycotic infections for neutropenic patients with acute leukemia: report of eighteen cases. *J Thorac Cardiovasc Surg* 1998;115(1):63-8; discussion 8-9.

[121] Giles FJ. Monocyte-macrophages, granulocyte-macrophage colony-stimulating factor, and prolonged survival among patients with acute myeloid leukemia and stem cell transplants. *Clin Infect Dis* 1998;26(6):1282-9.

[122] Roilides E, Holmes A, Blake C, Venzon D, Pizzo PA, Walsh TJ. Antifungal activity of elutriated human monocytes against Aspergillus fumigatus hyphae: enhancement by granulocyte-macrophage colony-stimulating factor and interferon-gamma. *J Infect Dis* 1994;170(4):894-9.

[123] Roilides E, Sein T, Holmes A, et al. Effects of macrophage colony-stimulating factor on antifungal activity of mononuclear phagocytes against Aspergillus fumigatus. *J Infect Dis* 1995;172(4):1028-34.

[124] Rowe JM, Andersen JW, Mazza JJ, et al. A randomized placebo-controlled phase III study of granulocyte-macrophage colony-stimulating factor in adult patients (> 55 to 70 years of age) with acute myelogenous leukemia: a study of the Eastern Cooperative Oncology Group (E1490). *Blood* 1995;86(2):457-62.

[125] Ozer H, Armitage JO, Bennett CL, et al. 2000 update of recommendations for the use of hematopoietic colony-stimulating factors: evidence-based, clinical practice guidelines. American Society of Clinical Oncology Growth Factors Expert Panel. *J Clin Oncol* 2000;18(20):3558-85.

[126] Roilides E, Uhlig K, Venzon D, Pizzo PA, Walsh TJ. Prevention of corticosteroid-induced suppression of human polymorphonuclear leukocyte-induced damage of Aspergillus fumigatus hyphae by granulocyte colony-stimulating factor and gamma interferon. *Infect Immun* 1993;61(11):4870-7.
[127] Nagai H, Guo J, Choi H, Kurup V. Interferon-gamma and tumor necrosis factor-alpha protect mice from invasive aspergillosis. *J Infect Dis* 1995;172(6):1554-60.
[128] Safdar A. Strategies to enhance immune function in hematopoietic transplantation recipients who have fungal infections. *Bone Marrow Transplan*t 2006;38(5):327-37.
[129] Safdar A, Rodriguez G, Ohmagari N, et al. The safety of interferon-gamma-1b therapy for invasive fungal infections after hematopoietic stem cell transplantation. *Cancer* 2005;103(4):731-9.
[130] Price TH, Bowden RA, Boeckh M, et al. Phase I/II trial of neutrophil transfusions from donors stimulated with G-CSF and dexamethasone for treatment of patients with infections in hematopoietic stem cell transplantation. *Blood* 2000;95(11):3302-9.
[131] Sherertz RJ, Belani A, Kramer BS, et al. Impact of air filtration on nosocomial Aspergillus infections. Unique risk of bone marrow transplant recipients. *Am J Med* 1987;83(4):709-18.
[132] Mattiuzzi GN, Kantarjian H, O'Brien S, et al. Intravenous itraconazole for prophylaxis of systemic fungal infections in patients with acute myelogenous leukemia and high-risk myelodysplastic syndrome undergoing induction chemotherapy. *Cancer* 2004;100(3):568-73.
[133] Ullmann AJ, Cornely OA. Antifungal prophylaxis for invasive mycoses in high risk patients. *Curr Opin Infect Dis* 2006;19(6):571-6.
[134] Ullmann AJ, Lipton JH, Vesole DH, et al. Posaconazole or fluconazole for prophylaxis in severe graft-versus-host disease. *N Engl J Med* 2007;356(4):335-47.
[135] Nucci M, Marr KA, Queiroz-Telles F, et al. Fusarium infection in hematopoietic stem cell transplant recipients. *Clin Infect Dis* 2004;38(9):1237-42.
[136] Boutati EI, Anaissie EJ. Fusarium, a significant emerging pathogen in patients with hematologic malignancy: ten years' experience at a cancer center and implications for management. *Blood* 1997;90(3):999-1008.
[137] Gaziev D, Baronciani D, Galimberti M, et al. Mucormycosis after bone marrow transplantation: report of four cases in thalassemia and review of the literature. *Bone Marrow Transplant* 1996;17(3):409-14.
[138] Maertens J, Demuynck H, Verbeken EK, et al. Mucormycosis in allogeneic bone marrow transplant recipients: report of five cases and review of the role of iron overload in the pathogenesis. *Bone Marrow Transplant* 1999;24(3):307-12.
[139] Costa SF, Alexander BD. Non-Aspergillus fungal pneumonia in transplant recipients. *Clin Chest Med* 2005;26(4):675-90, vii.
[140] Groll AH, Walsh TJ. Uncommon opportunistic fungi: new nosocomial threats. Clin Microbiol Infect 2001;7 Suppl 2:8-24.
[141] Jahagirdar BN, Morrison VA. Emerging fungal pathogens in patients with hematologic malignancies and marrow/stem-cell transplant recipients. *Semin Respir Infect* 2002;17(2):113-20.
[142] Sampathkumar P, Paya CV. Fusarium infection after solid-organ transplantation. *Clin Infect Dis* 2001;32(8):1237-40.

[143] Castiglioni B, Sutton DA, Rinaldi MG, Fung J, Kusne S. Pseudallescheria boydii (Anamorph Scedosporium apiospermum). Infection in solid organ transplant recipients in a tertiary medical center and review of the literature. *Medicine* (Baltimore) 2002;81(5):333-48.

[144] Berenguer J, Rodriguez-Tudela JL, Richard C, et al. Deep infections caused by Scedosporium prolificans. A report on 16 cases in Spain and a review of the literature. Scedosporium Prolificans Spanish Study Group. *Medicine* (Baltimore) 1997;76(4):256-65.

[145] Espinel-Ingroff A. In vitro fungicidal activities of voriconazole, itraconazole, and amphotericin B against opportunistic moniliaceous and dematiaceous fungi. *J Clin Microbiol* 2001;39(3):954-8.

[146] Husain S, Munoz P, Forrest G, et al. Infections due to Scedosporium apiospermum and Scedosporium prolificans in transplant recipients: clinical characteristics and impact of antifungal agent therapy on outcome. *Clin Infect Dis* 2005;40(1):89-99.

[147] Trifilio S, Singhal S, Williams S, et al. Breakthrough fungal infections after allogeneic hematopoietic stem cell transplantation in patients on prophylactic voriconazole. *Bone Marrow Transplant* 2007.

[148] Page RL, 2nd, Schwiesow J, Hilts A. Posaconazole as salvage therapy in a patient with disseminated zygomycosis: case report and review of the literature. *Pharmacotherapy* 2007;27(2):290-8.

[149] Glenn TJ, Blair JE, Adams RH. Coccidioidomycosis in hematopoietic stem cell transplant recipients. *Med Mycol* 2005;43(8):705-10.

[150] Goodrich JM, Reed EC, Mori M, et al. Clinical features and analysis of risk factors for invasive candidal infection after marrow transplantation. *J Infect Dis* 1991;164(4):731-40.

[151] Stringer JR, Beard CB, Miller RF, Wakefield AE. A new name (Pneumocystis jiroveci) for Pneumocystis from humans. *Emerg Infect Dis* 2002;8(9):891-6.

[152] Rodriguez M, Sifri CD, Fishman JA. Failure of low-dose atovaquone prophylaxis against Pneumocystis jiroveci infection in transplant recipients. *Clin Infect Dis* 2004;38(8):e76-8.

[153] Torre-Cisneros J, De la Mata M, Pozo JC, et al. Randomized trial of weekly sulfadoxine/pyrimethamine vs. daily low-dose trimethoprim-sulfamethoxazole for the prophylaxis of Pneumocystis carinii pneumonia after liver transplantation. *Clin Infect Dis* 1999;29(4):771-4.

[154] Marras TK, Sanders K, Lipton JH, Messner HA, Conly J, Chan CK. Aerosolized pentamidine prophylaxis for Pneumocystis carinii pneumonia after allogeneic marrow transplantation. *Transpl Infect Dis* 2002;4(2):66-74.

[155] De Castro N, Neuville S, Sarfati C, et al. Occurrence of Pneumocystis jiroveci pneumonia after allogeneic stem cell transplantation: a 6-year retrospective study. *Bone Marrow Transplant* 2005;36(10):879-83.

[156] Torres HA, Chemaly RF, Storey R, et al. Influence of type of cancer and hematopoietic stem cell transplantation on clinical presentation of Pneumocystis jiroveci pneumonia in cancer patients. *Eur J Clin Microbiol Infect Dis* 2006;25(6):382-8.

[157] Ison MG, Fishman JA. Cytomegalovirus pneumonia in transplant recipients. *Clin Chest Med* 2005;26(4):691-705, viii.

[158] Meyers JD, Flournoy N, Thomas ED. Nonbacterial pneumonia after allogeneic marrow transplantation: a review of ten years' experience. *Rev Infect Dis* 1982;4(6):1119-32.
[159] Crawford SW, Bowden RA, Hackman RC, Gleaves CA, Meyers JD, Clark JG. Rapid detection of cytomegalovirus pulmonary infection by bronchoalveolar lavage and centrifugation culture. *Ann Intern Med* 1988;108(2):180-5.
[160] Blacklock HA, Griffiths P, Stirk P, Prentice HG. Specific hyperimmune globulin for cytomegalovirus pneumonitis. *Lancet* 1985;2(8447):152-3.
[161] Taplitz RA, Jordan MC. Pneumonia caused by herpesviruses in recipients of hematopoietic cell transplants. *Semin Respir Infect* 2002;17(2):121-9.
[162] Konoplev S, Champlin RE, Giralt S, et al. Cytomegalovirus pneumonia in adult autologous blood and marrow transplant recipients. *Bone Marrow Transplant* 2001;27(8):877-81.
[163] Shepp DH, Dandliker PS, de Miranda P, et al. Activity of 9-[2-hydroxy-1-(hydroxymethyl)ethoxymethyl]guanine in the treatment of cytomegalovirus pneumonia. *Ann Intern Med* 1985;103(3):368-73.
[164] Boeckh M, Leisenring W, Riddell SR, et al. Late cytomegalovirus disease and mortality in recipients of allogeneic hematopoietic stem cell transplants: importance of viral load and T-cell immunity. *Blood* 2003;101(2):407-14.
[165] Junghanss C, Boeckh M, Carter RA, et al. Incidence and outcome of cytomegalovirus infections following nonmyeloablative compared with myeloablative allogeneic stem cell transplantation, a matched control study. *Blood* 2002;99(6):1978-85.
[166] Ljungman P, Aschan J, Lewensohn-Fuchs I, et al. Results of different strategies for reducing cytomegalovirus-associated mortality in allogeneic stem cell transplant recipients. *Transplantation* 1998;66(10):1330-4.
[167] Reusser P. Cytomegalovirus infection and disease after bone marrow transplantation: epidemiology, prevention, and treatment. Bone Marrow Transplant 1991;7 Suppl 3:52-6.
[168] Enright H, Haake R, Weisdorf D, et al. Cytomegalovirus pneumonia after bone marrow transplantation. Risk factors and response to therapy. *Transplantation* 1993;55(6):1339-46.
[169] Holmberg LA, Boeckh M, Hooper H, et al. Increased incidence of cytomegalovirus disease after autologous CD34-selected peripheral blood stem cell transplantation. *Blood* 1999;94(12):4029-35.
[170] Leung AN, Gosselin MV, Napper CH, et al. Pulmonary infections after bone marrow transplantation: clinical and radiographic findings. *Radiology* 1999;210(3):699-710.
[171] Franquet T, Lee KS, Muller NL. Thin-section CT findings in 32 immunocompromised patients with cytomegalovirus pneumonia who do not have AIDS. *AJR Am J Roentgenol* 2003;181(4):1059-63.
[172] Tamm M, Traenkle P, Grilli B, et al. Pulmonary cytomegalovirus infection in immunocompromised patients. *Chest* 2001;119(3):838-43.
[173] Sakamaki H, Yuasa K, Goto H, et al. Comparison of cytomegalovirus (CMV) antigenemia and CMV in bronchoalveolar lavage fluid for diagnosis of CMV pulmonary infection after bone marrow transplantation. *Bone Marrow Transplant* 1997;20(2):143-7.

[174] Michaelides A, Liolios L, Glare EM, et al. Increased human cytomegalovirus (HCMV) DNA load in peripheral blood leukocytes after lung transplantation correlates with HCMV pneumonitis. *Transplantation* 2001;72(1):141-7.

[175] Westall GP, Michaelides A, Williams TJ, Snell GI, Kotsimbos TC. Human cytomegalovirus load in plasma and bronchoalveolar lavage fluid: a longitudinal study of lung transplant recipients. *J Infect Dis* 2004;190(6):1076-83.

[176] Humar A, Lipton J, Welsh S, Moussa G, Messner H, Mazzulli T. A randomised trial comparing cytomegalovirus antigenemia assay vs screening bronchoscopy for the early detection and prevention of disease in allogeneic bone marrow and peripheral blood stem cell transplant recipients. *Bone Marrow Transplant* 2001;28(5):485-90.

[177] Leruez-Ville M, Ouachee M, Delarue R, et al. Monitoring cytomegalovirus infection in adult and pediatric bone marrow transplant recipients by a real-time PCR assay performed with blood plasma. *J Clin Microbiol* 2003;41(5):2040-6.

[178] Reinke P, Prosch S, Kern F, Volk HD. Mechanisms of human cytomegalovirus (HCMV) (re)activation and its impact on organ transplant patients. *Transpl Infect Dis* 1999;1(3):157-64.

[179] Bordon V, Bravo S, Van Renterghem L, et al. Surveillance of cytomegalovirus (CMV) DNAemia in pediatric allogeneic stem cell transplantation: incidence and outcome of CMV infection and disease. *Transpl Infect Dis* 2007.

[180] Bacigalupo A, Bregante S, Tedone E, et al. Combined foscarnet -ganciclovir treatment for cytomegalovirus infections after allogeneic hemopoietic stem cell transplantation (Hsct). *Bone Marrow Transplant* 1996;18 Suppl 2:110-4.

[181] Bowden RA, Slichter SJ, Sayers M, et al. A comparison of filtered leukocyte-reduced and cytomegalovirus (CMV) seronegative blood products for the prevention of transfusion-associated CMV infection after marrow transplant. *Blood* 1995;86(9):3598-603.

[182] Nichols WG, Price TH, Gooley T, Corey L, Boeckh M. Transfusion-transmitted cytomegalovirus infection after receipt of leukoreduced blood products. *Blood* 2003;101(10):4195-200.

[183] Zaia JA. Prevention and treatment of cytomegalovirus pneumonia in transplant recipients. *Clin Infect Dis* 1993;17 Suppl 2:S392-9.

[184] Goodrich JM, Bowden RA, Fisher L, Keller C, Schoch G, Meyers JD. Ganciclovir prophylaxis to prevent cytomegalovirus disease after allogeneic marrow transplant. Ann Intern Med 1993;118(3):173-8.

[185] Walter EA, Greenberg PD, Gilbert MJ, et al. Reconstitution of cellular immunity against cytomegalovirus in recipients of allogeneic bone marrow by transfer of T-cell clones from the donor. *N Engl J Med* 1995;333(16):1038-44.

[186] Lujan-Zilbermann J, Benaim E, Tong X, Srivastava DK, Patrick CC, DeVincenzo JP. Respiratory virus infections in pediatric hematopoietic stem cell transplantation. *Clin Infect Dis* 2001;33(7):962-8.

[187] Roghmann M, Ball K, Erdman D, Lovchik J, Anderson LJ, Edelman R. Active surveillance for respiratory virus infections in adults who have undergone bone marrow and peripheral blood stem cell transplantation. *Bone Marrow Transplant* 2003;32(11):1085-8.

[188] van Kraaij MG, van Elden LJ, van Loon AM, et al. Frequent detection of respiratory viruses in adult recipients of stem cell transplants with the use of real-time polymerase chain reaction, compared with viral culture. Clin Infect Dis 2005;40(5):662-9.
[189] Chemaly RF, Ghosh S, Bodey GP, et al. Respiratory viral infections in adults with hematologic malignancies and human stem cell transplantation recipients: a retrospective study at a major cancer center. *Medicine* (Baltimore) 2006;85(5):278-87.
[190] Bowden RA. Respiratory virus infections after marrow transplant: the Fred Hutchinson Cancer Research Center experience. *Am J Med* 1997;102(3A):27-30; discussion 42-3.
[191] Franquet T, Rodriguez S, Martino R, Gimenez A, Salinas T, Hidalgo A. Thin-section CT findings in hematopoietic stem cell transplantation recipients with respiratory virus pneumonia. *AJR Am J Roentgenol* 2006;187(4):1085-90.
[192] Whimbey E, Englund JA, Couch RB. Community respiratory virus infections in immunocompromised patients with cancer. Am J Med 1997;102(3A):10-8; discussion 25-6.
[193] Raboni SM, Nogueira MB, Tsuchiya LR, et al. Respiratory tract viral infections in bone marrow transplant patients. *Transplantation* 2003;76(1):142-6.
[194] Bredius RG, Templeton KE, Scheltinga SA, Claas EC, Kroes AC, Vossen JM. Prospective study of respiratory viral infections in pediatric hemopoietic stem cell transplantation patients. *Pediatr Infect Dis J* 2004;23(6):518-22.
[195] Nichols WG, Corey L, Gooley T, Davis C, Boeckh M. Parainfluenza virus infections after hematopoietic stem cell transplantation: risk factors, response to antiviral therapy, and effect on transplant outcome. *Blood* 2001;98(3):573-8.
[196] Garcia R, Raad I, Abi-Said D, et al. Nosocomial respiratory syncytial virus infections: prevention and control in bone marrow transplant patients. *Infect Control Hosp Epidemiol* 1997;18(6):412-6.
[197] Hall CB. Nosocomial respiratory syncytial virus infections: the "Cold War" has not ended. Clin Infect Dis 2000;31(2):590-6.
[198] Ghosh S, Champlin RE, Ueno NT, et al. Respiratory syncytial virus infections in autologous blood and marrow transplant recipients with breast cancer: combination therapy with aerosolized ribavirin and parenteral immunoglobulins. *Bone Marrow Transplant* 2001;28(3):271-5.
[199] Abdallah A, Rowland KE, Schepetiuk SK, To LB, Bardy P. An outbreak of respiratory syncytial virus infection in a bone marrow transplant unit: effect on engraftment and outcome of pneumonia without specific antiviral treatment. *Bone Marrow Transplant* 2003;32(2):195-203.
[200] Small TN, Casson A, Malak SF, et al. Respiratory syncytial virus infection following hematopoietic stem cell transplantation. *Bone Marrow Transplant* 2002;29(4):321-7.
[201] Ljungman P. Respiratory virus infections in bone marrow transplant recipients: the European perspective. *Am J Med* 1997;102(3A):44-7.
[202] Falsey AR, Walsh EE. Respiratory syncytial virus infection in adults. *Clin Microbiol Rev* 2000;13(3):371-84.
[203] Barton TD, Blumberg EA. Viral pneumonias other than cytomegalovirus in transplant recipients. *Clin Chest Med* 2005;26(4):707-20, viii.
[204] Escuissato DL, Gasparetto EL, Marchiori E, et al. Pulmonary infections after bone marrow transplantation: high-resolution CT findings in 111 patients. *AJR Am J Roentgenol* 2005;185(3):608-15.

[205] Englund JA, Piedra PA, Whimbey E. Prevention and treatment of respiratory syncytial virus and parainfluenza viruses in immunocompromised patients. *Am J Med* 1997;102(3A):61-70; discussion 5-6.

[206] Community-acquired respiratory viruses. *Am J Transplant* 2004;4 Suppl 10:105-9.

[207] Ottolini MG, Curtis SR, Mathews A, Ottolini SR, Prince GA. Palivizumab is highly effective in suppressing respiratory syncytial virus in an immunosuppressed animal model. *Bone Marrow Transplant* 2002;29(2):117-20.

[208] Boeckh M, Englund J, Li Y, et al. Randomized controlled multicenter trial of aerosolized ribavirin for respiratory syncytial virus upper respiratory tract infection in hematopoietic cell transplant recipients. *Clin Infect Dis* 2007;44(2):245-9.

[209] Whimbey E, Vartivarian SE, Champlin RE, Elting LS, Luna M, Bodey GP. Parainfluenza virus infection in adult bone marrow transplant recipients. *Eur J Clin Microbiol Infect Dis* 1993;12(9):699-701.

[210] Elizaga J, Olavarria E, Apperley J, Goldman J, Ward K. Parainfluenza virus 3 infection after stem cell transplant: relevance to outcome of rapid diagnosis and ribavirin treatment. *Clin Infect Dis* 2001;32(3):413-8.

[211] McCurdy LH, Milstone A, Dummer S. Clinical features and outcomes of paramyxoviral infection in lung transplant recipients treated with ribavirin. *J Heart Lung Transplant* 2003;22(7):745-53.

[212] Nichols WG, Guthrie KA, Corey L, Boeckh M. Influenza infections after hematopoietic stem cell transplantation: risk factors, mortality, and the effect of antiviral therapy. *Clin Infect Dis* 2004;39(9):1300-6.

[213] Vu D, Peck AJ, Nichols WG, et al. Safety and tolerability of oseltamivir prophylaxis in hematopoietic stem cell transplant recipients: a retrospective case-control study. *Clin Infect Dis* 2007;45(2):187-93.

[214] Symeonidis N, Jakubowski A, Pierre-Louis S, et al. Invasive adenoviral infections in T-cell-depleted allogeneic hematopoietic stem cell transplantation: high mortality in the era of cidofovir. *Transpl Infect Dis* 2007;9(2):108-13.

[215] Myers GD, Bollard CM, Wu MF, et al. Reconstitution of adenovirus-specific cell-mediated immunity in pediatric patients after hematopoietic stem cell transplantation. *Bone Marrow Transplant* 2007;39(11):677-86.

[216] Shields AF, Hackman RC, Fife KH, Corey L, Meyers JD. Adenovirus infections in patients undergoing bone-marrow transplantation. *N Engl J Med* 1985;312(9):529-33.

[217] Adenovirus. Am J Transplant 2004;4 Suppl 10:101-4.

[218] Hassan IA, Chopra R, Swindell R, Mutton KJ. Respiratory viral infections after bone marrow/peripheral stem-cell transplantation: the Christie hospital experience. *Bone Marrow Transplant* 2003;32(1):73-7.

[219] Buchbinder S, Elmaagacli AH, Schaefer UW, Roggendorf M. Human herpesvirus 6 is an important pathogen in infectious lung disease after allogeneic bone marrow transplantation. *Bone Marrow Transplant* 2000;26(6):639-44.

[220] Hentrich M, Oruzio D, Jager G, et al. Impact of human herpesvirus-6 after haematopoietic stem cell transplantation. *Br J Haematol* 2005;128(1):66-72.

[221] Gorak E, Geller N, Srinivasan R, et al. Engraftment syndrome after nonmyeloablative allogeneic hematopoietic stem cell transplantation: incidence and effects on survival. *Biol Blood Marrow Transplant* 2005;11(7):542-50.

[222] Spitzer TR. Engraftment syndrome following hematopoietic stem cell transplantation. *Bone Marrow Transplant* 2001;27(9):893-8.

[223] Maiolino A, Biasoli I, Lima J, Portugal AC, Pulcheri W, Nucci M. Engraftment syndrome following autologous hematopoietic stem cell transplantation: definition of diagnostic criteria. *Bone Marrow Transplant* 2003;31:393-7.

[224] Karlin L, Darmon M, Thiery G, et al. Respiratory status deterioration during G-CSF-induced neutropenia recovery. *Bone Marrow Transplan*t 2005;36:245-50.

[225] Capizzi SA, Kumar S, Huneke NE, et al. Peri-engraftment respiratory distress syndrome during autologous hematopoietic stem cell transplantation. *Bone Marrow Transplant* 2001;27:1299-303.

[226] Lee CK, Gingrich RD, Hohl RJ, Ajram KA. Engraftment syndrome in autologous bone marrow and peripheral stem cell transplantation. *Bone Marrow Transplant* 1995;16:175-82.

[227] Marin D, Berrade J, Ferra C, et al. Engraftment syndrome and survival after respiratory failure post-bone marrow transplantation. *Intensive Care Med 1*998;24:732-5.

[228] Afessa B, Tefferi A, Litzow MR, Krowka MJ, Wylam ME, Peters SG. Diffuse alveolar hemorrhage in hematopoietic stem cell transplant recipients. *Am J Respir Crit Care Med* 2002;166(5):641-5.

[229] Afessa B, Tefferi A, Litzow MR, Peters SG. Outcome of diffuse alveolar hemorrhage in hematopoietic stem cell transplant recipients. *Am J Respir Crit Care Med* 2002;166(10):1364-8.

[230] Robbins RA, Linder J, Stahl MG, et al. Diffuse alveolar hemorrhage in autologous bone marrow transplant recipients. *Am J Med* 1989;87:511-8.

[231] Majhail NS, Parks K, Defor TE, Weisdorf DJ. Alveolar hemorrhage following allogeneic hematopoietic cell transplantation using reduced-intensity conditioning. *Bone Marrow Transplant* 2006;38:765-8.

[232] Agusti C, Ramirez J, Picado C, et al. Diffuse alveolar hemorrhage in allogeneic bone marrow transplantation. A postmortem study. *Am J Respir Crit Care Med* 1995;151:1006-10.

[233] Metcalf JP, Rennard SI, Reed EC, et al. Corticosteroids as adjunctive therapy for diffuse alveolar hemorrhage associated with bone marrow transplantation. University of Nebraska Medical Center Bone Marrow Transplant Group. *Am J Med* 1994;96:327-34.

[234] Raptis A, Mavroudis D, Suffredini A, et al. High-dose corticosteroid therapy for diffuse alveolar hemorrhage in allogeneic bone marrow stem cell transplant recipients. *Bone Marrow Transplant* 1999;24:879-83.

[235] Lewis ID, DeFor T, Weisdorf DJ. Increasing incidence of diffuse alveolar hemorrhage following allogeneic bone marrow transplantation: cryptic etiology and uncertain therapy. *Bone Marrow Transplant* 2000;26:539-43.

[236] Wanko SO, Broadwater G, Folz RJ, Chao NJ. Diffuse alveolar hemorrhage: retrospective review of clinical outcome in allogeneic transplant recipients treated with aminocaproic acid. *Biol Blood Marrow Transplant* 2006;12:949-53.

[237] Clark JG, Hansen JA, Hertz MI, Parkman R, Jensen L, Peavy HH. NHLBI workshop summary. Idiopathic pneumonia syndrome after bone marrow transplantation. *Am Rev Respir Dis* 1993;147:1601-6.

[238] Kantrow SP, Hackman RC, Boeckh M, Myerson D, Crawford SW. Idiopathic pneumonia syndrome: changing spectrum of lung injury after marrow transplantation. *Transplantation* 1997;63:1079-86.
[239] Afessa B, Litzow MR, Tefferi A. Bronchiolitis obliterans and other late onset non-infectious pulmonary complications in hematopoietic stem cell transplantation. *Bone Marrow Transplant* 2001;28(5):425-34.
[240] Fukuda T, Hackman RC, Guthrie KA, et al. Risks and outcomes of idiopathic pneumonia syndrome after nonmyeloablative and conventional conditioning regimens for allogeneic hematopoietic stem cell transplantation. *Blood* 2003;102:2777-85.
[241] Crawford SW, Longton G, Storb R. Acute graft-versus-host disease and the risks for idiopathic pneumonia after marrow transplantation for severe aplastic anemia. *Bone Marrow Transplant* 1993;12:225-31.
[242] Yanik GA, Ho VT, Levine JE, et al. The impact of soluble tumor necrosis factor receptor etanercept on the treatment of idiopathic pneumonia syndrome after allogeneic hematopoietic stem cell transplantation. *Blood* 2008;112:3073-81.
[243] Yanik G, Hellerstedt B, Custer J, et al. Etanercept (Enbrel) administration for idiopathic pneumonia syndrome after allogeneic hematopoietic stem cell transplantation. *Biol Blood Marrow Transplant* 2002;8:395-400.
[244] Chien JW, Martin PJ, Flowers ME, Nichols WG, Clark JG. Implications of early airflow decline after myeloablative allogeneic stem cell transplantation. *Bone Marrow Transplant* 2004;33:759-64.
[245] Santo Tomas LH, Loberiza FR, Jr., Klein JP, et al. Risk factors for bronchiolitis obliterans in allogeneic hematopoietic stem-cell transplantation for leukemia. Chest 2005;128:153-61.
[246] Yoshihara S, Tateishi U, Ando T, et al. Lower incidence of Bronchiolitis obliterans in allogeneic hematopoietic stem cell transplantation with reduced-intensity conditioning compared with myeloablative conditioning. *Bone Marrow Transplant* 2005;35:1195-200.
[247] Paz HL, Crilley P, Patchefsky A, Schiffman RL, Brodsky I. Bronchiolitis obliterans after autologous bone marrow transplantation. *Chest* 1992;101:775-8.
[248] Frankovich J, Donaldson SS, Lee Y, Wong RM, Amylon M, Verneris MR. High-dose therapy and autologous hematopoietic cell transplantation in children with primary refractory and relapsed Hodgkin's disease: atopy predicts idiopathic diffuse lung injury syndromes. *Biol Blood Marrow Transplant* 2001;7:49-57.
[249] Ohnuma K, Toyoda Y, Ishida Y, et al. Fatal obstructive lung disease after haploidentical sibling cord blood transplantation. *Bone Marrow Transplant* 1998;21:939-41.
[250] Endo M, Furukawa H, Aramaki T, et al. Unusual late pulmonary complication in a child after umbilical cord blood transplantation: high-resolution CT-pathologic correlation. *J Thorac Imaging* 2005;20:103-6.
[251] Clark JG, Schwartz DA, Flournoy N, Sullivan KM, Crawford SW, Thomas ED. Risk factors for airflow obstruction in recipients of bone marrow transplants. *Ann Intern Med* 1987;107:648-56.
[252] Payne L, Chan CK, Fyles G, et al. Cyclosporine as possible prophylaxis for obstructive airways disease after allogeneic bone marrow transplantation. *Chest* 1993;104:114-8.

[253] Chien JW, Martin PJ, Gooley TA, et al. Airflow obstruction after myeloablative allogeneic hematopoietic stem cell transplantation. *Am J Respir Crit Care Med* 2003;168(2):208-14.
[254] Holland HK, Wingard JR, Beschorner WE, Saral R, Santos GW. Bronchiolitis obliterans in bone marrow transplantation and its relationship to chronic graft-v-host disease and low serum IgG. *Blood* 1988;72:621-7.
[255] Schwarer AP, Hughes JM, Trotman-Dickenson B, Krausz T, Goldman JM. A chronic pulmonary syndrome associated with graft-versus-host disease after allogeneic marrow transplantation. *Transplantation* 1992;54:1002-8.
[256] Nakane T, Nakamae H, Kamoi H, et al. Prognostic value of serum surfactant protein D level prior to transplant for the development of bronchiolitis obliterans syndrome and idiopathic pneumonia syndrome following allogeneic hematopoietic stem cell transplantation. *Bone Marrow Transplant* 2008;42:43-9.
[257] Hildebrandt GC, Granell M, Urbano-Ispizua A, et al. Recipient NOD2/CARD15 variants: a novel independent risk factor for the development of bronchiolitis obliterans after allogeneic stem cell transplantation. *Biol Blood Marrow Transplant* 2008;14:67-74.
[258] Ringden O, Remberger M, Ruutu T, et al. Increased risk of chronic graft-versus-host disease, obstructive bronchiolitis, and alopecia with busulfan versus total body irradiation: long-term results of a randomized trial in allogeneic marrow recipients with leukemia. Nordic Bone Marrow Transplantation Group. *Blood* 1999;93:2196-201.
[259] Marras TK, Chan CK, Lipton JH, Messner HA, Szalai JP, Laupacis A. Long-term pulmonary function abnormalities and survival after allogeneic marrow transplantation. *Bone Marrow Transplant* 2004;33:509-17.
[260] Chan CK, Hyland RH, Hutcheon MA, et al. Small-airways disease in recipients of allogeneic bone marrow transplants. An analysis of 11 cases and a review of the literature. *Medicine* (Baltimore) 1987;66:327-40.
[261] Epler GR. Bronchiolitis obliterans and airways obstruction associated with graft-versus-host disease. *Clin Chest Med 1988*;9:551-6.
[262. Yousem SA. The histological spectrum of pulmonary graft-versus-host disease in bone marrow transplant recipients. *Hum Pathol* 1995;26:668-75.
[263] Ditschkowski M, Elmaagacli AH, Trenschel R, et al. T-cell depletion prevents from bronchiolitis obliterans and bronchiolitis obliterans with organizing pneumonia after allogeneic hematopoietic stem cell transplantation with related donors. *Haematologica* 2007;92:558-61.
[264] Panoskaltsis-Mortari A, Tram KV, Price AP, Wendt CH, Blazar BR. A new murine model for bronchiolitis obliterans post-bone marrow transplant. *Am J Respir Crit Care Med* 2007;176:713-23.
[265] Holler E, Kolb HJ, Moller A, et al. Increased serum levels of tumor necrosis factor alpha precede major complications of bone marrow transplantation. *Blood* 1990;75:1011-6.
[266] Rowbottom AW, Riches PG, Downie C, Hobbs JR. Monitoring cytokine production in peripheral blood during acute graft-versus-host disease following allogeneic bone marrow transplantation. *Bone Marrow Transplant* 1993;12:635-41.
[267] Wyatt SE, Nunn P, Hows JM, et al. Airways obstruction associated with graft versus host disease after bone marrow transplantation. *Thorax* 1984;39:887-94.

[268] Clark JG, Crawford SW, Madtes DK, Sullivan KM. Obstructive lung disease after allogeneic marrow transplantation. Clinical presentation and course. Ann Intern Med 1989;111:368-76.

[269] Yokoi T, Hirabayashi N, Ito M, et al. Broncho-bronchiolitis obliterans as a complication of bone marrow transplantation: a clinicopathological study of eight autopsy cases. Nagoya BMT Group. *Virchows Arch* 1997;431:275-82.

[270] Dudek AZ, Mahaseth H, DeFor TE, Weisdorf DJ. Bronchiolitis obliterans in chronic graft-versus-host disease: analysis of risk factors and treatment outcomes. *Biol Blood Marrow Transplant* 2003;9:657-66.

[271] Sakaida E, Nakaseko C, Harima A, et al. Late-onset noninfectious pulmonary complications after allogeneic stem cell transplantation are significantly associated with chronic graft-versus-host disease and with the graft-versus-leukemia effect. *Blood* 2003;102:4236-42.

[272] Philit F, Wiesendanger T, Archimbaud E, Mornex JF, Brune J, Cordier JF. Post-transplant obstructive lung disease ("bronchiolitis obliterans"): a clinical comparative study of bone marrow and lung transplant patients. *Eur Respir J* 1995;8:551-8.

[273] Marras TK, Chan CK. Obliterative bronchiolitis complicating bone marrow transplantation. *Semin Respir Crit Care Med* 2003;24:531-42.

[274] Schultz KR, Green GJ, Wensley D, et al. Obstructive lung disease in children after allogeneic bone marrow transplantation. *Blood* 1994;84:3212-20.

[275] Palmas A, Tefferi A, Myers JL, et al. Late-onset noninfectious pulmonary complications after allogeneic bone marrow transplantation. *Br J Haematol* 1998;100:680-7.

[276] Soubani AO, Uberti JP. Bronchiolitis obliterans following haematopoietic stem cell transplantation. *Eur Respir J* 2007;29(5):1007-19.

[277] Erard V, Chien JW, Kim HW, et al. Airflow decline after myeloablative allogeneic hematopoietic cell transplantation: the role of community respiratory viruses. *J Infect Dis* 2006;193(12):1619-25.

[278] Krowka MJ, Rosenow EC, 3rd, Hoagland HC. Pulmonary complications of bone marrow transplantation. *Chest* 1985;87:237-46.

[279] Quabeck K. The lung as a critical organ in marrow transplantation. *Bone Marrow Transplant* 1994;14 Suppl 4:S19-28.

[280] Galanis E, Litzow MR, Tefferi A, Scott JP. Spontaneous pneumomediastinum in a patient with bronchiolitis obliterans after bone marrow transplantation. *Bone Marrow Transplant* 1997;20:695-6.

[281] Cazzadori A, Di Perri G, Bonora S, Lanzafame M, Allegranzi B, Concia E. Fatal pneumothorax complicating BAL in a bone marrow transplant recipient with bronchiolitis obliterans. *Chest* 1997;111:1468-9.

[282] Jung JI, Jung WS, Hahn ST, Min CK, Kim CC, Park SH. Bronchiolitis obliterans after allogenic bone marrow transplantation: HRCT findings. Korean J Radiol 2004;5:107-13.

[283] Garg K, Lynch DA, Newell JD, King TE, Jr. Proliferative and constrictive bronchiolitis: classification and radiologic features. *AJR Am J Roentgenol* 1994;162:803-8.

[284] Padley SP, Adler BD, Hansell DM, Muller NL. Bronchiolitis obliterans: high resolution CT findings and correlation with pulmonary function tests. *Clin Radiol* 1993;47:236-40.

[285] Bankier AA, Van Muylem A, Knoop C, Estenne M, Gevenois PA. Bronchiolitis obliterans syndrome in heart-lung transplant recipients: diagnosis with expiratory CT. *Radiology* 2001;218:533-9.

[286] Filipovich AH, Weisdorf D, Pavletic S, et al. National Institutes of Health consensus development project on criteria for clinical trials in chronic graft-versus-host disease: I. Diagnosis and staging working group report. *Biol Blood Marrow Transplant* 2005;11:945-56.

[287] Pandya CM, Soubani AO. Bronchiolitis obliterans following hematopoietic stem cell transplantation: a clinical update. *Clin Transplant*;24:291-306.

[288] Sirithanakul K, Salloum A, Klein JL, Soubani AO. Pulmonary complications following hematopoietic stem cell transplantation: diagnostic approaches. *Am J Hematol* 2005;80:137-46.

[289] Sanchez J, Torres A, Serrano J, et al. Long-term follow-up of immunosuppressive treatment for obstructive airways disease after allogeneic bone marrow transplantation. *Bone Marrow Transplant* 1997;20:403-8.

[290] Duncan CN, Buonanno MR, Barry EV, Myers K, Peritz D, Lehmann L. Bronchiolitis obliterans following pediatric allogeneic hematopoietic stem cell transplantation. *Bone Marrow Transplant* 2008;41:971-5.

[291] Crawford SW, Clark JG. Bronchiolitis associated with bone marrow transplantation. *Clin Chest Med* 1993;14:741-9.

[292] Crawford SW. Supportive care in bone marrow transplantation: pulmonary complications. *Cancer Treat Res* 1997;77:231-54.

[293] Patriarca F, Skert C, Sperotto A, et al. Incidence, outcome, and risk factors of late-onset noninfectious pulmonary complications after unrelated donor stem cell transplantation. *Bone Marrow Transplant* 2004;33:751-8.

[294] Sullivan KM, Storek J, Kopecky KJ, et al. A controlled trial of long-term administration of intravenous immunoglobulin to prevent late infection and chronic graft-vs.-host disease after marrow transplantation: clinical outcome and effect on subsequent immune recovery. *Biol Blood Marrow Transplant* 1996;2:44-53.

[295] Ishii T, Manabe A, Ebihara Y, et al. Improvement in bronchiolitis obliterans organizing pneumonia in a child after allogeneic bone marrow transplantation by a combination of oral prednisolone and low dose erythromycin. *Bone Marrow Transplant* 2000;26:907-10.

[296] Gerhardt SG, McDyer JF, Girgis RE, Conte JV, Yang SC, Orens JB. Maintenance azithromycin therapy for bronchiolitis obliterans syndrome: results of a pilot study. *Am J Respir Crit Care Med* 2003;168:121-5.

[297] Verleden GM, Vanaudenaerde BM, Dupont LJ, Van Raemdonck DE. Azithromycin reduces airway neutrophilia and interleukin-8 in patients with bronchiolitis obliterans syndrome. *Am J Respir Crit Care Med* 2006;174:566-70.

[298] Gottlieb J, Szangolies J, Koehnlein T, Golpon H, Simon A, Welte T. Long-term azithromycin for bronchiolitis obliterans syndrome after lung transplantation. *Transplantation* 2008;85:36-41.

[299] Siddiqui J. Immunomodulatory effects of macrolides: implications for practicing clinicians. *Am J Med* 2004;117 Suppl 9A:26S-9S.

[300] Khalid M, Al Saghir A, Saleemi S, et al. Azithromycin in bronchiolitis obliterans complicating bone marrow transplantation: a preliminary study. *Eur Respir J* 2005;25:490-3.

[301] Whitford H, Walters EH, Levvey B, et al. Addition of inhaled corticosteroids to systemic immunosuppression after lung transplantation: a double-blind, placebo-controlled trial. Transplantation 2002;73:1793-9.

[302] Zheng L, Walters EH, Wang N, et al. Effect of inhaled fluticasone propionate on BAL TGF-beta(1) and bFGF concentrations in clinically stable lung transplant recipients. *J Heart Lung Transplant* 2004;23:446-55.

[303] Bashoura L, Gupta S, Jain A, et al. Inhaled corticosteroids stabilize constrictive bronchiolitis after hematopoietic stem cell transplantation. *Bone Marrow Transplant* 2008;41:63-7.

[304] Foss FM. Extracorporeal photopheresis in the treatment of graft-vs-host disease. *J Cutan Med Surg* 2003;7(4 Suppl):13-7.

[305] Foss FM, DiVenuti GM, Chin K, et al. Prospective study of extracorporeal photopheresis in steroid-refractory or steroid-resistant extensive chronic graft-versus-host disease: analysis of response and survival incorporating prognostic factors. *Bone Marrow Transplant* 2005;35:1187-93.

[306] Dall'Amico R, Rossetti F, Zulian F, et al. Photopheresis in paediatric patients with drug-resistant chronic graft-versus-host disease. *Br J Haematol* 1997;97:848-54.

[307] Oyan B, Koc Y, Emri S, Kansu E. Improvement of chronic pulmonary graft-vs-host disease manifesting as bronchiolitis obliterans organizing pneumonia following extracorporeal photopheresis. *Med Oncol* 2006;23:125-9.

[308] Alcindor T, Gorgun G, Miller KB, et al. Immunomodulatory effects of extracorporeal photochemotherapy in patients with extensive chronic graft-versus-host disease. *Blood* 2001;98:1622-5.

[309] Couriel DR, Hicks K, Giralt S, Champlin RE. Role of tumor necrosis factor-alpha inhibition with inflixiMAB in cancer therapy and hematopoietic stem cell transplantation. *Curr Opin Oncol* 2000;12:582-7.

[310] Majhail NS, Schiffer CA, Weisdorf DJ. Improvement of pulmonary function with imatinib mesylate in bronchiolitis obliterans following allogeneic hematopoietic cell transplantation. *Biol Blood Marrow Transplant* 2006;12:789-91.

[311] Shapira MY, Abdul-Hai A, Resnick IB, et al. Alefacept treatment for refractory chronic extensive GVHD. *Bone Marrow Transplant* 2009;43:339-43.

[312] Miano M, Cuzzubbo D, Terranova P, et al. Daclizumab as useful treatment in refractory acute GVHD: a paediatric experience. *Bone Marrow Transplant* 2009;43:423-7.

[313] Rabitsch W, Deviatko E, Keil F, et al. Successful lung transplantation for bronchiolitis obliterans after allogeneic marrow transplantation. *Transplantation* 2001;71:1341-3.

[314] Curtis DJ, Smale A, Thien F, Schwarer AP, Szer J. Chronic airflow obstruction in long-term survivors of allogeneic bone marrow transplantation. Bone Marrow Transplant 1995;16:169-73.

[315] Freudenberger TD, Madtes DK, Curtis JR, Cummings P, Storer BE, Hackman RC. Association between acute and chronic graft-versus-host disease and bronchiolitis

obliterans organizing pneumonia in recipients of hematopoietic stem cell transplants. *Blood* 2003;102:3822-8.

[316] Yoshihara S, Yanik G, Cooke KR, Mineishi S. Bronchiolitis obliterans syndrome (BOS), bronchiolitis obliterans organizing pneumonia (BOOP), and other late-onset noninfectious pulmonary complications following allogeneic hematopoietic stem cell transplantation. *Biol Blood Marrow Transplant* 2007;13:749-59.

[317] Afessa B, Peters SG. Chronic lung disease after hematopoietic stem cell transplantation. *Clin Chest Med* 2005;26:571-86

[318] Williams LM, Fussell S, Veith RW, Nelson S, Mason CM. Pulmonary veno-occlusive disease in an adult following bone marrow transplantation. Case report and review of the literature. *Chest* 1996;109:1388-91.

[319] Hackman RC, Madtes DK, Petersen FB, Clark JG. Pulmonary venoocclusive disease following bone marrow transplantation. *Transplantation* 1989;47:989-92.

[320] Mandel J, Mark EJ, Hales CA. Pulmonary veno-occlusive disease. *Am J Respir Crit Care Med* 2000;162:1964-73.

[321] Curtis RE, Travis LB, Rowlings PA, et al. Risk of lymphoproliferative disorders after bone marrow transplantation: a multi-institutional study. *Blood* 1999;94:2208-16.

[322] Benkerrou M, Jais JP, Leblond V, et al. Anti-B-cell monoclonal antibody treatment of severe posttransplant B-lymphoproliferative disorder: prognostic factors and long-term outcome. *Blood* 1998;92:3137-47.

[323] Stevens SJ, Verschuuren EA, Verkuujlen SA, Van Den Brule AJ, Meijer CJ, Middeldorp JM. Role of Epstein-Barr virus DNA load monitoring in prevention and early detection of post-transplant lymphoproliferative disease. Leuk Lymphoma 2002;43:831-40.

[324] Gottschalk S, Heslop HE, Roon CM. Treatment of Epstein-Barr virus-associated malignancies with specific T cells. *Adv Cancer Res* 2002;84:175-201.

[325] Peters A, Manivel JC, Dolan M, Gulbahce HE, Baker KS, Verneris MR. Pulmonary cytolytic thrombi after allogeneic hematopoietic cell transplantation: a further histologic description. *Biol Blood Marrow Transplant* 2005;11:484-5.

[326] Morales IJ, Anderson PM, Tazelaar HD, Wylam ME. Pulmonary cytolytic thrombi: unusual complication of hematopoietic stem cell transplantation. *J Pediatr Hematol Oncol* 2003;25:89-92.

[327] Castellano-Sanchez AA, Poppiti RJ. Pulmonary cytolytic thrombi (PCT). A previously unrecognized complication of bone marrow transplantation (BMT). *Am J Surg Pathol* 2001;25:829-31.

[328] Woodard JP, Gulbahce E, Shreve M, et al. Pulmonary cytolytic thrombi: a newly recognized complication of stem cell transplantation. *Bone Marrow Transplant* 2000;25:293-300.

[329] Sundar KM, Carveth HJ, Gosselin MV, Beatty PG, Colby TV, Hoidal JR. Granulomatous pneumonitis following bone marrow transplantation. Bone Marrow Transplant 2001;28:627-30.

[330] Heyll A, Meckenstock G, Aul C, et al. Possible transmission of sarcoidosis via allogeneic bone marrow transplantation. *Bone Marrow Transplant* 1994;14:161-4.

[331] Bhagat R, Rizzieri DA, Vredenburgh JJ, Chao NJ, Folz RJ. Pulmonary sarcoidosis following stem cell transplantation: is it more than a chance occurrence? *Chest* 2004;126:642-4.

[332] Hallstrand TS, Sprenger JD, Agosti JM, Longton GM, Witherspoon RP, Henderson WR, Jr. Long-term acquisition of allergen-specific IgE and asthma following allogeneic bone marrow transplantation from allergic donors. *Blood* 2004;104:3086-90.

[333] Dirksen U, Hattenhorst U, Schneider P, et al. Defective expression of granulocyte-macrophage colony-stimulating factor/interleukin-3/interleukin-5 receptor common beta chain in children with acute myeloid leukemia associated with respiratory failure. *Blood* 1998;92:1097-103.

[334] Cordonnier C, Fleury-Feith J, Escudier E, Atassi K, Bernaudin JF. Secondary alveolar proteinosis is a reversible cause of respiratory failure in leukemic patients. *Am J Respir Crit Care Med* 1994;149(3 Pt 1):788-94.

[335] Tomonari A, Shirafuji N, Iseki T, et al. Acquired pulmonary alveolar proteinosis after umbilical cord blood transplantation for acute myeloid leukemia. *Am J Hematol* 2002;70:154-7.

In: Hematopoietic Stem Cells: New Research
Editors: Wesley G. Montgomery and Heather I. Burton
ISBN 978-1-62257-468-1

Chapter 2

HEMATOPOIETIC STEM CELLS: POTENTIAL NEW APPLICATIONS FOR TRANSLATIONAL MEDICINE

***Hady Felfly*[1,*] *and Gabriel G. Haddad*[2,3]**
[1]University of California San Francisco, California, US
[2]University of California San Diego, California, US
[3]Rady's Children's Hospital, San Diego, California, US

ABSTRACT

Hematopoietic stem cells (HSC) are multipotent cells that produce the various lineages of blood and HSC transplantations (HSCT) are widely used to reconstitute damaged bone marrow (BM). Over time, HSCT has evolved for the treatment of non-blood diseases as well, brain in particular. However, HSCT required total myeloablation through irradiation and/or chemotherapy for the treatment of BM-related diseases, and HSCs are difficult to safely deliver in large amounts into the brain. In blood disorders, for a minimal myelosuppression to be sufficient and allow donor cells to engraft, it is necessary to determine the minimal percentage of normal BM cells needed to achieve phenotypic correction. Recent studies on animal models of β-thalassemia and sickle cell disease (SCD), through Competitive Repopulation Assay (CRA) following lethal irradiation of recipients, demonstrated that an average of 25% normal BM cells allows the production of enough normal red blood cells to significantly correct the β-thalassemia and SCD phenotypes, at the levels of BM, blood, histology, and survival, with normal donor cells contributing to 50-60% of peripheral red blood cells. Further assays using mild myelosuppression showed that long term sustained phenotypic correction can be obtained for both diseases through a novel transplantation strategy based on modulating four parameters: dose of irradiation/myelosuppression, number of transplanted cells, timing of cell injections, and number of cell doses. Through a minimal dose of irradiation of 1Gy (100 Rads) or 2Gy, two injections of BM cells within the first 24h after myelosuppression resulted in engraftment in 100% of mice and a sustained therapeutic mixed chimerism in β-thalassemia, while three to four injections were needed to achieve

* Corresponding author: hadyfelfly@gmail.com; 513 Parnassus Avenue, HSE1509, San Francisco, CA 94143-0442, US.

a similar outcome in SCD. Following the success of these trials, we modified this novel HSCT strategy and applied it to determine whether we can protect mice from lethal stroke induced through the Middle Cerebral Artery Occlusion (MCAO). Ischemia/reperfusion resulted in a major infarct that propagated over time to encompass ~70% of the affected hemisphere. When two doses of HSCs were injected at 2h and 24h after the reperfusion, 40% of mice survived, visible neurological defects disappeared, and the infarct size was reduced by two to four fold. Histological examination of brains in surviving mice revealed very few donor cells in the recipient brains, decreased total neurons count and increased glial cell numbers. These data suggest that the neuro-protection was not dependent on cell-supplementation, but rather the protection is manifested likely through growth factor secretion. Combined, these studies create a novel HSCT approach that has proved efficient for the treatment of various disorders. A "window of opportunity" exists for each disease where the donor cells should be administered, and multiple injections of donor HSCs can rescue diseases that would otherwise not be treatable. We hypothesize that the initial injection primes the affected tissue, and subsequent ones help in repair. This new strategy has opened the way for a new era of HSCT for the potential treatments and possibly cures of many diseases.

I. Introduction

Hematopoietic stem cells (HSCs) are multipotent stem cells naturally generating the cellular elements circulating in blood (red blood cells, white blood cells, and platelets). They reside mainly in the bone marrow, and a low number of HSCs circulates in the peripheral blood, and enters various organs, including the spleen. It is hypothesized that these circulating HSCs replenish various organs with cells and participate in repairs [Lanzkron *et al.*, 1999; Zhao *et al.*, 2000].

HSCs are the most characterized stem cells. They are defined by various cell surface markers that allow their purification and use for transplantations. HSC transplantation (HSCT) is a widely performed transplantation originally aimed to cure blood diseases. Over-time, however, applications of HSCT for non-hematopoietic diseases have emerged. Currently, HSCT is practiced for a wide variety of diseases, including thalassemias, sickle cell disease, leukemias, metabolic diseases, and neurological diseases, including stroke.

While many HSCT are successful, those performed on blood diseases are often associated with side effects related to the irradiation and/or chemotherapy used to prepare the subject to accept the graft, known as myeloablation. HSCT aimed to cure neurological diseases where delivery of stem cells is needed to the central nervous system, are faced with difficulties of delivering sufficient stem cells to the damaged area without causing much trauma. Given all these factors, it became crucial to establish new transplantation strategies that could treat blood diseases with minimal myelosuppression, and to generate a new strategy to safely deliver stem cells into the brain efficiently enough to allow treatment. Here we discuss the case of three diseases, two hematopoietic and one neural: β-thalassemia, sickle cell disease (SCD), and stroke. We will review the basic pathophysiology of each and describe the most recent advances in their treatment using mouse models, strategies that can be applied in the clinical arena.

I.1. Stem Cells of the Hematopoietic System

I.1.1. Definition and Types

Stem cells are immature non-differentiated cells, characterized by three properties: proliferation, self-renewal, and capacity to differentiate [Hillman & Finch, 1996]. There are at least three different types of stem cells that exist in the hematopoeitic tissue: hematopoietic stem cell (HSC), epithelial stem cell (ESC), and mesenchymal stem cell (MSC). HSC and ESC are believed to arise from a common precursor stem cell known as hemangioblast [Choi *et al.*, 1998; Keller *et al.*, 2001; Robertson *et al.*, 2000; Sabin, 1920]. These cells can be distinguished by various morphological and functional characteristics.

- Hematopoietic stem cells (HSCs)

  Hematopoietic stem cells are pluripotent stem cells that give rise to blood cellular elements (RBCs, WBCs, and platelets) and they can repopulate a recipient host after lethal irradiation. Two major subpopulations of HSCs could be distinguished: long-term repopulating HSCs and short-term repopulating HSCs, based on their ability to repopulate irradiated hosts for long-term and short term, respectively [Lanzkron *et al.*, 1999; Zhao *et al.*, 2000].

  The purification of HSCs usually leads to a cell suspension enriched in HSCs. HSCs are usually defined by their ability to regenerate all of the hematopoietic lineages in vivo. Purification of cell populations capable of such repopulation is usually done on the basis of particular cell surface markers. Yet, the results obtained suggest that even such populations are not 100% pure HSCs [Osawa *et al,* 1996; Wagers *et al.*, 2002]. Therefore, depending on the particular combination of markers used, subpopulation with various purities of HSCs could be obtained. The majority of human hematopoietic cells capable of producing multlineage hematopoietic engraftment in myeloablated recipients express the CD34 ($CD34^+$) [Zanjani *et al.*, 1997; *Larochelle et a*l., 1996; Andrews *et al.*, 1992], and human HSCs are usually considered negative for lineage markers (Lin^-), $CD34^+$, $CD38^-$ [Hogan *et al.*, 2002; Verstegen *et al.*, 1998; Mazurier *et al.*, 2003]. Murine HSCs are usually considered Lin^-, $cKit^+$, $Sca1^+$ [Spangrude *et al.*, 1998; Osawa *et al.*, 1996], but mouse HSCs also express the CD34 although its regulation is different from humans [Okuno *et al,* 2002; Morel *et al.*, 1998]. However, studies both in mouse and humans indicate that CD34 is a marker of activated and/or cycling stem cells, and that $CD34^+$ stem cells can revert to quiescent $CD34^-$ state [Sato *et al.*, 1998; Dao *et al.*, 2003; Zanjani *et al.*, 2003]. Some reports have indicated that the most primitive murine HSCs are $CD34^-$, $cKit^+$, $Sca1^+$, and Lin^- [Osawa *et al.*, 1996a; Smith *et al.*, 1991; Spangrude *et al.*, 1995; Uchisda *et al.*, 1996; Matsuzaki *et al.*, 2004], while reports on whether human $CD34^-$ $CD38^-$ population is more primitive than the $CD34^+$ $CD38^-$ population are still controversial [Verfaillie *et al.*, 2000; Uchida *et al.*, 2001]. A subpopulation of stem cells was identified based on its ability to extrude the Rhodamine 123 or the Hoechst 33341, and called side population (SP), both in mice [Goodell *et al.*, 1996] and humans [Goodell *et al.*, 1997]. A high-purity HSCs is positive for side-population (SP^+), $CD34^+$, $CD38^-$ in humans (Uchida *et al.*, 2001), while the cells that have the strongest efflux activity (``Tip`` SP cells) have the phenotype $CD34^-$, $cKit^+$, $Sca1^+$, Lin^- in the mouse [Matsuzaki *et al.*, 2004].

- Epithelial stem cells (ESCs)

  Also called endothelial progenitor cells or angioblasts, these cells can give rise to mature endothelial cells in vessels. [Asahara *et al.*, 1999; Lin *et al.*, 2000; Shi *et al.*, 1998; Kocher *et al.*, 2001].
- Mesenchymal stem cells (MSCs)

  Also called stromal cells [Phinney *et al.*, 1999; Prockop, 1997; Pittenger *et al.*, 1999], MSCs can differentiate into many cell types including adipocytes, chondrocytes, osteocytes and muscle cells [Prockop, 1997; Pittenger *et al.*, 1999].

I.1.2. Hematopoietic Stem Cell Niche

The control of stem cell properties is affected by the localization of HSCs themselves [Croizat *et al.*, 1970; Gidali & Lajtha, 1972]. The niche hypothesis, formulated by Schofield [Schofield, 1978] suggested that true HSCs exist in association with one or more other supporting cells and would therefore, in essence, be fixed tissue cells. These microenvironmental cells were postulated to form a specific niche that, when in close association with the HSC, confer on it the attribute of indefinite self-renewal capacity, while effectively inhibiting differentiation and maturation of the cell. HSCs exhibit selective lodgment in the hypoxic area at the endosteal region [Nilsson *et al.*, 1997 & 2001; Cipolleschi *et al.*, 1993; Lord 1992], as opposed to the proliferating and maturing progenitors which tend to be closer to blood vessels in areas with more oxygen [Cipolleschi *et al.*, 1993; Lord 1992].

I.1.3. Hematopoietic Stem Cell Homing

Homing is the process by which stem cells reach the bone marrow after intra-venous injection into recipient hosts. It involves many complex processes such as cell adhesion, rolling, passage through the bone marrow endothelium [Mazo *et al.*, 1999; Zanjani *et al.*, 1999; Kollet *et al.*, 2001; Peled *et al.*, 2000; Lapidot *et al.*, 2005; Quesenberry *et al.*, 2005] and entering the BM extravascular tissue [Calvi *et al.*, 2003; Avecilla *et al.*, 2004; Sorrentino, 2004; Zhang *et al.*, 2003; Kopp *et al.*, 2005]. Following the entry into the BM other processes take place, including interaction with BM stromal cells [Quesenberry & Becker, 1998], endolgement in one of the extravascular bone marrow niches [Calvi *et al.*, 2003; Avecilla *et al.*, 2004] where they interact with the endosteal niche and vascular niche [Calvi *et al.*, 2003; Avecilla *et al.*, 2004; Zhang *et al.*, 2003; Kopp *et al.*, 2005] and proliferate in the bone marrow microenvironment. All of the different classes of cell adhesion receptors appear to play a role in anchoring hematopoietic cells within the marrow or in promoting hematopoietic differentiation [Carlos & Harlan, 1994; Long, 1992; Lewishon *et al.*, 1990; Yong *et al.*, 1998; Long *et al.*, 1992; Bruno *et al.*, 1995; Quesenberry *et al.*, 1998; Aizawa & Tavassoli, 1987].

I.2. Erythropoiesis

The term erythropoiesis refers to the entire process by which RBCs (erythrocytes) are produced [Dessypris, 1998; Bull *et al.*, 1995]. In response to erythropoietin, a growth factor that stimulates the erythroid precursors, erythropoiesis occurs in the central sinus beds of medullary marrow over a period of about 5-7 days through at least 3 successive reduction divisions from proerythroblast to basophilic erythroblast, then to polychromatophilic erythroblast, and finally to orthochromatophilic erythroblast. With successive developmental stages, the following changes occur: reduction in cell volume, condensation of chromatin, decrease in the nucleus-to-cytoplasm (N:C) ratio, loss of nucleoli, decrease in ribonucleic acid (RNA) in the cytoplasm, decrease in mitochondria, and gradual increase in synthesis of hemoglobin [Dessypris, 1998; Bull *et al.*, 1995]. The nucleus of the orthochromatophilic erythroblast is eventually extruded, leaving a non-nucleated polychromatophilic erythrocyte (reticulocyte) which is released into the circulating blood to mature in 1 to 2 days. Progressive cellular divisions of one proerythroblast results in the production of 14 to 16 RBCs [Dessypris, 1998].

II. Hematopoietic Diseases

β-thalassemias and sickle cell disease (SCD) are among the most common single gene disorders associated with high mortality and morbidity. They are both related to abnormalities affecting the β-globin chain of hemoglobin. While β-thalassemias is due to a quantitative defect in hemoglobin, SCD is caused by a qualitative abnormality of hemoglobin. In severe cases, both diseases are associated with multi-organ damage in addition to severe anemia.

II.1. β-Thalassemia

β-thalassemias is characterized by an imbalance in the ratio of α- to β-globin chains of hemoglobin due to a decreased or absence of β-globin chain synthesis, resulting in anemia of various severity [Thein, 1999; Harrison, 2002]. The severity of the disease depends on the degree of this imbalance, and the excess α-globin chains form aggregates inside the red blood cells (RBCs) resulting in the so called Heinz bodies which precipitate in the RBC membrane causing increased rigidity of the RBC membrane and decreased RBC half-life, aggravating the anemia [Shinar *et al.*, 1987, 1989; Aljurf *et al.*, 1996; Advani *et al.*, 1992; Yuan *et al.*, 1992;, Wyrick-Glatzel & Hugues, 2002; Harrison, 2002]. This disease is also associated with other morphological abnormalities of the RBCs including hypochromia, microcytosis, anisocytosis [Bunyaratvej *et al.*, 1985; Bessis, 1973; Schreir, 1989; Harrison, 2002], Patients with severe β-thalassemia develop, in addition to anemia, iron accumulation in various tissues due to excessive erythroid destruction and blood transfusions [Oliveri & Brittenham, 1997; Du *et al.*, 1997; Gullo *et al.*, 1993; Skalr *et al.*, 1987; Sonakul *et al.*, 1988; Bothwell *et al.*, 1979; Link *et al.*, 1985; Harrison, 2002], erythroid hyperplasia and extramedullary erythroipoiesis and splenomagaly, and pathologies in other organs such as liver and kidneys.

II.2. Sickle Cell Disease (SCD)

A single point mutation in the 6th codon of the β-globin gene leads to substitution of glutamic acid by valine, resulting in an abnormal globin: β^S. This leads to the formation of "sickle hemoglobin", or HbS ($\alpha_2\beta^S{}_2$). The conformational change that HbS undergoes when deoxygenated exposes the substituted valine on the molecular surface of β^S globin, instead of the polar glutamic acid. This allows intermolecular hydrophobic interactions between β^S of adjacent hemoglobin molecules (in contrast to normal hemoglobins where no such interactions occur), ultimately resulting in the polymerization of HbS [Wang, 2004; Lukens, 2004]. This is the molecular hallmark of sickle cell disease [Bunn, 1997]. As a consequence, the normally pliable RBC assumes a rigid non-deformable sickled shape, with ensuing erythrocyte membrane damage and hemolysis. The rigidity of these cells contributes to the overall process of microvascular occlusion that leads to tissue ischemia and organ dysfunction and decreased life span, as well as to an excessive degradation of RBC/decreased RBC half-life [Herrick, 1910; Wang, 2004; Lukens, 2004; Bunn, 1997; Kaul *et al.*, 1996; Glader, 1994]. In heterozygotes individuals, symptoms are precipitated by decreased oxygen levels, like during exercise or at high altitude, while in homozygous patients symptoms are severe starting from the first year of life, dying at a very early age if untreated.

Hereditary persistence of fetal hemoglobin (HPFH) is a condition characterized by continuation of fetal hemoglobin (HbF) synthesis in the adult stage of erythropoiesis. The importance of this condition is clearly demonstrated by the striking amelioration of the phenotype of individuals homozygous for sickle cell disease who also coinherit a HPFH determinant producing relatively large amounts of HbF, since HbF has anti-sickling properties [Thein and Weatherall, 1989; Cappellini *et al.*, 1989].

II.3. Available Therapy

II.3.1. β-Thalassemia

Patients with severe anemia receive regular blood transfusions [Cazzola *et al.*, 1995; Piomelli, 1995]; with time, however, iron accumulates, and could cause intoxication or hemochromatosis, necessitating iron chelation [Olivieri & Brittenham, 1997; Kontoghiorghes *et al.*, 1990; Wonke *et al.*, 1998], and reducing iron absorption from the gut (Urbinati, 2006). The therapy of β-thalassemia also includes HbF induction with agents like butyrate, 5-azacytidine, hydroxyurea, and erythropoietin, which are administered for long periods, with potential toxicities and variable outcome [Zeng *et al.*, 1995; Alberto *et al.*, 1998; Arruda *et al.*, 1997; Olivieri *et al.*, 1992; Dover, 1998; Collins *et al.*, 1995; Ley *et al.*, 1982]. β-thalassemia therapy also includes the use of anti-oxidants: protecting the cell membrane [Grinberg *et al.*, 1994, 1997], as well as other supportive and symptomatic therapies [Urbinati, 2006]. Hematopoietic stem cell transplantations (HSCT) provide the means to cure β-thalassemia. Many HSCT are being done in human clinics with variable degrees of success [Vellodi *et al.*, 1994; Boulad *et al.*, 1998; Walters *et al.*, 1994].

II.3.2. Sickle Cell Disease

The therapy for SCD includes blood transfusions [Steinberg, 1999; Embury *et al.*, 1994; Adams *et al.*, 1998; Wang *et al.*, 1991], and iron chelation for the treatment of hemochromatosis [Vichinsky *et al.*, 2007]. It also includes the use of agents that induce HbF such as hydroxyurea, erythropoietin, butyrate, and 5-azacytidine with variable outcome and toxicities [Steinberg, 2003; Saleh & Hillen, 1997; Blau *et al.*, 1993; Keefer *et al*, 2006; Atweh *et al.*, 1999].

SCD treatment also includes agents that decrease RBC dehydration like clotrimazole and magnesium [Brugnara, 2003; Stocker 2003; Muzyamba *et al.*, 2006; DeFranceschi *et al.*, 2000; Rust *et al.*, 2007], or relief from vaso-occlusion using vaso-dilators such as nitric oxide [Machado, 2007; Dasgupta *et al.*, 2006; Montero-Huerta *et al.*, 2006]. The prevention and treatment of infections is also performed by chronic antibiotic administration [Steinberg, 1999; Gaston *et al.*, 1986]).

As with β-thalassemia, hematopoietic stem cell transplantation (HSCT) represents the curative option. Variable degree of success is observed in the HSCT done in human clinics. [Bernaudin *et al.*, 1993; Abboud *et al.*, 1994; Locatelli *et al.*, 2003; Kalinyak *et al.*, 1995; Ferster *et al.*, 1993; Vermylen & Cornu, 1994].

II.4. Unsolved Problems

Patients with severe thalassemia and SCD depend on regular transfusions. However, this results in excessive iron accumulation/hemochromatosis overtime and is life-threatening in the absence of continuous iron chelation. Bone marrow transplantation (BMT) or hematopoietic stem cell transplantation (HSCT) from an allogenic source or using genetically corrected stem cells provides an alternative. Suitable histo-compatible donor is required for allogenic BMT, and the patient is vulnerable to graft versus host disease and early mortality. This can be avoided through autologous BMT, but that requires proper genetic modification of the patient stem cells and sufficient expression levels of the therapeutic transgene. In both cases, total replacement of the patient's bone marrow was thought needed to achieve correction. However, the possibility of achieving a cure with mixed rather than total chimerism, and therefore with partial rather than total replacement of the patient's bone marrow, was supported by occasional cases of transfusion-independent patients with stable mixed chimerism. This resulted in recent studies on mouse models which culminated in devising new transplantation strategies that allowed phenotype correction of both β-thalassemia and SCD in mouse models, through mixed chimerism achieved by BMT following mild myelosuppression and multiple stem cell injections.

III. Stroke

III.1. Description

Stroke is a pathology where brain cells die in large numbers following the absence of blood flow to a brain region for a certain period of time. The dead area of variable size is the infarct. Depending on the brain region affected, the length of time of blood interruptions and the size of the infarct, the consequence of a stroke can vary from silent (no symptoms), to a variety of disabilities (motor and sensory losses), to lethal. Once an infarct has formed, it is made up of two zones: a central zone or "core" with <15% blood supply [Kuroda and Bulloch, 1992] and mostly dead cells, and a peripheral zone or "penumbra" with 30-40%

blood supply and cells are suffering from low blood supply and will survive for a short period of time [Hakim, 1998]. An infarct core grows outwards, whereby cells in the penumbra would eventually die if blood supply is not reestablished early enough. Stroke is among the most common cause of mortality and morbidities in developed countries [Davenport and Dennis, 2000].

III.2. Available Therapies and Technical Hindrances

Stem cell transplantation provide a means of preventing the propagation of infarct size and protecting the brain from damage, which would allow the patient to avoid all or most of the consequences of stroke. These transplantations have been performed with variable outcomes both in humans and animals. These studies used different types of stem cells, including neural stem cells, mesenchymal stem cells, embryonic stem cells, and hematopoietic stem cells, and the outcome of these studies was variable, with some studies showing decreased infarct after transplantations. While most of these studies focused on studying the fate of donor cells, optimization of the transplantations to increase survival of recipients remained lacking.

One of the major obstacles in the stem cell transplantations for stroke is the delivery of the cells; while intrabrain injection yields the highest delivery, it creates physical damage during the injection which could result in additional neurological damage. Intravenous injections are safer, but the cells will have to pass through the brain blood barrier (BBB). Studies have shown that the BBB's permeability increases following stroke, allowing more stem cells to cross from the blood into the brain, a finding which could be utilized for the delivery of stem cells. Optimizing the process, however, is needed.

IV. HSCT for Erythroid Blood Diseases: Mixed Chimerism, Normal Erythroid Amplification, and the Competitive Repopulation Assay

The first pre-requisite for an efficient therapy with minimal mylosuppression is the ability to achieve a therapeutic level of HSCs/RBCs through BMT following a mild myelosuppression. Therefore, the first step was to test various percentages of normal BM cells/HSCs and measure the level of normal RBCs in peripheral blood that results from each, and determine the degree of phenotype improvement that goes with each level of normal HSCs/RBCs. This allows to determine whether a long term "correction" of the phenotype can be achieved with a mixed chimerism, and the level of that chimerism. Furthermore, this 'therapeutic" level of chimerism is not to be expected to necessarily yield 100% correction of all disease paramenters, but rather, enough correction to improve major parameters, decrease morbidity and prolong survival; a 100% phenotype correction might not even be possible with 100% donor chimerism anyway, because of some irreversible damage that would have affected certain organs. To this end, the "Competitive Repopulation Assay (CRA)" transplantation method has to be applied.

To determine the level of chimerism of donor and recipient, or of normal versus pathologic cells, markers are used. The X/Y chromosome [Quesenberry *et al*, 2001], where the two cell population (donor/recipient) are of opposite sex, and the Ly5.1/Ly5.2 cell surface markers [Yokoi *et al*, 2011; Quesenberry *et al*, 2001] allow only the detection of nucleated cells/white blood cells, but not that of RBCs. The third method, based on the use of cells with different isotypes of glucose phosphate isomerase (Gpi1a and Gpi1b) [Robinson *et al*, 2000] allows the detection of both RBCs and WBCs since it is present in all cells, and can be assayed by membrane electrophoresis and quantified. The studies described below used the Gpi marker.

First described by David Harrisson [Harrisson *et al*, 1993] CRA is based on a differential ability of two hematopoietic cell population to survive and proliferate. It is a transplantation strategy whereby recipients will receive a lethal dose of myeloablation (irradiation and/or chemotherapy) and the donor cells will consist of two populations of stem/bone marrow cells: one normal and one pathologic, for example thalassemic (thal), in reciprocal proportions, such as, 0% normal-100% thal, 5% normal, 95% thal, 10% normal, 90% thal.....100% normal-0% thal. Donor cells will reach the bone marrow (BM) and compete for the repopulation of this "myeloablated" space. Since in β-thalassemia (and SCD) the abnormality is at the level of the erythopoietic lineage, there will be no expected competition at the level of HSCs, but rather, at the level of the cells of the erythoipoietic lineage, when progenitors of the red cells start forming; since thalassemic erythroid cells have a survival disadvantage and will be dying excessively in the bone marrow, the normal erythroid cells should be able to expand more at the expense of the dying thalassemic cells. This will result in more normal erythroid cells in the bone marrow, at a percentage that is expected to be higher than the percentage of normal stem cells. This is the first level of amplification of normal erythroid cells, within the bone marrow.

Next, these erythroid cells will lead to RBCs that will be released in the peripheral blood. At this level, there is a second amplification step of normal RBCs: while thalassemic RBCs have a shortened half-life, the normal RBCs live longer and will expand further at the expense of the fast-dying thalassemic RBCs. This will result in an additional increase in the percentage of normal RBCs in peripheral blood relative to the percentage of injected normal stem cells. The normal white blood cells (WBCs) are expected to remain at a percentage similar to that of the normal injected stem cells, and therefore the percentage of normal WBCs in peripheral blood is an approximate reflection of the percentage of the normal stem cells in the bone marrow of the recipient.

This level of amplification results from both the intravascular hemolysis of thalassemic RBCs and their excessive destruction in the spleen.

During a CRA for β-thalassemia, the percentage of normal RBC and WBC will be measured in the peripheral blood using markers, and for each percentage of normal WBCs the corresponding percentage of normal RBC will be charted, and the disease parameters analyzed. The minimal level of normal WBC/RBC that provides significant phenotype correction with prolonged survival and decreased organ damage and anemia will be considered the minimal level of normal HSCs/BM cells needed to achieve phenotype correction (mixed chimerism).

In the studies we describe later in this chapter, the CRA approach is followed by assays aimed to achieve that minimal level of normal WBC/RBC, however, using a minimal myelosuppression of thalassemic recipients, and donor cells consisting only of normal BM cells/HSCs. This requires testing various levels of myelosuppression of recipients in combination with different numbers of donor cells, until a particular combination of parameters yields desired outcome, i.e. therapeutic level of donor cells.

This approach has been applied for β-thalassemia and SCD and allowed to determine both the therapeutic level of donor cells, as well as the minimal dose of irradiation/myelosuppression needed to achieve that therapeutic level.

V. Stem Cell Therapy for Β-Thalassemia

V.1. Mouse Models for β-thalassemia

To perform transplantation studies aimed for future clinical applications, appropriate animal models must be used. Many models for β-thalassemia have been generated, and there are six murine models that reproduce various severities of the human β-thalassemia. One is naturally occurring, while the remaining five are experimentally generated.

- **$Hbb^{th\text{-}1}$**

  The first mouse model for β-thalassemia resulted from a naturally occurring deletion of the adult β^{maj} globin gene and its promoter and was described by Skow in 1983 [Skow *et al.*, 1983]. Most mice homozygous for the deficiency survived to adulthood and reproduced but were smaller at birth than their littermates and demonstrated a hypochromic, microcytic anemia with severe anisocytosis, poikylocytosis and reticulocytosis. Heinz bodies are observed in a high proportion of circulating RBCs. Mice heterozygous for the deficiency demonstrated a mild reticulocytosis but were not clinically anemic.
- **$Hbb^{th\text{-}2}$**

  The second model for β-thalassemia was generated by Shehee [Shehee *et al.*, 1993] by a disruption of the adult β^{maj} globin gene in mouse embryonic stem cells using homologous recombination to insert selectable sequences into the gene. Mice homozygous for this insertional disruption are severelly anemic and die perinatally, while heterozygotes show severe thalassemia *intermedia* phenotype.
- **$Hbb^{th\text{-}3}$**

  In this model generated by Yang [Yang *et al.*, 1995], both adult cis β-globin genes have been deleted. Mice homozygous for this deletion die perinatally, similar to the most severe form of Cooley's anemia in humans. Mice heterozygous for the deletion show hematologic indices characteristics typical of severe thalassemia. Tissue and organ damage typical of β-thalassemia, such as bone deformities and splenic enlargement due to increased hematopoiesis are present. Spontaneous iron overload in the spleen, liver and kidneys, are also seen in the heterozygous animals.
- **Hbb^{0}/Hbb^{S}**

  This thalassemic model is the one selected for this study described below. In this model generated by Ciavatta [Ciavatta *et al.*, 1995], both adult cis β-globin genes, β^{maj} and β^{min}, have been deleted. Homozygous animals die in utero, however, heterozygous mice are fertile and transmit the deleted allele to progeny.

Heterozygous animals reproduce the human β-thalassemia *intermedia.* That includes severe anemia with dramatically reduced hemoglobin levels, abnormal red cell morphology (microcytosis, anisocytosis, poikylocytosis, hypochromia), splenomegaly and markedly increased reticulocyte counts and many histological abnormalities.

- **$Hbb^{th\text{-}4}$**

    In this model generated by Lewis [Lewis *et al.*, 1998], two murine adult cis β-globin genes were replaced with a human β-globin gene containing a splice site mutation that results in no functional human β-globin chain. No homozygous mice survived postnatally, and heterozygotes showed classic signs of β-thalassemia including anisocytosis and poikylocytosis. Typical thalassemic anomalies are found in many organs including liver, spleen, heart and kidneys, as well as iron deposition.

- **$DH^{\Delta 4bp}$**

    Generated by Jamsai [Jamsai *et al.*, 2005], this model consists of a double heterozygous for a mutant human β-globin gene containing a 4bp deletion and the $Hbb^{th3+/-}$ model. Mice are very anemic and have characteristic damage of severe β-thalassemia.

V.2. Amplification of Normal Erythoid Component in Transplant-recipient Mice after CRA

When mice were subjected to CRA with different percentages of normal and thalassemic BM cells, peripheral blood analysis of chimerism revealed that the percentage of normal RBCs was significantly amplified relative to that of normal WBCs, almost two fold when the percentage of normal WBCs was between 10% and 39%, and was almost 100% for WBC percentages greater than 39% (Figure 1). The wide range of normal RBC chimerism allows to pinpoint the window where a significant phenotype correction can be obtained by studying the RBC parameters, BM and organ pathology, and survival of mice in all these categories. This allows determining the minimal percentage of normal BM cells that help achieve that, and whether this percentage is low enough to be reasonably obtained with a mild myelosuppression.

V.3. Analysis of Disease Parameters Reveals Optimal Window for Phenotype Correction

Once the level of normal peripheral blood RBCs obtained from each percentage of normal WBC/BM cells was determined, the next step was to study the disease parameters at all groups of chimerism, and determine accordingly which is the optimal therapeutic window. The disease parameters can be divided into three categories: peripheral blood parameters, bone marrow/erythropoiesis parameters, and organ pathology.

V.3.1. Peripheral Blood Parameters

Many parameters need to be examined to verify peripheral RBC improvement, including RBC count, hemoglobin levels, percentage of hypochromic cells, mean cellular hemoglobin level, RBC morphology, volume, and percentage of RBC containing α-globin chain precipitate (Heinz bodies), RBC half-life and reticulocyte count.

There was an improvement of most RBC parameters with 10% normal WBCs, with noticeable improvement of RBC morphology and decreased frequency of fragmented and abnormal RBCs [Felfly *et al*, 2007]. However, with 19% normal WBCs (~50% normal RBCs), RBC morphology correction was more pronounced with three-fold decrease of cell fragments and 2.7 fold decrease in the percentage of RBCs with visible Heinz bodies, and there was a two-fold increase in RBC count and hemoglobin levels, >50% decrease in the percentage of hypochromic cells, correlating with respective improvement of mean RBC volume and hemoglobin content. In addition, while chimeric mice with 0% normal RBCs (100% thalassemic) have an RBC half-life of 4.2±2.4 days, roughly three-fold lower than normal controls (12.9 ±1.6 days), mice with increasing percentage of chimerism showed a progressive improvement of RBC half-life, with mice in the groups of chimerism of 10% and 19% showing RBC half-life of 7.0±2.6 days and 7.3±0.6 days, respectively. Furthermore, starting 31% normal WBC chimerism, there was a significant reduction of the percentage of reticulocytes, an indirect evidence of improved erythropoiesis. These parameters indicate that starting 19% normal WBCs (~50% normal RBCs) there is a substantial improvement of most peripheral blood RBC parameters [Felfly *et al*, 2007].

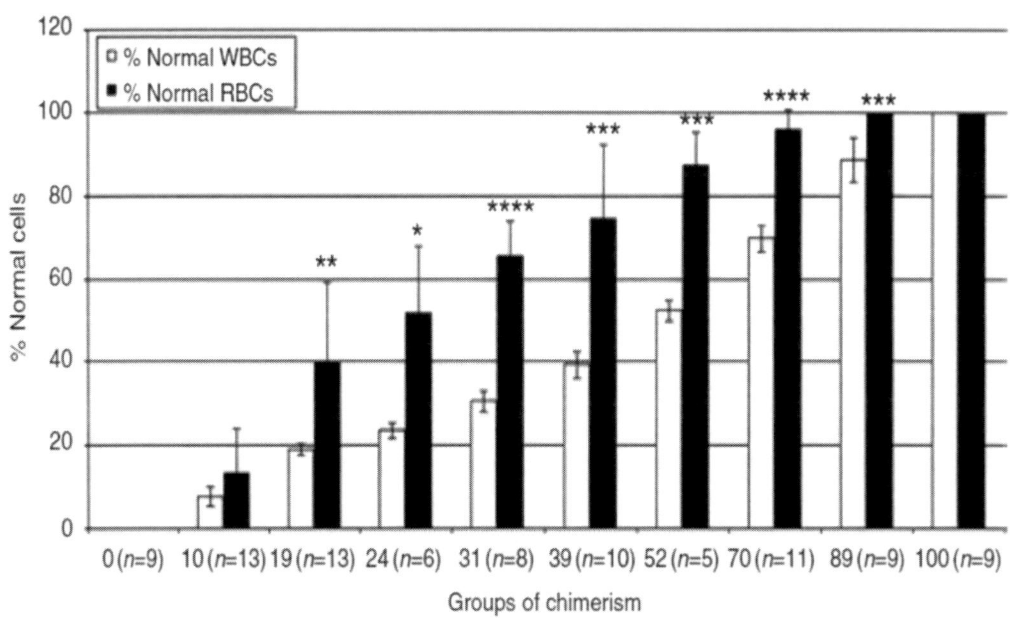

Figure 1. Chimerism in hemi-βthal mice. Comparison of engraftment levels of normal white blood cells (WBCs) (open bars) and normal red blood cells (RBCs) (black bars) for each of the 10 groups of chimeric mice at 7 months after transplantation. The n beside each group indicates the number of mice in the group. In hemi-βthal hematopoietic chimeric mice, amplification of the normal erythroid cell lineage relative to WBC was observed systematically. Data represent the mean values and standard

deviation for each group of mice. t-test analysis of percentage of normal WBCs versus percentage of normal RBCs, *, $p<0.01$, **$p<0.003$, ***$p<0.0003$, **** $p<3 \times 10^{-6}$. (Adapted from Felfly et al, 2007).

V.3.2. Normalization of Erythropoiesis Efficiency

Severe β-thalassemia is characterized by an ineffective erythropoiesis, whereby erythroid progenitors have an excessive premature death in the bone marrow before reaching the mature stage of RBCs, which reduces the number of RBCs released into the peripheral blood from the medullary erythroid lineage. Furthermore, in β-thalassemia there is an increased splenic extramedullay erythroipoiesis, whereby the spleen tries to compensate for the decreased medullary erythropoiesis, however, this is also inefficient and does not result in improving peripheral blood parameters.

In the bone marrow of thalassemic mice there was a mild increase in erythroid progenitors, while in their spleen there was an average of ~11-fold increase of these progenitors; however, with 10% normal WBCs, this percentage went down to normal range, indicating that with only around 20% normal RBCs circulating in peripheral blood, erythropoietic stress decreases enough so that the spleen no more needs to increases its erythropoiesis for compensation [Felfly *et al*, 2007].

The next step in evaluating erythropoiesis is to determine the percentage of the various populations of erythroid progenitors in bone marrow and spleen. There are four populations, from least to most mature these are: proerythroblast, basophilic erythroblast, polychromatophylic erythroblast and orthochromatophilic erythroblast, which is the stage that directly precedes the formation of reticulocytes. In bone marrow of thalassemic mice, there was a strong increase in the percentage of basophilic erythroblast in an attempt to compensate for the anemia, however, most of these cells die in subsequent stages before reaching the stage of orthochromatophilic erythroblasts, and that is the inefficient erythropoiesis. In chimeric mice, starting 24% normal WBCs, there was a significant decrease in basophilic and increase in orthochromatophilic erythroblast, indicative of a significant improvement of medullary erythroipoieisis. A similar improvement was observed in the spleens of these mice with the 24% normal WBCs [**Figure 2**; Felfly *et al*, 2007].

V.3.3. Improvement of Pathologic Parameters and Increased Lifespan in the Range of 19-24% Normal WBCs

β-thalassemia is characterized by many organ pathologies. The spleen is enlarged (splenomegaly) due to retention of abnormal RBCs and extramedullary erythropoiesis, resulting in increased spleen-to-body weight ratio. This also results in loss of splenic architecture with disorganized while pulp and expansion of red pulp. Iron is deposited in multiple organs, in particular spleen, liver and kidney, and a little in the heart. There is also hyperplasia of the liver Kupffer cells [Felfly *et al*, 2007].

The spleen-to-body weight ratio was significantly reduced even with 10% normal WBCs (~20% normal RBCs) suggesting a high RBC clearance ability of the spleen, so high that if the percentage of abnormal RBCs is 80% or less, the spleen is able to clear most of them without much enlargement, and this ratio became normal with 19% normal WBC (Figure 3).

Iron deposits in spleen, kidney and heart were reduced starting 10% normal WBCs, and substantially reduced between 19 and 24% normal WBCs, while liver iron deposits decreased more than two-fold starting 19% normal WBCs along with normalization of Kupffer cell in the range of 19-24% normal WBCs [Figure 3; Felfly *et al*, 2007].

To evaluate the overall impact of these improvements of the global physiology of the mice, the lifespan was measured. Mice with 10% normal WBCs had a significant improvement of lifespan and those with 19% normal WBCs had a normal lifespan [Felfly *et al*, 2007].

Altogether, the data of this study revealed that in the range of 19-24% normal WBCs, equivalent of 19-24% normal BM cells/HSCs, which results in ~50% normal RBCs in peripheral blood, is sufficient to provide significant long term correction of the β-thalassemic phenotype. Therefore, the 19-24% normal HSCs constitutes the minimal percentage of normal HSC/BM cells needed for phenotype correction and therefore, is the "therapeutic threshold" for the clinical and biological correction of β-thalassemia in mouse models.

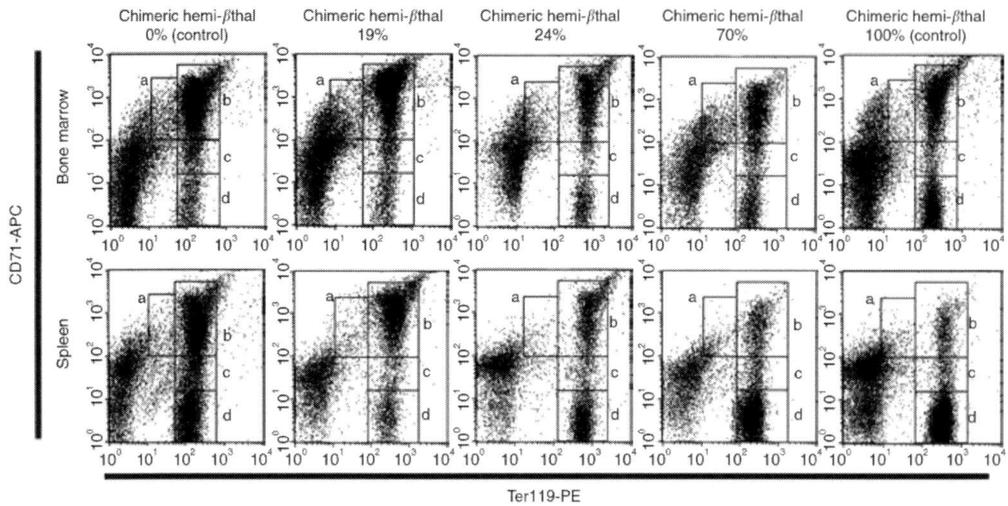

Figure 2. Analysis of erythroid cell precursor maturation in chimeric hemi-β thal mice.
Flow cytometry analysis of single erythroid cell from bone marrow (BM) (above) and spleen (bottom). Four regions are delineated by squares representing cell subpopulations: a, $Ter119^{med}CD71^{high}$ proerythroblast; b, $Ter119^{high}CD71^{high}$ basophilic erythroblast; c, $Ter119^{high}CD71^{med}$ polychromatophilic erythroblast; d, $Ter119^{high}CD71^{low}$ orthochromatophilic erythroblast. The 24% chimeric group displayed marked improvement in early to late erythroid precursors in BM and spleen, when compared with controls having 0% chimeric hemi-βthal (Adapted from Felfly et al, 2007).

V.3.4. Achieving the Therapeutic Threshold for β-thalassemia by BMT Following Minimal Myelosuppression

The ability to correct the phenotype with only 19-24% normal BM cells indicated that a total replacement of the diseased BM is not necessary for the correction, and that a partial replacement of the thalassemic BM allows the needed improvements and increased lifespan. Therefore, total myeloablation of the recipient BM is not needed, but rather a partial myelosuppression is expected to be sufficient to prepare the recipient BM so that normal donor BM/HSCs can efficiently engraft. For this purpose, 4 parameters needed optimization, in combination: minimal dose of myelosuppression/irradiation, minimal number of normal donor BM cells, timing of donor cell injection, and the number of cell injections. By the time this study was conducted, there were two reports showing that transplant-recipient mice could engraft after partial myelosuppression, providing further hints that correcting a disease phenotype could be possible by BMT/HSCT after partial myelosuppression.

The goal of any strategy aimed to correct the disease with minimal myslosuppression is to minimize the damage that can happen to the patient from irradiation/chemotherapy, while delivering just enough to allow sufficient engraftment. Various cell numbers have to be tested. In addition, the engraftment/homing efficiency of injected cells is very low, <10% often 1-5% in irradiated hosts [Cui *et al*, 1999; Szillvassy *et al*, 1999; Cerny *et al*, 2002; Van der Loo & Ploemacher, 1995; Van Hennil *et al*, 1999; Cahman & Eaves, 2000], therefore to minimize the loss of cells and increase the homing efficiency and result in the use of minimal amounts of cells, fractionating the same amount of cells into multiple injections of equal cell number need to be tested, and at various times after the irradiation.

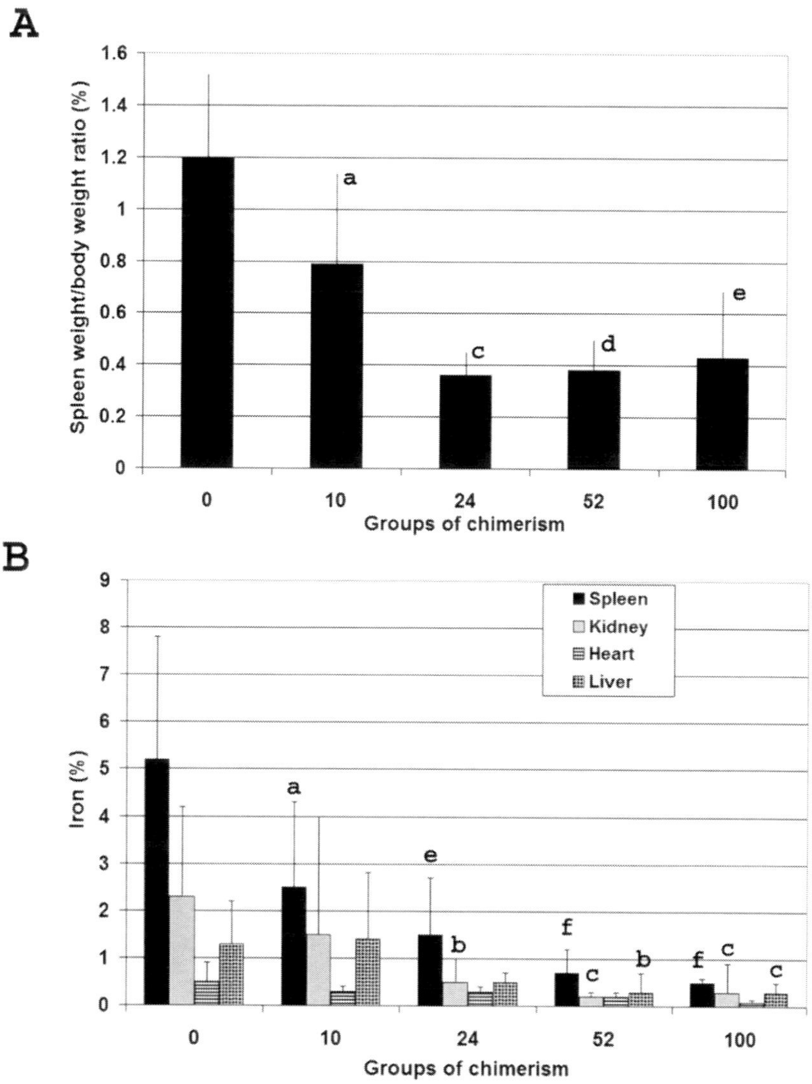

Figure 3. Pathological assessment in chimeric hemi-βthal mice.
A, spleen-to-body weight ratio; B, iron deposits in tissues measured as percentage of surface area examined (Iron deposits in kidney were measured in cortex) t-test: sample vs chimeric 0%; a, $p \leq 0.05$; b, $p \leq 0.04$; c, $p<0.03$; d, $p<0.02$; e, $p<0.01$; f, $p<0.005$ (Adapted from data in Felfly et al, 2007).

To this end, two low levels of irradiation were used: 1Gy (100 Rads) and 2 Gy (200 Rads). (Table 1). For each irradiation dose, two different amounts of donor BM cells were transplanted: 40 and 60 million total BM cells after 1Gy, and 20 and 40 million cells after 2Gy. Cells were transferred either in one dose 4h after irradiation, or in two equal doses 4h and 28h after irradiation. While donor cells did not engraft in all transplant-recipient mice, the percentage of mice with engrafted donor cells increased both with the number of donor cells and the number of cell injections. Furthermore, the level of donor chimerism increased in parallel with the number of cells and number of injections, and was higher after 2Gy irradiation (Table **1**). So the next step to increase the engraftment efficiency was to fractionate the donor cells into two injections of equal numbers. After 1Gy irradiation followed by 2 injections of a total of 60 million donor BM cells, all recipients engrafted, and the percentage of normal WBC in peripheral blood averaged at 40% , though with high variability, while after 2Gy, two injections of a total of 40 million donor cells allowed engraftment in all recipient mice, with an average of normal WBCs in peripheral blood ~80%. In both cases, hematologic parameters showed an improvement similar to what was observed with equivalent normal WBC chimerism after total myeloablation (Table 1).

Table 1. Engraftment and chimerism of hemi-βthal mice with minimal myeloablation

Irr. Level	Cells	Dose	n	n	% Chimerism	
(Gy)	(10^7)	(#)	(total)	(engr)	WBC	RBC
2	2	1	8	4	**36.2** ±23.2	**77.3** ±29.3
	4	1	7	6	**61.5** ±34.9[a]	**87.1** ±28.8
	1	2	5	4	**63.3** ±25.7	**96.0** ± 4.7
	2	2	5	5	**82.5** ±21.7[a]	**100.0** ± 0.0
1	4	1	6	0	**0**	**0**
	6	1	7	3	**23.1** ±17.3	**65.0** ±31.1
	2	2	7	3	**48.1** ±38.8	**68.8** ±54.1
	3	2	6	6	**40.2** ±20.6[b]	**76.3** ±38.7

Abbreviations: WBC, white blood cell; RBC, red blood cell. Data of chimeric levels at 7 months after transplantation. n (total), total number of transplanted mice; n (engr), number of transplanted mice engrafted; dose (#), number of infusion dose. t-test : a, Level of chimerism at 2Gy in 1 or 2 doses versus 1Gy (2 doses) $P \leq 0.02$, $P \leq 0.001$ respectively b, Level of chimerism (1Gy 1 vs 2 doses) $P \leq 0.02$; (Adapted from Felfly et al, 2007).

Therefore, two injections of donor BM cells proved substantially more efficient that one injection of a similar cell number (Table 1). We hypothesize that the first injection somehow "primes" the recipient BM with donor cells, while the second injection provides a 'booster" that increases donor chimerism and allows therapeutic levels of WBC/RBC in peripheral blood. While the mechanism is not clear, one injection might result in some cells seeding the bone marrow without enough ability to expand sufficiently, while with two injections, the second injection provides the additional "supply" of normal donor cells needed to overcome the increased proliferative status of the thalassemic erythropoietic lineage and allows therapeutic levels of normal WBC/RBC in peripheral blood. Although a one-injection strategy contains the same load of cells as two injections, the number of cells reaching the recipient BM might be less than in two-injection strategy; alternatively, changes within the recipient BM over time after irradiation might make it unfavorable for donor cell engraftment and/or proliferation after one injection: at 4h, there might not be enough space within the BM to receive all homing donor cells, and at 28h, the permeability of the blood-bone marrow barrier might have decreased and wouldn't allow all homing cells to penetrate the BM either; two injections at these two time points each carrying half the amount of cells would overcome these possible recipient-related low responsiveness.

VI. Stem Cell Therapy for Sickle Cell Disease (SCD)

VI.1. Mouse Models for SCD

A panoply of animal models for sickle cell disease exists. They could be broadly divided in two groups, based on whether or not they produce murine globin chains.

Models Producing Both Murine and Human Globin Chains

The first models expressing moderately high levels of both human α- and β^S-globin chains were reported by Greaves [Greaves *et al.*, 1990] and Ryan [Ryan *et al.*, 1990]. The former could not reproduce and the only reported characteristic is the presence of irreversibly sickled cells in 0.1% frequency. The latter was reported to present slight anemia and RBC sickling when crossed to thalassemic mice. Subsequently, many different lines of mice with variable degrees of severity reproduced, allowing more detailed studies of pathology.

- *SAD-1 mouse*

  This is the model used in the current thesis project. Generated by Trudel [Trudel *et al.*, 1991, 1994] and extensively characterized [Trudel *et al.*, 1991, 1994; Blouin *et al.*, 1999; DePaepe & Trudel, 1994], this mouse expresses the human β^{SAD} and α-globin transgenes. β^{SAD} induces strong hemoglobin polymerization, and results in the formation of a new form of hemoglobin, human HbSAD ($\alpha_2^h\ \beta_2^{SAD}$), which has a high polymerization potential when diluted by the endogenous mouse hemoglobin. The β^{SAD} gene carries three mutations: β^S, $\beta^{S\text{-}Antilles}$, and $\beta^{DLos\text{-}Angeles}$, where the latter two exacerbate polymerization. The level of human HbSAD is at 19% [Trudel *et al.*, 1991]. This model closely reproduces the human SCD on molecular, biological, pathological and clinical levels. That includes the presence of an ineffective erythropoiesis, increased RBC turnover, vaso-occlusions, organ damage, and shortened lifespan.
- *The Costantini-Fabry-Nagel (NYC1) model*

  Generated by Fabry [Fabry *et al.*, 1992a, b] this model, in which 75% of all β-like chains are human β^S, expresses murine β^{minor}, but not β^{major} which is achieved by breeding a mouse line carrying a deletion of β^{major} [Skow *et al.*, 1983] into the transgenic line. This model exhibits mild biological and clinical features of SCD [Fabry *et al.*, 1992a, 1992b, Lutty *et al.*, 1994; Shear *et al.*, 1993]
- *The S + S-Antilles model (Fabry et al., 1995).*

  This model is an NYC-1 mouse with the addition of the β^S-Antilles transgene [Rubin *et al.*, 1991] and homozygous deletion of mouse β^{major}. The product of the $\beta^{S\text{-}Antilles}$ gene is a hemoglobin with the sickle mutation coupled to a second mutation that enhances polymerization and reduces the oxygen affinity [Montplaisir *et al.*,

1986]. The phenotype is more severe than the NYC1 model with homozygous β^{major} deletion. There is no adult anemia, but the model exhibits severe anomalies characteristic of SCD

Models Producing Exclusively Human Globin Chains

These models are also called knock-out models because the transgenic mice expressing the sickling globin has been crossed to mice heterozygote knock out for murine α- and β-globin genes, progressively resulting in mice that produce only human α- and β-globin chains.

- *Transgenic mice with thalassemic characteristics*

  Three models generated by Paszty (the Berkeley or BERK mouse) [Paszty *et al.*, 1997], Ryan [Ryan *et al.*, 1997], and Chang [Chang *et al.*, 1998] are all anemic with the presence of abundant irreversibly sickled cells. The organ damage reported is similar to the S + A-Antilles or SAD models. Human γ is incorporated into all three the knock-out mice aforementioned and is expressed at high levels during the fetal period. All three models present low mean corpuscular hemoglobin concentration (MCHC). The chain imbalance measured in the first model and the decrease in the mean corpuscular hemoglobin (MCH) in the other two models, strongly suggest the presence of thalassemic pathology [Fabry *et al.*, 1997], as has been described by Nagel [Nagel *et al.*, 2001]. The low MCHC protects against polymer formation and may be a factor which allows many of these mice to survive to adulthood.
- *Transgenic mice that are not thalassemic*

  The NYC-1 mouse line [Fabry *et al.*, 1992a] expressing the human α-globin gene and a β^S gene has also been bred to mouse expressing human γ-globin [Gilman *et al.*, 1995; Arcasoy *et al.*, 1997], then to heterozygote knock-out mice for the α- and β-globin genes, resulting in full knock-out transgenic mice. In these mice, γ-globin levels ranges from 4% to 37% [Fabry *et al.*, 1997; Fabry *et al.*, 1999]. The MCHC of many mice has an average value similar to control, and only that of the 37% γ-globin chain mice is elevated. Because of the higher MCHC, some of these mice are generally more severe than Berkeley mice [Fabry *et al.*, 1997; Fabry *et al.*, 1999].

VI.2. Therapeutic Threshold for SCD

Stem cell therapy for SCD was explored by the same investigators similarly to β-thalassemia. Through CRA, an amplification of the normal erythroid component was observed in peripheral blood of recipients, which was comparable to the one observed with β-thalassemia (Figure 4).

Like β-thalassemia, SCD has many parameters that have to be verified for phenotype correction. Blood parameters include in particular, the percentage of hyperchromic RBCs, the mean corpuscular hemoglobin concentration (CHCM), mean cell volume (MCV), hemoglobin level and RBC half-life. The SAD mouse model displays anemia in new born only but not in the adult stage and has only a mild decrease in MCV. However, all other disease parameters are severely impaired comparatively to the human disease. That includes increased number of progenitors in BM and spleen, splenomegaly, iron deposits in organs such as spleen and liver, fribrosis in spleen, liver, kidney and lungs, and glomerular hypertrophy in kidneys, ineffective erythropoiesis and decreased life span.

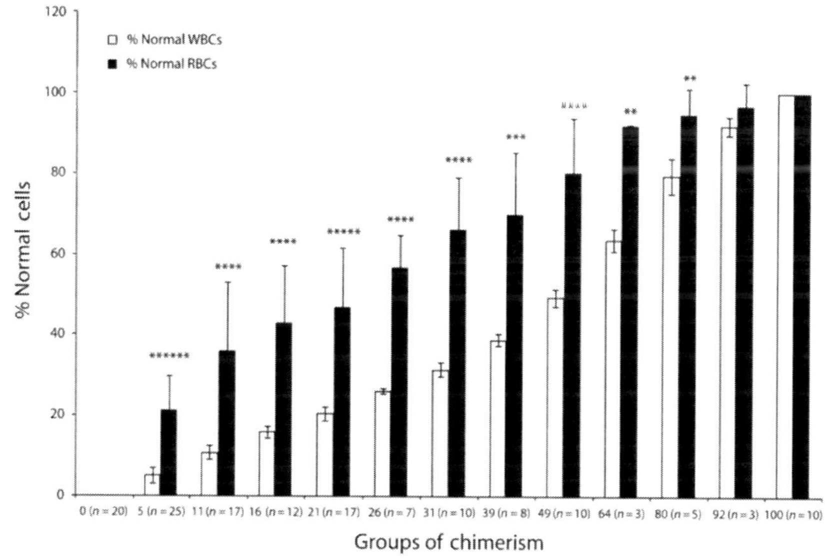

Figure 4. Chimerism in SAD mice.
Comparison between chimerism levels of normal WBCs (open bars) and normal RBCs (black bars) for each of the 13 groups of chimeric mice 7 months post-transplantation. The n below each group refers to the number of mice per group. Amplification of the normal erythroid cell population in peripheral blood of SAD chimeric mice relative to WBCs was observed systematically. t-test: p = normal RBCs vs normal WBCs; *, $p<0.05$; **, $p<0.004$; ***, $p<8 \times 10^{-4}$; ****, $p<6 \times 10^{-5}$; *****, $p<2 \times 10^{-6}$; ******, $p<3 \times 10^{-8}$ (Adapted from Felfly et al, 2009).

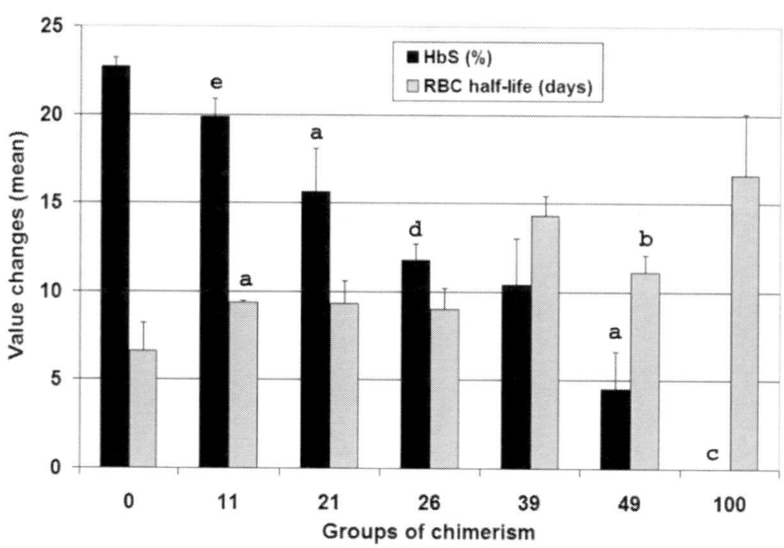

Figure 5. Red blood cell parameters in chimeric SAD mice. Abbreviations: RBC, red blood cells; HbS, hemoglobin SAD; t-test: sample vs chimeric 0%; a, $p<0.04$; b, $p<0.02$; c, $p<0.01$; d, $p<0.009$; e, $p<0.005$; (Adapted from data in Felfly et al, 2009).

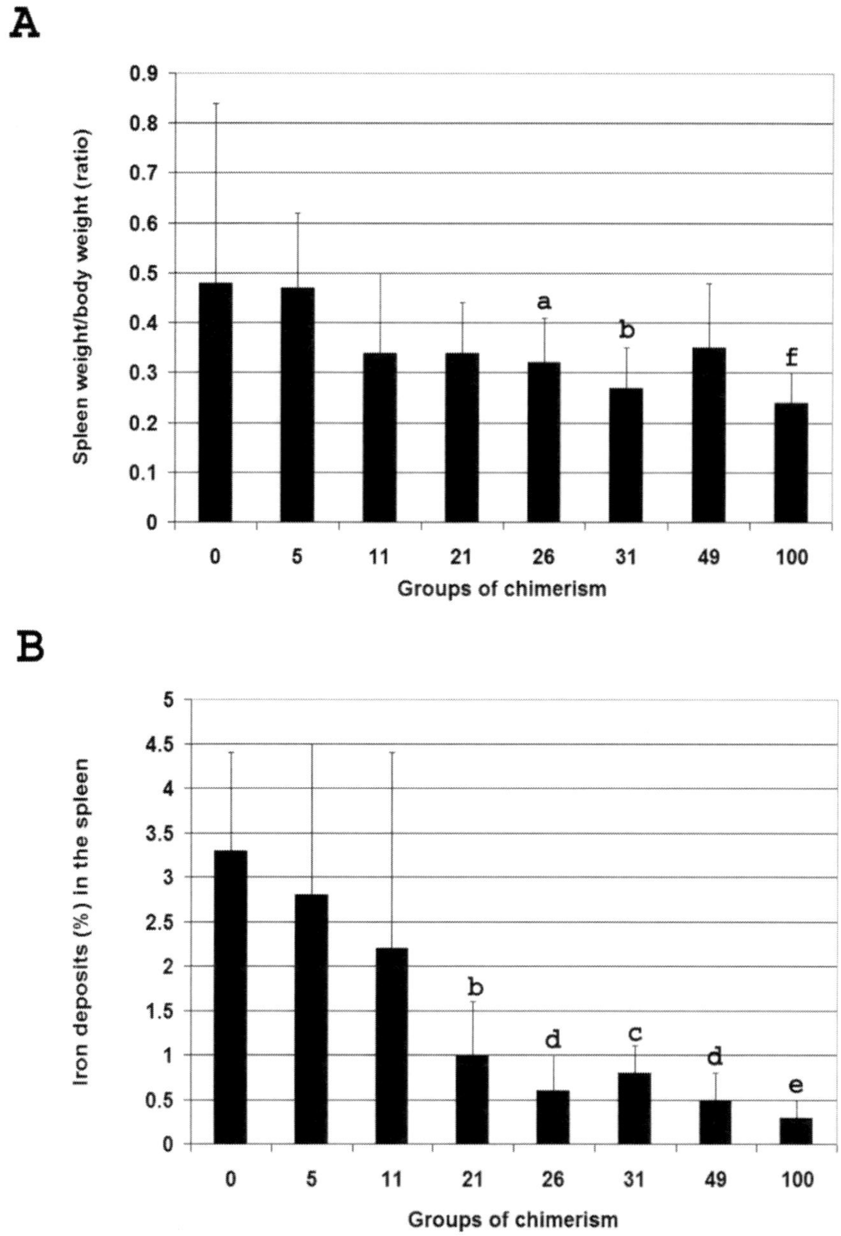

Figure 6. Pathological analysis of SAD chimeric mice.
Abbreviations: WBCs, white blood cells; wt, weight; t-test: sample vs chimeric 0%; a, p<0.05; b, p<0.02; c, p<0.006 d, p<0.004; e, p<0.003; f, p<0.0008 (Adapted from data in Felfly et al, 2009).

Peripheral blood parameters showed substantial improvement starting 31% normal WBCs (~60% normal RBCs), while the inefficient erythropoiesis showed significant improvement starting 16% normal WBCs and progenitor numbers were normalized by 16% normal WBCs. HbS levels in peripheral blood were decreased in parallel to the increase in the percentage of normal RBCs, and were inversely correlated with RBC half-life which increased with the percentage of normal RBCs (Figure 5).

Table 2A. Engraftment and chimerism of SAD mice with minimal myelosuppression and one cell dose

Irr. Level	Cells	Trans. Time	n	n	% Chimerism	
(Gy)	(10^7)	(h)	(total)	(engr)	**WBC**	**RBC**
2	2	4	21	4	**37.0** ±9.5	**84.2** ±15.1[d]
	4	4	12	5	**48.1** ±21.4**	**88.4** ±26.0[a]
	5	4	8	5	**76.6** ±11.1[A,B,C]	**97.3** ± 4.0[b]
	2	52	13	2	**38.3** ±14.6	**73.5** ± 9.2[e]
	5	52	8	3	**27.8** ±20.6	**50.1** ± 34.1
1	4	4	19	6	**21.1** ±15.5	**66.0** ±31.7[b]
	6	4	7	4	**21.7** ±14.0	**69.5** ±4.9[c]
	8	4	8	4	**52.6** ±14.4*[#]	**87.9** ±1.7[b]
	4	28	17	6	**32.0** ±20.6	**65.7** ±23.6[a]
	8	28	10	4	**59.1** ±32.2	**90.7** ±18.6

Abbreviations: WBC, white blood cells,; RBC, red blood cells; n (total), total number of mice transplanted; n (engr), number of transplanted mice that engrafted.

t-test:

RBC vs WBC chimerism; a, $p<0.03$; b, $p<0.02$; c, $p<0.007$; d, $p<0.004$; e, $p<0.0001$.

Level of WBC chimerism, %WBC in one group vs %WBC in another group; *1Gy, 4h: 8 x 10^7 cells vs 4 x 10^7, $p<0.02$; #1Gy, 8 x 10^7 vs 6 x 10, $p<0.05^7$; **2Gy, 4h, 4 x 10^7 vs 1Gy, 4h, 4 10^7, $p<0.05$; A, 2Gy, 4h, 5 x 10^7 vs 2 x 10^7, $p<0.0008$; B, 2Gy, 4h, 5 x 10^7 vs 4 x 10^7, $p<0.04$; C, 2Gy, 5 x 10^7, 4h vs 52h, $p<0.04$; (Adapted from Felfly et al, 2009).

Between 16 and 26% normal WBCs there was a significant and substantial improvement of most histological parameters including decreased fibrosis and iron deposits in various organs, normalized spleen volume and cellularity, and correction of glomerular size in the kidneys, and mice lived to a normal life span by 26% normal WBCs [Figure 6; Felfly *et al*, 2009].

These parameters showed that the majority of the disease indices were corrected between 16 and 26% normal WBCs. However, a few peripheral blood parameters required a higher percentage of 31% normal WBCs for correction [Felfly *et al*, 2009]. Therefore the therapeutic threshold of SCD is considered in the 26-31% normal WBCs thus covering correction of all disease parameters.

To achieve 26-31% normal WBC chimerism after minimal myelosuppression, the same strategy used for β-thalassemia was applied for SCD. With one cell injection at 4h, 28h or 52h, very few animals showed donor chimerism, although in those mice, the percentage of normal WBCs in peripheral blood was within the therapeutic range for most of them. (Table 2A)

When multiple injections were assayed (Table 2B), after 1Gy irradiation and 60 million donor BM cells, while only one mouse of 7 engrafted after 2 injections, all mice (7/7) engrafted after 3 injections with an average donor WBC chimerism within the therapeutic threshold. After 2Gy irradiation, 6 of 7 mice engrafted after 2 injections, and all mice engrafted after 3 and 4 injections, and in all three groups, the average donor WBC chimerism was higher than the therapeutic threshold.

Table 2B. Engraftment and chimerism of SAD mice with minimal myelosuppression and multiple cell doses

Irr. Level	Cells	Inject	n	n	% Chimerism	
(Gy)	(10^7)	(#)	(total)	(engr)	WBC	RBC
2	4	2	7	6^b	**73.5** ±20.0	**89.5** ±10.8^a
		3	5	5	**50.7** ±26.0	**70.4** ±21.8
		4	6	6	**67.2** ±15.1	**90.4** ±8.3
1	6	2	7	1	**34.4**	**77.8**
		3	7	7	**28.7** ±20.6	**52.3** ±22.3

Abbreviations: WBC, white blood cells,; RBC, red blood cells; n (total), total number of mice transplanted; n (engr), number of transplanted mice that engrafted.

t-test: RBC vs WBC chimerism; a, $p<0.03$; b, 2Gy, 2 x 2 x 10^7 vs 1Gy 2 x 3 x 10^7, $p<0.03$ (Adapted from Felfly et al, 2009).

The new transplantation strategy thus proved effective for different blood diseases, and the decisive factor seems to be the number of cell injections along with the timing of the first injection, as one injection at 28h or 52h was, for the most part, less efficient that one injection at 4h, and multiple injections were more efficient than just one. SCD seems more demanding than β-thalassemia, with both the therapeutic threshold and the number of injections needed for optimal results were higher for SCD. However, the difference was mild, and SCD was corrected with the same low level of irradiation as β-thalassemia, and the therapeutic threshold was close to that of thalassemia; however, SCD required at least 3 injections for donor cells to engraft in all recipient mice, clearly indicating that SCD bone marrow microenvironment was more resilient. This might be due to the nature of the SCD pathologies.

VI.3. Correction of β-thalassemia and SCD: A Model

Based on the successful therapy for both diseases, and given the similarity in the transplantation requirements, a common model can be proposed. Mild irradiation of thalassemic or sickle mice increases the permeability of the blood-bone marrow barrier, and damages or "stuns" the recipient BM cells, weakening them and somehow decreasing their ability to compete for the stem cell niche. A first intravenous injection of normal donor BM cells within 4h after irradiation results seeds or "primes" the recipient BM with normal cells that will start to proliferate, yet unable to produce sufficient donor cells to contribute to recipient peripheral blood chimerism. These cells displace recipient stem cells and succeed in interacting with the stem cell niche. Additional "booster" injections of donor BM cells within the following 24h provide additional doses of normal cells that will produce enough erythroid cells that will compete with the recipient pathological and fast dying erythroid cells to yield donor cells in the peripheral blood. Depending on the dose of irradiation, the total number of cells injected and the number of injections, erythroid cells from the donor succeed in overcoming the recipient counterparts sufficiently enough to yield a therapeutic level of donor cells in recipient's peripheral blood.

VII. STEM CELL THERAPY FOR STROKE

Stroke poses a more challenging case for stem cell therapy for many reasons. 1-The brain is protected by blood-brain-barrier (BBB) separating the brain from the blood and making the intravenous delivery of stem cells of a low efficiency. Intra-brain injection could deliver cells directly, but physical damage to parts of the brain could happen during the actual injection, in addition to possibility of swelling that might cause further neurological damage; 2-The brain is not the natural environment of BM cells/HSCs; 3-Ischemic injury leads to infarct relatively quickly, and therefore the timing of cell delivery is crucial for the success and the "window" of time before full death occurs due to infarct must be precisely determined; 4-Severe stroke can be lethal, and therefore two issues are posed: protecting from death and protecting from neurological damage.

Many studies have investigated the intra-brain delivery of donor stem cells in animal models of stroke, however, the ideal method would be intravenous delivery with no exposure or physical damage to the brain. For this to be successful, many parameters have to be set: first, a reproducible mouse model for stroke has to be generated and its phenotype characterized in details; second, the time after ischemia where cell death is still minimal before reaching the stage of full infarct, has to be determined; third, the effect of various amounts of donor cells have to be tested; fourth, the timing of cell injection will have to be assayed for optimal delivery time after the infarct.,

VII.1. Animal Models for Stroke

Animal models for ischemic brain injury can be divided in two major categories based on whether the brain is exposed during the procedure or not. These are: models not requiring craniotomy, and models requiring craniotomy. [Durukan and Tatlisumak, 2007].

1. Models not requiring craniotomy,
   a) Thromboembolic strokes: these are lesions where multiple small ischemic areas can be induced by emboli. Autologous blood clots, artificial embolizing materials, such as silicone, collagen, or silver balls, or microspheres, are injected into a large artery leading to the brain. This results in occluding smaller arteries downstream. Leading to infarcts of various sizes and locations
   b) Middle Cerebral Artery Occusion (MCAO): in this approach, a filament is introduced into the Internal Carotid Artery (ICA) and advanced until it blocks the middle cerebral artery (MCA). In permanent occlusion the filament is kept in the artery; in transient occlusion, it is withdrawn after a certain length of time, resulting in occlusion/reperfusion model. Lesions can vary from microscopic to large infarct depending on the occlusion time.
   c) Endothelin-1 injection: endothelin-1 is a vaso-constrictor that allows the formation of lesions in various areas of the brain, but provides less control over duration and size of the affected area due to dose-dependency

2. Models requiring craniotomy:

   In these models, there is exposure of the brain to the atmosphere and the blood-brain barrier (BBB) is experimentally compromised. These approaches will directly occlude the MCA by a surgical approach

VII.2. Preliminary Trials and Suitable Models

The MCAO method became the most largely used approach because of the technical feasibility and the ability to obtain reproducible lesions. Using this method, many investigators generated stroke models in rodents and studied the effect of stem cell transplantation. Different types of stem cells, such as neural stem cells, mesenchymal stem cells, and human cord CD34+ cells. The results of these trials varied from no success [Nystedt *et al*, 2006] to decreasing the infarct size [Honna *et al*, 2006; Ukai *et al*, 2007], or improvement of some neurological aspects [Lee *et al*, 2007; Liu *et al*, 2006; Nystedt *et al*, 2006]. However, the variability of the infarct size between studies [Honna *et al*, 2006; Nystedt *et al*, 2006; Ukai *et al*, 2007] and the severity of the models as well as the variable and partial outcome raised challenges towards finding an actual reproducible and reliable stem cell transplantation that will correct all the aspects of the stroke.

The table below summarizes previous attempts to protect from or correct stroke after MCAO (Table 3).

To this end, Felfly and colleagues [Felfly *et al*, 2010], generated a stroke model that produced a large infarct, was reproducibly obtained, and affected mice showed neurological damage and shortened survival. This model was then used to assess multiple strategies of hematopoietic stem cell transplantations (HSCT) that opened in a new promising era of stroke therapy with stem cells.

A permanent occlusion of the MCA resulted in a large infarct occupying ~70% of the hemisphere, and all of these mice died in no more than 4 days. To allow intravenous stem cell delivery, however, reperfusion is needed. Various length of occlusion times followed by reperfusion were tested to assess the best time that will result in a strong reproducible infarct. With 30 minutes, 1h, and 1.5h occlusion, not all mice had macroscopic lesions, and the infarct size was not reproducible. With 2h occlusion or longer, all mice had lesions, and the infarct size was reproducible between individual mice, with longer occlusions resulting in a faster propagation of the lesion and shorter survival. Therefore, 2h occlusion followed by reperfusion was found to be the most suitable: it has a large (~70%) reproducible infarct, and the occluded vessel is reopened allowing reperfusion, as well as stem cell delivery to the affected area by IV injection. The amount of dead tissue in the infarct area increased overtime and was full at 16h after reperfusion. [Figure 7, adapted from Felfly *et al*, 2010]

Table 3. Preliminary stem cell transplantation trials for stroke therapy

Animals	MCAo	Cell Type	Cell No	Route	Inject No	Inject Time after MCAo	Assessed	Ref
Mouse	Perman	hCD34+	$5x10^5$	IV	1	48h	↑ angio, improve behavior, endogenous neurogenesis and neuronal survival	Taguchi A. *et al.* 2004, JCI 114(3): 330-338
Mouse	90min	Endothelial cells	$1.5x10^6$	IV	1	Pre-MCAo	BM cells differentiate into vessel endothelial cells in brain	Hess DC *et al.* 2002, Stroke 33:1362-1368
Rats	Perman	hCB CD34+	$5x10^5$ to $2x10^6$	IV	1	24h	A bit better memory recovery No change in infarct size, no functional recovery, no differntiation	Nystedt J *et al.*, 2006, Acta Neurobiol Exp 66(4): 293-300
Mouse	Perman	hUCB or PBPC	Abstract only	IV	1	24h	Prevented dvpt of severe motor asymmetry ↓ hyperactivity	Willing AE *et al.*, 2003, Cell Transplant 12(4): 449-454
Rat	3h	NSC ES-derived	10^6	Intra Carotid	1	48h	New neuronal sprouting	Jiang Q *et al.*, 2006, Neuroimage 32:1080-1089
Mouse	Perman	NSC ES-derived	10^5	Intra brain	1	1 wk	↓ hemisphere atrophy, 3/10 mice developed tumors	Comi AM *et al.*, 2008, Pediatric Neurology 38(2):86-92
Mouse	Intracerebral hemorrhage collagenase	hNSC line	$2x10^5$	Intra brain	1	1 wk	Improved functional recovery	Lee HJ *et* al., 2007, Stem Cells 25:1204-1212
Rat	1h	H fetal NSC	3 x 1. 10^5	Intra-brain	3	7 days	No change in lesion size Donor cells migrate and express markers of astrocytes and neurons	Kelly S *et al.,* 2004, PNAS 101(32):11839-11844
Mouse	2h + hypoxia 8% O2 20 min	NSC C17.2	3x 10^5	Intra Carotid	1	48h	Improve behavioral recovery	Guzman *R et al.*, 2008, Stroke 39: 1300-1306
Rat	2h	Neurotrophic factor	-	Intra brain	1	Days 2 thru 7	↑ cell proliferation in SVZ and neuron survival	Kobayashi *T et al.*, 2006, Stroke 37: 2361-2367

Table 3. (Continued)

Animals	MCAo	Cell Type	Cell No	Route	Inject No	Inject Time after MCAo	Assessed	Ref
Animals	MCAo	Cell Type	Cell No	Route	Inject No	Inject Time after MCAo	Assessed	Ref
Rat	1h	Murine neuroepithelial cells MHP36	$2x10^5$	Intra brain	1	2wk	Graft survived 2 wks later Low immunoreactivity of MHP36 cells	Modo M *et al*., 2002, Brain Research 958:70-82
Rat	Normal mice	NSC	N.I.	Intra brain	1	N.I.	Migrate and differentiate	Gage F *et al* 1995, PNAS 92:11879-11883
Rat	Perman	hMSC	10^7	IV	1	3h	↓ lesion size, functional recovery and ↑ vessels	Liu H *et al*., 2006, Brain 129:2734-2745
Rat	45 min	hMSC	$10^4 – 10^7$	IV	1	12h	↓ lesion size, functional recovery/ memory… correlate with No of cells injected	Honna T *et al*., 2006, Experimental Neurology 199:56-66
Rat	Perma	MSC	$5 x 10^6$	IV	1	3 days	↑ vessels	Zin'kova NN *et al*., 2007, Tsitologila 49(7):566-575
Rat	2h	MSC	$3 x 10^5$	Intra brain	1	24h	Improve function and recovery but no differentiation into neurons	Wei JJ *et al*., 2007, Zhonghua Yi Xue Za Zhi 87(3): 1874-189
Rat	Perman	MSC	10^6	IV	1	6h	↑ blood flow to affected areas, functional improvements, ↓ infarct size	Ukai R *et al*., 2007, J of Neurotrauma 24(3): 508-520
Rat	Perman	mES or ES-N	$120 x 10^3$	Intra brain	1 in 2 sites	7 days	↓ number of rotation, better on rotarod	Yanagisawa D *et al*., 2006, Neuroscience Letters 407: 74-79
Mouse	30 min	Primate ES-derived NSC	$5 to 20 x 10^4$	Intra brain	1	24	Donor cells survive, differentiate and network in mouse brain	Hayashi J *et al*., 2006, J of Cerebral Blood Flow & Metabolism 26 :906-914

Abbreviations : No, number ; IV, intra-venous ; NSCs, neural stem cells ; ES, embryonic stem cells ; h, human ; CB, cord blood ; UCB, umbilical cord blood ; PBPC, peripheral blood pluripotent cells ; MSC, mesenchymal stem cells ; N.I., not indicated ; h, hour ; wk, week ; Perman, permanent ; SVZ, sub-ventricular zone; Ref, references.

Table 4. Neurological scoring of MCAO mice

Mouse groups	Pre-HSCT (2h after MCAO)							Post-HSCT (7 days after transplantation)							14 d
	n (%)	Tors Tilt [1]	Circul motion [2]	Can't bare weight	Barrel rolling	Right reflex	Score	n (%)	Tors tilt	Circul motion	Can't bare weight	Barrel rolling	Right reflex	Score	Score
MCAO cont (A)	15 (71%)	1	2	3	0	+	6	4 (67%)	1	2	3	0	+	6	n/a
MCAO cont (B)	6 (29%)	1	2	3	4	+	10	2 (33%)	1	2	3	4	+	10	n/a
MCAO + 6 x 10^6 HSCs (C)	17 (59%)	1	2	3	0	+	6	5 (42%)	1*	2**	0	0	-	$3^{a,c}$	0
								4 (33%)	0	0	0	0	-	$0^{a,c}$	0
MCAO + 6 x 10^6 HSCs (D)	12 (42%)	1	2	3	4	+	10	2 (17%)	1*	2**	0	0	-	$3^{b,d}$	0
								1 (8%)	0	0	0	0	-	$0^{b,d}$	0
MCAO + 12 x 10^6 HSCs (E)	7 (70%)	1	2	3	0	+	6	3 (60%)	1*	2**	0	0	-	$3^{e,f}$	0
								1 (20%)	0	0	0	0	-	0	0
MCAO + 12 x 10^6 HSCs (F)	3 (30%)	1	2	3	4	+	10	1 (20%)	0	0	0	0	-	0	0

n, number of mice; %, percentage of mice; MCAO, middle cerebral artery occlusion; HSCT, hematopoietic stem cell transplantation; HSCs, hematopoietic stem cells; Naïve cont., control mice that were not subjected to MCAO; MCAO cont., control mice subjected to MCAO only; Tors tilt, torso turned towards the right; circul motion, circular motion towards the right; n/a, not applicable (mice were dead by that time); 14d, 14 days post HSCT.

Scoring: all signs but the righting reflex were given a score as previously described with slight modification (McCullogh et al, 2005). Different signs were given a different "grading" number and the total score was the sum of the grades of all the graded signs; 0, sign not detected; 1, 2, 3, 4, sign detected; Righting reflex was noted as impaired (+, i.e. mouse shakes/moves randomly before righting up), or normal (-, mouse right up immediately without any random movement).

Circular motion: mouse turns in a circular fashion instead of walking straight; Can't bare weight, mouse is leaning towards the paralyzed side and cannot hold up its body weight on that side; Barrel rolling; when placed on their back or slightly lifted by the tail, mice roll once or twice like a barrel; righting reflex; mice are placed on their back.

1, the torso is turned to the right in a pronounced way; *, the torso is slightly turned to the right; 2, circular motion 10-21 times per minute; **, circular motion ≤ 5 times per minute.

t-test: a, group C 2h vs. 7 days, $p<4 \times 10\text{-}8$; b, group D, 2h vs. 7 days, $p<0.02$; c, group A vs. C, 7 days, $p<0.004$; d, group D vs. B, 7 days, $p<0.02$; e, groups E & F, 2h 7 days, $p<0.0003$; f, groups E & F, 7 days vs. groups A & B, 7 days, $p<0.0008$ (Adapted from Felfly et al, 2010).

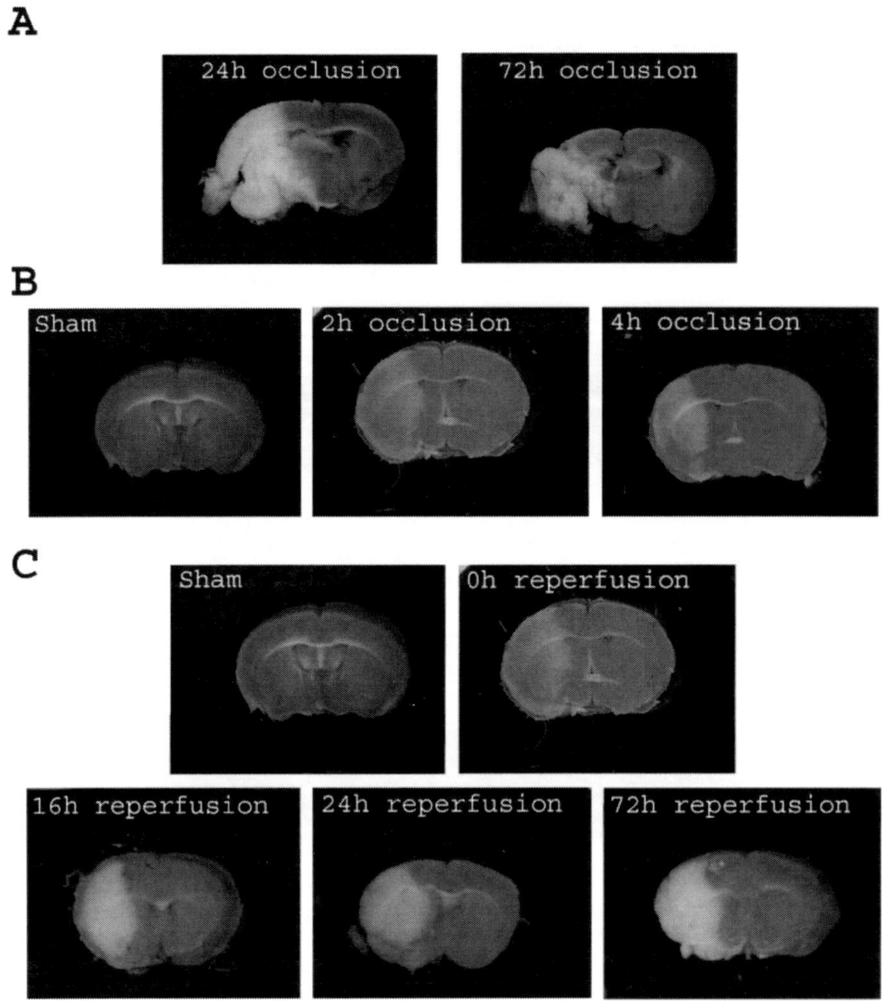

Figure 7. Generating the stroke model. Brains of control mice and mice subjected to stroke were sectioned and stained with 2,3,5 triphenyl tetrazolium chloride (TTC) to detect the infarct area. Intact tissue stained red while infarcted tissue appears white. A-After permanent occlusion, TTC-stained brains after 24 h and 72 h of MCAO revealed a major infarct area occupying most of the hemisphere, and liquefying at 72 h. B-Permanent occlusion of only 2 h or 4 h resulted in a clear infarct, more severe with a longer occlusion time, and respectively occupying 69.7±6.5% and 65.2±7.1% of the ipsilateral hemisphere as shown in the histogram. C-Mice were subjected to 2 h MCAO followed by reperfusion and TTC staining at variable times afterwards (16 h, 24 h and 72 h). The infarct area appeared a mix of white and pink in color just after 2 h. Overtime, the color became fully white in the affected area suggesting complete death of the tissue in the affected area (Adapted from Felfly et al, 2010).

These mice also showed many signs of neurological impairment (Table 4). All mice showed a rotational motion in the cage as soon as they woke up, and this was considered an inclusion criterion; mice not showing this motion were excluded from the study. Mice also showed unilateral paralysis of the limb and inability to hold their own weight. The torso was arched toward one side, and some mice displayed a barrel rolling motion when lifted by the tail. When mice were placed on their back, they took ~2 seconds to turn back, while controls turned back immediately. Furthermore, >99% of mice died within 12 days after the surgery.

VII.3. BM Cells vs Enriched HSCs

The MCAO model described above was then subjected to HSCT, in attempts to find a successful stem cell therapy for stroke. Since total bone marrow (BM) cells contains at least three types of stem cells [Chao and Hirschi, 2010]: hematopoietic stem cell (HSC), mesenchymal stem cell (MSC) and endothelial stem cell (ESC), BM cells were first selected as therapeutic cells with the assumption that they will have the combined benefit of the three stem cell types.

These trials used transplantation strategies that modulated 3 parameters: cell number, timing of injections of the stem cells after the reperfusion, and the number of injections. The number of cells varied from 70 million to 500 million cells. The timing of the injection varied from 2h post-reperfusion, to 24h or 48h after reperfusion. The number of injections was 1, 2 or 3. These studies revealed an optimal window for transplantation to be ~2h after reperfusion. This is concordant with the histological observations of the infarct area where immediately after reperfusion not all the tissue is dead, while 16h later, all the infarct area is dead [Figure 7, adapted from Felfly *et al*, 2010]. This means that the cells have to be delivered during a narrow window before all the tissue is dead, otherwise, the protective effect would not be significant. One injection of cells 2h after reperfusion, however, did not allow the mice to survive much longer than control. A second injection the next day prolonged the survival up to 7 days. This was the best survival obtained in all the strategies tested. Clearly, this was still not satisfactory. One reason might be that the total BM cells included a lot of inflammatory cells that might have a negative effect, which is why the mice did not live too long. However, this indicated that the optimal time for transplantation is within 2h after reperfusion as “window of opportunity”, and that two injections could be needed: the first injection provided an initial protective effect that slowed the progression of cell death in the brain, and the second injection functioned as a booster to enhance the recovery. This also meant that it would be advisable possibly to remove inflammatory cells, and use an enriched population of HSC [Felfly *et al*, 2010].

HSC can be selected for using cell surface markers. One way is to purify HSC by positive selection. HSC are double positive for Sca1, c-Kit, and negative for lineage differentiation markers, such as CD4, CD8, Ter119, Gr1, B220, Mac1, CD3, etc. [Schroeder 2010; Ciriza and Garcia-Ojeda 2010]. By labeling BM cells with these markers, cells that are Sca1+ and c-Kit+ and negative for all the lineage markers are made up of the HSC population. Another way is to obtain a population of cells that is enriched in HSC, and that is by positive selection using only one marker, such as Sca1 or c-Kit. This results is a mixture of cells that has lost most inflammatory cells, but still retain progenitor cells and HSCs [Wilson *et al*, 2007]. Using this enrichment approach, we selected for Sca1+ cells which allowed 7-fold enrichment in HSCs. By having less inflammatory cells, this population was expected to have the beneficial effects of HSCs without the potentially detrimental effects of the inflammatory cells. Increasing amounts of Sca1+ cells injected IV 2h after the reperfusion, starting from 500000 cells and up, showed a progressive prolongation of survival with increasing cell numbers, and starting 3 million cells, a few mice lived beyond 2 weeks. Adding a second injection of another 3 million cells 18h later resulted in the protection of ~40% of transplant-recipient mice which survived for all the duration of the study (>5 months) and did not show the neurological deficit observed in non-transplanted controls. Doubling the number of cells per injection resulted in a similar protection, but not more, suggesting that the effect of HSC might have reached a plateau [Figure 8, adapted from Felfly *et al*, 2010]

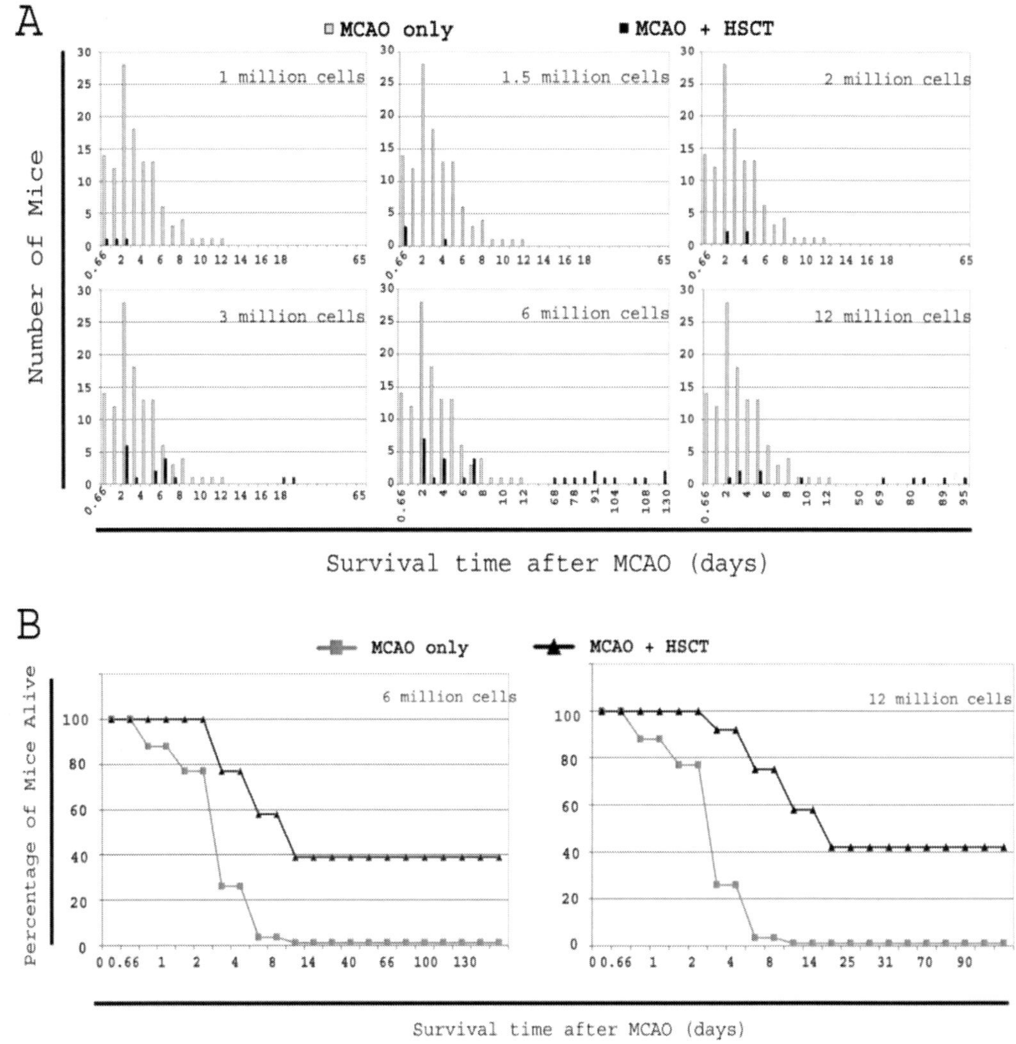

Figure 8. Increasing numbers of cells transplanted into recipient mice that were subjected to stroke progressively increases survival. Grey bars: controls (stroke only); Black bars, experimental (mice subjected to stroke + HSCT). Transplantation of 6 million or 12 million HSCs protects 40% of mice subjected to lethal stroke (Adapted from Felfly et al, 2010).

VII.4. Neurological and Histological Improvements in Surviving Mice

The transplant-recipient mice that survived >2 weeks showed a progressive decline in the neurological deficit starting few days after the transplantation, and the recovery was complete by 2 weeks (Table 4). However, in this study, other functions such as memory or advanced motor skills were not assessed. The brains of these mice were dissected and stained for the detection of infarct using triphenyl tetrazolium chloride (TTC), a vital stain that turns red in live tissues, but appears white in dead tissues. 5 days after the stroke induction, control mice presented a large infarct of ~70% of the hemisphere, while the transplant-recipient mice showed only 30% infarct, a clear indication of protective effect of the HSCs. 5 months after transplantation, brains of the mice showed up to 15% smaller hemisphere indicative of tissue loss. This loss, however, is minimal compared to the original infarct size of 70% [Figure 9, adapted from Felfly *et al*, 2010]. It indicates that the HSCs were able to protect the majority of the hemisphere; this protection, however, was not complete, and part of the brain tissue did die and was lost.

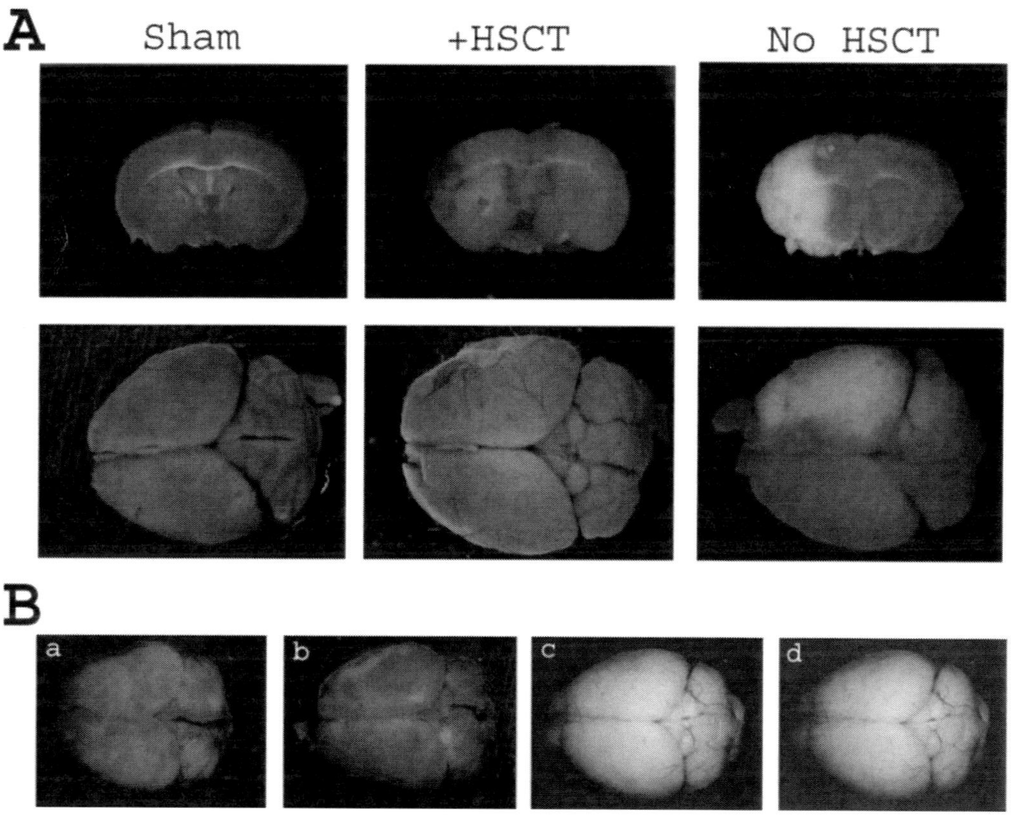

Figure 9. Rescue of brain tissue after Sca1+ bone marrow cell transplantation (HSCT). At various times after Sca1+ cell transplantation, MCAO mice were sacrificed and their TTC stained brains were used to evaluate the infarct. A — 5 days after 2 h transient occlusion, the infarct had a volume of 68.7%±5.15% of the affected hemisphere (right column) and became fully white, while transplant-recipient mice (middle column) showed a clear regression of the infarct size to almost one-half to one-fourth (17.73%±11.00%). B — Transplant-recipient MCAO mice surviving past 2 months after the MCAO were sacrificed at 5 months after the transplantation. TTC Staining did not reveal any infarcted region, suggesting an elimination of the dead tissue overtime. The gross morphology of the brains revealed shrinkage of the affected hemisphere, clearly noticeable in 50% of animals analyzed, as shown in panels a and b. The amount of brain tissue lost ranged from 7.76% to 15.38% of ipsilateral hemisphere (Adapted from Felfly et al, 2010).

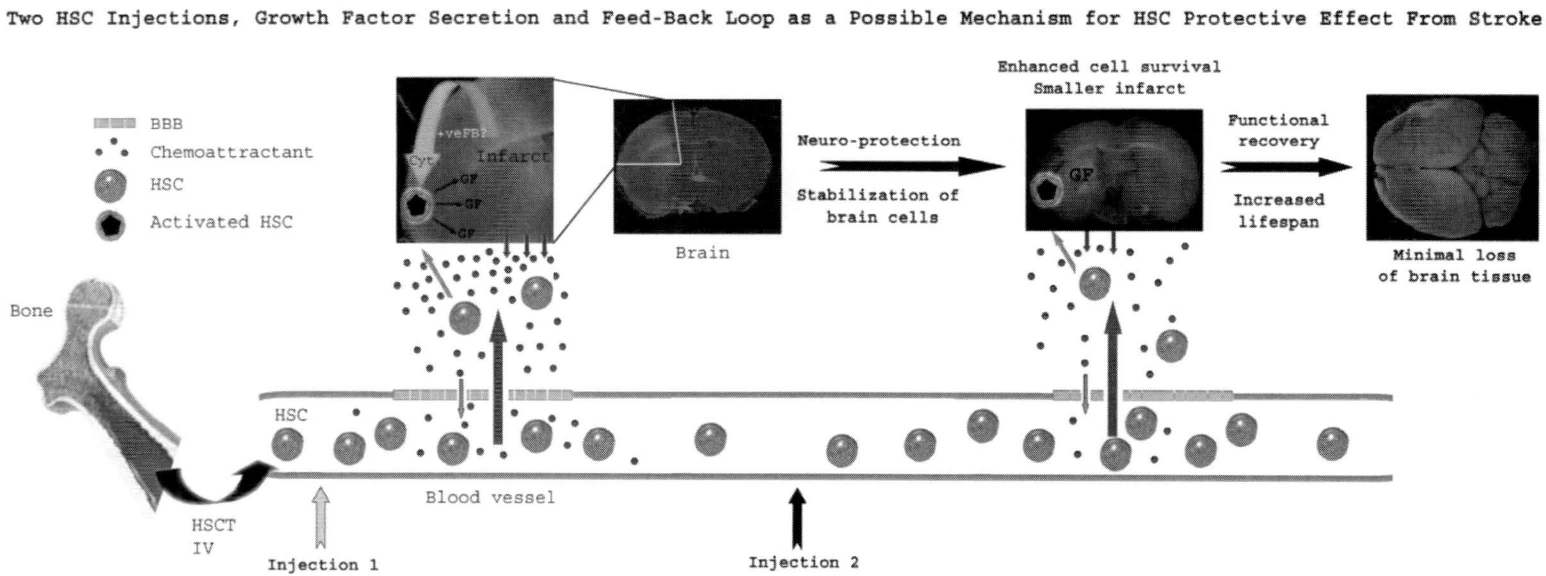

Figure 10. A proposed model for the protective effect of hematopoietic stem cell transplantation on brain infarct. HSCs are obtained from the bone marrow and enriched, then injected intravenously (IV) into mice subjected to stroke (ischemia/reperfusion). The first injection takes place within ~2h after reperfusion. HSCs circulate in the bloodstream and they are attracted toward the infarct tissue through soluble chemo-attractant secreted by the injured brain, such as SDF-1. At the area of the highest levels of chemo-attractant, near the brain tissue, HSCs extravasate and cross the blood brain barrier (BBB) which is impaired in ischemic brain injury. Once in the brain, HSCs are activated by cytokines secreted by the dying tissue; in return, activated HSCs secrete some growth factors that help stabilize the surviving brain cells, therefore limiting the propagation of the infarct. A positive feed-back loop therefore exists between the donor HSCs and the recipient ischemic brain tissue. A second injection of HSCs 18h later, results in further stabilizing brain cells, allows functional recovery, prevents infarct propagation and allows mice to live longer. Together, both injections also results in only a minimal loss of brain tissue.

VII.5. Fate of Donor Cells and Recipient's Brain Cells after HSCT Following MCAO

Tracing experiments where donor cells contained a marker are transplanted into mice subjected to MCAO are an important tool to understanding the fate of donor cells and provides a mechanistic view as to how donor cells protect recipient brains. These experiments revealed that donor cells could be observed 2h after the second stem cell injection, but their number was very low, indicating that the protection observed is not due to cell supplementation. A plausible explanation is that donor cells secreted growth factors that protect brain cells.

Another parameter in understanding the effect of donor cells on recipient brains is determining whether the numbers of neurons and glial cells are affected. The normal proportion of neurons vs. non-neurons is ~1:1 [Banderia *et al*, 2009; Azevedo *et al*, 2009]. The affected brain hemispheres of the mice showed ~25% less neurons and twice more glia compared to the contra-lateral hemispheres, suggestimg that neurons were more vulnerable to blood vessel occlusion/reperfusion, and that glial cells are induced/activated following stroke, which might be a mechanism by which the brain tries to compensate for cell loss. This also suggests that the HSCs transplanted did not have any "additive" effects on brain cells since there are less neurons; the effect of the HSCs was more protective that regenerative. While one cannot exclude the possibility that some HSCs might have generated a few brain cells, if any, this is minimal since the number of brain cells in the affected hemisphere did decrease.

VII.6. Neuro-protection Following HSCT: Potential Mechanism

Donor cells were found to constitute only 1 in 10000 in brains of recipient mice after HSCT, excluding any additive effect on the brain. These cells were also distributed mostly at cortical and subcortical regions, roughly corresponding to the penumbra, suggesting no direct contact with the dying infarct core. Therefore, the most plausible mode of action becomes growth factor based: donor cells could have secreted some soluble growth factors that diffused in the brain and stabilized the brain cells, therefore preventing cell death of a large proportion of brain cells. Cases where stem cells secrete growth factors in contact with infarct extract has been shown for mesenchymal stem cells (MSCs) [Chen *et al*, 2002]. We therefore propose a mechanistic model explaining how IV-injected HSCs reach the brain and provide their protective effect (Figure 10). Following an ischemia/reperfusion lesion, the blood-brain barrier (BBB) increases its permeability and the ischemic brain releases stromal derived factor (SDF) as chemo-attractant for circulating HSCs [Cui *et al*, 2009; Cui *et al*, 2007]. HSCs injected intravenously within 2h of the reperfusion will be attracted by SDF-1 gradient and cross the BBB. Once near the brain tissue, these cells get stimulated by cytokines produced by the dying ischemic cells and get activated and in turn, secrete some yet to be determined growth factors that will stabilize recipient brain cells and protect them from cell death, therefore slowing the progression of the lesion. A second injection of HSCs 16-20h later provides a booster that will help keep the cells protected by the first injection alive, and allow some functional recovery. Therefore a positive feed-back loop develops between the dying brain cells and the HSCs. Two cell doses appear crucial as the first injection provides temporary protection while the second injection stabilizes them further and allows functional recovery and prolonged survival.

CONCLUSION

Hematopoietic stem cells (HSCs) have proven useful for the treatment of a variety of diseases. As described in this chapter, HSC transplantation (HSCT) allowed the treatment of unrelated diseases: hematopoietic and neurological. The application of HSCT also showed that the simple injection of HSCs is not sufficient to obtain an improvement of the phenotype; rather, optimizing various parameters associated with the tansplantation is needed for successful therapy. What is common for all three diseases, is that all required more than one cell injection to obtain a recovery. Furthermore, the timing of the injections is also crucial: for blood diseases requiring irradiation prior to the HSCT, the first injection has to be within 4h after irradiation and not 24h or more later, and for stroke, it should be within 2h. However, as desscibed by Felfly [Felfly *et al*, 2010], the infarct propagates and cell death becomes full after 16h following reperfusion, indicating that the "window of opportunity" for stroke therapy is not restricted to 2h after repersufion, but likely ~4-6h while the death is still minimal, providing a broader "safe zone" for preparing the cells.

It is interesting to know why two or more injections within 24h allow recovery, while a single injection of the same amount of cells is not sufficient. This is likely due to the host and the stem cell niche rather than the stem cells themselves. The HSCs are the same, but the status of the irradiated recipient bone marrow or ischemic brain is not. Understanding the changes occurring in the bone marrow and the ischemic brain area overtime will give a better insight into the interactions needed between donor HSCs and the recipient tissue. In addition, the brain and bone marrow are quite different and the behavior of donor cells is expected to be different between those two areas, and yet, the outcome was comparable and the requirements were similar, providing further prove to the ability of HSCs to help repair damaged organs.

Thinking of clinical applications of these strategies, one would imagine they should be quite feasible, especially that transplantations for such diseases are already carried out on patients. What is ground breaking in these studies is providing long term survival after the HSCT and correction of most disease parameters, with minimal cellular requirements. These studies also highlight the importance of the transplantation strategy itself rather than just the number of cells. Furthermore, there was no reported donor stem cell-induced cancer in these mice, which works in favor of clinical applications: irradiation was minimal for blood diseases, and no irradiation was needed for stroke. The various injections are also not very spaced from each other, and therefore, patients would not be required to spend long periods at the hospital.

The success of these studies opens the way for applications on a variety of other diseases, knowing that slight modification of the transplantation conditions for each the of disease might be all that is needed for successful theray.

REFERENCES

Abboud,M.R., Jackson,S.M., Barredo,J., Beatty,J., and Laver,J. (1994). Bone marrow transplantation for sickle cell anemia *Am J Pediatr Hematol Oncol* 16(1):86-89.

Adams,R.J., McKie,V.C., Hsu,L., Files,B., Vichinsky,E., Pegelow,C., Abboud,M., Gallagher,D., Kutlar,A., Nichols,F.T., Bonds,D.R., and Brambilla,D. (1998). Prevention of a first stroke by transfusion in children with sickle cell anemia and abnormal results on transcranial Doppler ultrasonography. *N Engl J Med* 339:5-11.

Advani,R., Sorenson,S., Shinar,E., Lande,W., Rachmilewitz,R.A., and Shrier,S.L. (1992). Characterization and comparison of the red blood cell membrane damage in severe human α- and β-thalassemia. *Blood* 79:1058-1063.

Aizawa,S. and Tavassoli,M. (1987). In vitro homing of hematopoietic stem cells is mediated by a recognition system with galactosyl and mannosyl specificities. *Proc. Natl. Acad. Sci. USA*. 84:4485-4489.

Alberto,F.L., Arruda,V.R., Lima,C.S.P., Bordin,S., Martins,J., Saad,S.T.O., Costa,F.F. (1998). Long-term hydroxyurea therapy in thalassemia intermedia and thalassemia major patients. *Blood* 92(1):366.

Aljurf,M., Ma,L., Angelucci,E., Lucarelli,G., Snyder,L.M., Kiefer,C.R., Yuan,J., and Schriere,S.L. (1996). Abnormal assembly of membrane proteins in erythroid progenitors of patients with β-thalassemia major. *Blood* 87(5):2049-2056.

Andrews,R.G., Bryant,E.M., Bartelmez,S.H., Muirhead,D.Y., Knitter,G.H., Bensinger,W., Strong,D.M. (1992). CD34+ marrow cells, devoid of T and B lymphocytes, reconstitute stable lymphopoiesis and myelopoiesis in lethally irradiated allogenic baboons. *Blood* 80:1693-1701.

Arcasoy,M.O., Romana,M., Fabry,M.E, Scarpidi,E., Nagel,R.L. and Forget,B.G. (1997). High level of human γ-globin gene expression in adult mice carrying a transgene of deletion-type hereditary persistence of fetal hemoglobin. *Molecular and Cellular Biology*. 17:2076-2098.

Arruda,V.R., Lima,C.S., Saad,S.T., Costa,F.F. (1997). Successful use of hydroxyurea in beta-thalassemia major (letter). *N Engl J Med* 336:964.

Asahara,T., Takahashi,T., Masuda,H., Kalka,C., Chen,D., Twaguro,H., Inai,Y., Silver,M. and Isner,J.M. (1999). VEGF contributes to postnatal neovascularization by mobilizing bone marrow-derived endothelial progenitor cells. *EMBO J.* 18:3964-3972.

Atweh,G., Sutton,M., Nassif,I., Boosalis,V., Dover,G., Wallenstein,S. (1999). Sustained induction of fetal hemoglobin by pulse butyrate therapy in sickle cell disease. *Blood* 91(6):1790-1797.

Avecilla,S., Hattori,K., Heissig,B., Tejada,R., Liao,F., Shido,K., Jin,D.K., Dias,S., Zhang,E., Hartman,T.E., Hackett,N.R., Crystal,R.G., Witte,L., Hicklin,D.J., Bohlen,P., Eaton,D., Lyden,D., de Sauvage,F. and Rafii,S. (2004). Chemokine-mediated interaction of hematopoietic progenitors with the bone marrow vascular niche is required for thrombopoiesis. *Nat Med.* 10:64-71.

Bernaudin,F., Souillet,G., Vannier,J.P., Plouvier,E., Lemerle,S., Michel,G., Bordigoni,P., Lutz,P., Kuentz,M. (1993). Bone marrow transplantation (BMT) in 14 children with severe sickle cell disease (SCD): the Frenchexperience GEGMO. *Bone Marrow Transplantation* 12 Suppl 1:118-121.

Bessis,M. (1973). *Red cell shapes. An illustrated classification and its rationale in red cell shape*. New York, Springer-Verlag.

Blau,C.A., Constantoulakis,P., Shaw,C.M., Stamatoyannopoulos,G. (1993). Fetal hemoglobin induction with butyric acid: efficacy and toxicity. *Blood* 81(2):529-537.

Blouin,M.J., De Paepe,M.E., and Trudel,M. (1999). Altered hematopoiesis in sickle cell disease. *Blood*. 94:1451-1459.

Bothwell,T., Charlton,R., Cook,J., and Finch,C. (1979). *Iron Metabolism in Man*. Blackwell Scientific Publications. Oxford. London.

Boulad,M., Giardina,P., Gillio,A., Kernan,N., Small,T., Brochstein,J., Van Syckle,K., George,D., Szabolcs,O., O`Reilly,R.J. (1998). Bone marrow transplantation for homozygous beta-thalassemia-the Memorial Sloan-Kettering Cancer Center experience. *Ann NY Acad Sci*. 850:498-502.

Brugnara,C. (2003). Sickle cell disease: from membrane pathophysiology to novel therapies for prevention of erythrocyte dehydration. *J Pediatr Hematol Oncol* 25(12):927-933.

Bruno,E., Luikart,S.D., Long,M.W., and Hoffman,R. (1995). Marrow-derived heparin sulfate proteoglycan mediates the adhesion of hematopoietic progenitor cells to cytokines. *Experimental Hematology*. 23:1212-1217.

Bunn,H.F. (1997). Pathogenesis and treatment of sickle cell disease. *N Engl J Med*. 337:762-769.

Bunyaratvej,A., Sahaphong,S., Bhamarapravati,N., Wasi,P. (1985). Quantitative changes in red blood cell shapes in relation to clinical features in β-thalassemia/HbE disease. *Am J Clin Pathol* 83:555-559.

Calvi,L., Adams,G., Weibrecht,K, Weber,J.M., Olson,D.P., Knight,M.C., Martin,R.P., Schipani,E., Divieti,P., Bringhurst,F.R., Milner,L.A., Kronenberg,H.M., Scadden,D.T. (2003). Osteoblastic cells regulate the hematopoietic stem cell niche. *Nature* 425:841-846.

Carlos,T.M. and Harlan,J.M. (1994). Leukocyte endothelial adhesion molecules. *Blood*. 84:2068-2101.

Cashman, J., Eaves, C.J. 2000. High marrow seeding efficiency of human lymphomyeloid repopulating cells in irradiated NOD/SCID mice. *Blood*. 96:3979-3981.

Cazzola,M., De Stefano,P., Poncho,F., Locatelli,Y., Beguin,Y. (1995). Relationship between transfusion regimen and suppression of erythropoiesis in beta-thalassemia major. *Br J Hematol* 89:473-478.

Cerny, J., Doomer, M., McAuliffe, C., Habibian, H., Stencil, K., Berrios, V., Reilly, J., Carlson, J., Cerny, A.M., d' Hondt, L., Benoit, B., Lambert, J.F., Colvin, G., Nilsson, S., Becker, P., and Quesenberry, P. 2002. Homing of purified murine lymphohematopoietic stem cells: a cytokine-induced defect. Journal *of Hematology & Stem Cell Research*. 11(6):913-922.

Choi,K., Kennedy,M., Kazarov,M., Papadimitriou,J.C., Keller,G. (1998). A common precursor for hematopoietic and endothelia cells. *Development* 125:725-732.

Ciavatta,D.J., Ryan,T.M., Farmer,S.F., and Townes,T.M. (1995). Mouse model of human β^0-thalasemia: Targeted deletion of the mouse β^{maj}- and β^{min}-globin genes in embryonic stem cells. *Proc. Natl. Acad. Sci. USA*. 92:9259-9263.

Cipolleschi,M.G., Dello,S., and Olivotto,M. (1993). The role of hypoxia in the maintenance of hematopoietic stem cells. *Blood* 82:2031-2037.

Collins,A.F., Pearson,H.A., Giardina,P., McDonagh,K.T., Brusilow, S.W., Dover, G.J. (1995). Oral sodium phenylbutyrate therapy in homozygous beta thalassemia: a clinical trial. *Blood* 85:43-49.

Comi AM, Cho E, Mulholland JD, Hooper A, Li Q, Qu Y, Gary DS, McDonals JW, Johnston MV. 2008. Neural stem cells reduce brain inury after unilateral carotid ligation. *Pediatric neurology* 38:86-92.

Croizat,H., Frindel,E., and Tubiana,M. (1970). Proliferative activity of the stem cells in the bone-marrow of mice after single and multiple irradiations (total- or partial-body exposure). *Int J Radiat Biol Relat Stud Phys Chem Med* 18:347-358.

Cui, J., Wahi R.L., Shen, T., Fisher, S.J., Becker, E., Ginsberg, D., and Liong, M.W. 1999. Bone marrow cell trafficking following intravenous administration. *British Journal of Haematology*. 107:895-902.

Dao,M., Arevalo,J., Nolta,J.A. (2003). Reversibility of CD34 expression on human hematopoietic stem cells that retain the capacity for secondary reconstitution. *Blood* 101:4201-4208.

Dasgupta,T., Hebbel,R.P., and Kaul,D.K (2006). Protective effect of arginine on oxidative stress in transgenic sickle mouse models. *Free Radic Biol Med* 41(12):1771-1780.

DeFranceschi,L., Bachir,D., Galacteros,F., Tchernia,G., Cynober,T., Neuberg,D., Beuzard,Y., Brugnara,C. (2000). Oral magnesium pidolate: effects of long-term administration in patients with sickle cell disease. *Br J Hematol* 108(2):284-289.

DePaepe, ME, Trudel, M. 1994. The transgenic SAD mouse: a model of human sickle cell glomerulonephropathy. *Kidney International* 46(5):1337-1345.

Dover,G.J. (1998). Hemoglobin switching protocols in thalassemia: experience with sodium phenylbutyrate and hydroxyurea. *Ann NY Acad Sci* 850:80-86.

Du,Z.D., Roguin,N., Milgram,E., Saab,K., Koren,A. (1997). Pulmonary hypertension in patients with thalassemia major. *Am Heart J* 134:532-537.

Embury,S.H. and Steinberg, MH. (1994). Genetic modulators of disease. In:Embury H, Hebbel RP, Mohandas N, Steinberg H (eds). Sickle cell disease: basic principles and practice. New York: Raven Press. pp279-298.

Fabry,M.D., Costantini,F.D., Pachnis,A., Suzuka,S.M., Bank,N., Aynedjian,H.S., Factor,S., and Nagel,R.L. (1992a). High expression of human β^S and α-globin in transgenic mice: (II) red cell abnormalities, organ damage, and the effect of hypoxia. *Proc. Natl. Acad. Sci. USA*. 89:12155-12159.

Fabry,M.E., Nagel,R.L., Pachnis,A., Suzuka,S.M., and Costantini,F.D. (1992b). High expression of human β^S and α-globin in transgenic mice: (I) hemoglobin composiioon and hematological consequences. *Proc. Natl. Acad. Sci. USA* 89:12150-12154.

Fabry,M.E., Suzuka,S.M., Costantini,E.D., Paszty,C., Smithies,O., and Nagel,R.L. (1997). Sickle transgenic mice with exclusively human genes: unexpected features. *Blood*. 90:124a.

Fabry,M.E., Suzuka,S.M., Gilman,J.G., Costantini,E.D., Paszty,C., Smithies,O., and Nagel,R.L. (1999). Second generation knock-out mice are useful for validation of gene therapy strategies. *Blood*. 94:645a.

Ferster,A., Bujan,W., Corazza,F., Devalick,C., Fondu,P., Toppet,M., Verhas,M., Sariban,E. (1993). Bone marrow transplantation corrects splenic reticuloendothelial dysfunction in sickle cell anemia. *Blood* 81(4):1102-1105.

Gage FH, Coates PW, Palmer TD, Kuhn HG, Fisher LJ, Suhonen JO, Peterson DA, Duhr ST, Ray J. (1995). Survival and differentiation of adult neuronal progenitor cells transplanted to the adult brain. PNAS 92:11879-11883.

Gaston,M.H, Verter,J.L., Woods,G., Pegelow,C., Kelleher,J., Presbury,G., Zarkowsky,H., Vichinsky,E., Iyer,R., Lobel,J.S., *et al.* (1986). Prophylaxis with oral penicillin in children with sickle cell anemia: A randomized trial. *N Engl J Med* 314:1593.

Gidali,J. and Lajtha,L.G. (1972). Regulation of hemopoietic stem cell turnover in partially irradiated mice. *Cell Tissue Kinet* 5:147-157.

Gilman,J.G., Fabry,M.E., Suzuka,S.M. and Nagel,R.L. (1995). Human Gγ:Aγ ratios switch during prenatal development in transgenic mice with HS4-$^{G}\gamma$(-158T)-$^{A}\gamma$. *Blood*, 86:648a.

Glader,B.E. (1994). Anemia. In: Embury H, Hebbel RP, Mohandas N, Steinberg MH (eds). Sickle cell disease: basic principles and practice. *New York: Raven Press*. Pp:545-553.

Goodell,M.A., Brose,K., Paradis,G., Conner,A.S., Mulligan,R.C. (1996). Isolation and functional properties of murine hematopoietic stem cells that are replicating in vivo. *J Exp. Med.* 183:1797-1806.

Goodell,M.A., Rosenzweig,M., Kim,H., Marks,D.F., DeMaria,M., Paradis,G., Grupp,S.A., Sieff,C.A., Mulligan,R.C., Johnson,R.P. (1997). Dye efflux studies suggest that hematopoietic stem cells expressing low or undetectable levels of CD34 antigen exist in multiple species. *Nat Med* 3:1337-1345.

Greaves,D.R., Fraser,P., Vidal,M.A., Hedges,M.J., Ropers,D., Luzzatto,L., and Grosveld,E. (1990). A transgenic mouse model of sickle cell disorder. *Nature*. 343:183-185.

Grinberg,L.N., Newmark,H., Kitrossky,N., Rahamin,E., Chevion,M., Rachmilewitz, E.A. (1997). Protective effects of tea polyphenols against oxidative damage to red blood cells. *Biochemical Pharmacology* 54:973-978.

Grinberg,L.N., Rachmilewitz,E.A., Newmark,H. (1994). Protective effects of rutin against hemoglobin oxidation. *Biochemical Pharmacology* 48:643-649.

Gullo,L., Corcioni,E., Brancati,C, Bria,M., Pezzilli,R., Sprovieri,G. (1993). Morphologic and functional evaluation of the exocrine pancreas in β-thalassemia major. *Pancreas* 8:176-180.

Guzman R, De Los Angeles A, Cheshier S, Choi R, Hoang S, Liauw J, Schaar B, and Steinberg G. (2008). Intracarotid injection of fluorescence activated cell-sorted CD49d-positive neural stem cells improves targeted cell delivery and behavior after in stroke in a mouse stroke model. *Stroke* 39:1300-1306.

H. Felfly & M. Trudel. (2007). Long-term Correction of β-Thalassemia with minimal cellular requirements and transplantation modalities. *Molecular Therapy*. 15(9):1701-1709.

H. Felfly & M. Trudel. (2009). Successful correction of murine Sickle Cell Disease with reduced stem cell requirements reinforced by fractionated marrow infusions. *British Journal of Hematology* 148:646-658.

H. Felfly, Alysson Muotri, Hang Yao, Gabriel G. Haddad. (2010). Hematopoietic stem cell transplantation protects mice from lethal stroke. *Experimental Neurology* 225:284-293.

Harrison, D. E., Jordan, C. T., Zhong, R. K., and Astle, C. M. (1993). Primitive hemopoietic stem cells: direct assay of most productive populations by competitive repopulation with simple binomial, correlation and covariance calculations. *Exp Hematol* 21: 206-219.

Harrisson,C.R. (2002). Hemolytic anemias: intracorpuscular defects IV – Thalassemia. In Harmening DM, (ed.), *Clinical Hematology and Fundamentals of Hemostasis*, ed. 4. FA Davis Company, Philadelphia, PA, pp186-200.

Hayashi J, Takagi Y, Fuduka H, Imazato T, Nishimura M, Fujimoto M, Takahashi J, Hashimoto N, Nozaki K. (2006). Primate embryonic stem cell-derived neuronal progenitors transplanted into ischemic brain. *J Cereb Blood Flow Metab* 26:906-914.

Herrick,J.B. (1910). Peculiar elongated and sickle-shaped red blood corpuscules in a case of severe anemia. *Arch Intern Med.* 6:517-521.

Hess DC, Hill WD, Martin-Studdard A, carroll J, Brailer J, and Carothers J. (2002). Bone marrow as a source of endothelial cells and NeuN-expressing cells after stroke. *Stroke* 33:1362-1368.

Hillman,R.S. and Finch,C.A. (1996). *Red Cell Manual*, ed 7. FA Davis, Philadelphia, pp. 2.

Hogan,C.J., Shpall,E.J., Keller,G. (2002). Differential long-term and multilineage engraftment potential from subfractions of human CD34+ cord blood cells transplanted into NOD/SCID mice. *PNAS USA* 99:413-418.

Honma T, Honmou O, Lihoshi S, Harada K, Houkin K, Hamada H, Kocsis JD. (2006). Intravenous infusion of immortalized human mesenchymal stem cells protects against injury in a cerebral ischemia model in adult rat. *Experimental Neurology* 199:56-66.

Jamsai,D., Zaibak,F., Khongnium,W., Vadolas,J., Voullaire,L., Fowler,K.J., Gazeas,S., Fucharoen,S., Williamson,R., Ioannou,P.A. (2005). A Humanized mouse model for a common β0-thalassemia mutation. *Genomics* 85:453-461.

Jiang Q, Zhang ZG, Ding GL, Silver B, Zhang L, meng H, Lu M, Pourabdillah-Nejed D, Wang L, et al. (2006). MRI detects white matter reorganization after neural -progenitor cell treatment of stroke. *Neuroimage* 32:1080-1089.

Kalinyak,K.A., Morris,C., Ball,W.S., Ris,M.D., Harris,R., Rucknagel,D. (1995). Bone marrow transplantation in a young child with sickle cell anemia. *Am J Hematol* 48(4):256-261.

Kaul,D.K., Fabry,M.E., Nagel,R.L. (1996). The pathophysiology of vascular obstruction in sickle syndromes. *Blood Rev.* 10:29-44.

Keefer,J.R., Schneidereith.T.A., Mays.A., Purvis,S.H., Dover,G.J., and Smith,K.D. (2006). Role of cyclic nucleotide in fetal hemoglobin induction in cultured CD34+ cells. *Exp Hematol* 34(9):1151-1161.

Keller,G.A., Webb,S., and Kenney,M. (2001) Hematopoietic development of ES cells in culture. In: Clug,C.A. and Jordan,C.T. eds. *Hematopoietic Stem Cell Protocols. Totowa, NJ: Humana* Press.

Kelly S, Bliss TM, Shah AK, Sun GH, Ma M, Foo WC, Masel J, Yenari MA, Weissman IL, Uchida N, Palmer T, Steinberg GK. (2004). Transplamted human fetal neural stem cellssurvive, migrate, and differentiated in ischemic rat cerebral cortex. *PNAS* 101:11839-11844.

Kobayashi T, Ahlenius H, Thored P, Kobayashi R, Kokaia Z, and Lindvall O. (2006). Intracerebral infusion of glial cell line-derived neurotrophic factor promotes striatal neurogenesis after stroke in adult rats. *Stroke* 37:2361-2367.

Kocher,A.A., Schuster,M.D., Szabolcs,M.J., Takuma,S., Burkhoff,D., Wang,J., Homma,S., Edwards,N.M., Itescu,S. (2001). Neovascularization of ischemic myocardium by human bone-marrow-derived angioblasts prevents cardiomyocytes apoptosis, reduces remodeling and improves cardiac function. *Nat Med.* 7:430-436.

Kollet,O., Spiegel,A., Peled,A., Petit,I., Byk,T., Hershkovitz,R, Guetta,O., Barkai,G., Nagler,A., Lapidot,T. (2001). Rapid and efficient homing of human CD34(+)CD38(-

/low)CXCR4(+) stem and progenitor cells to the bone marrow and spleen of NOD/SCID and NOD/SCID/β2 (null) mice. *Blood* 97:3283-3291.

Kontoghiorghes,G.J., Bartlett,A.N., Hoffbrand,A.V., Goddard,J.G., Sheppard,L., Barr,J., Nortey,P. (1990). Long-term trial with the oral iron chelator 1,2 dimethyl-3-hydroxypyid-4-one (L1). *Br J Hematol* 76:295-300.

Kopp,H., Avecilla,S., Hooper,A., Shmelkov,S.V., Ramos,C.A., Zhang,F., Rafii,S. (2005). Tie2 activation contributes to hemangiogenic regeneration after myelosuppression. *Blood* 106:505-513.

Lanzkron,S.M., Collector,M.I., Sharkis,S.J. (1999). Hematopoeitic stem cell tracking in vivo: a comparison of short-term and long-term repopulating cells. *Blood.* 93:1916-1921.

Lanzkron,S.M., Collector,M.I., Sharkis,S.J. (1999). Hematopoeitic stem cell tracking in vivo: a comparison of short-term and long-term repopulating cells. *Blood.* 93:1916-1921.

Lapidot,T., Dar,A., Kollet,O. (2005). How do stem cells find their way home? *Blood* 106:1901-1910.

Larochelle,A., Vormoor,J., Hanenberg,H., Wang,J.C.Y., Bhatia,M., Lapidot,T., Moritz,T., Murdoch,B., Xiao,X.L., Kato,I., Williams,D.A., Dick,J.E. (1996). Identification of primitive human hematopoietic cells capable of repopulating NOD/SCID mouse bone marrow: implications for gene therapy. *Nat Med.* 2:1329-1336.

Lee HJ, Kim KS, Kim EJ, Choi HB, Lee KH, Park IH, Ko Y, jeong SW, Su K. (2007). Brain transplantation of immortalized human neural stem cells promotes functional recovery in mouse intracerebral hemorrhage stroke model. *Stem cells* 25:1204-1212.

Lee HJ, kim KS, Kim EJ, Choi HB, Lee KH, Park IH, Ko Y, Jeong SW, Kim SU. (2007). Brain transplantation of immortalized human neural stem cells promotes functional recovery in mouse intracerebral hemorrhage strole model. *Stem Cells* 25:1204-1212.

Lewis,J., Yang,B., Kim,R., Sierakowska,H., Kole,R., Smithies,O., Maeda,N. (1998). A Common human β-globin splicing mutation modeled in mice. *Blood* 91(6):2152-2156.

Lewishon,D.M., Nagler,A., Ginzton,N., Greenberg,P, Butcher,E.C. (1990). Hematopoietic progenitor cell expression of the H-CAM (CD44) homing associated adhesion molecule. *Blood.* 75:589-595.

Ley,T.J., DeSimone,J., Anagnou,N.P. *et al.* (1982). 5-Azacytidine selectively increases gamma-globin synthesis in a patient with beta+ thalassemia. *N Engl J Med.* 307:1469-1475.

Lin,Y., Weisdorf,D.J., Solovey,A., Hebbel,R.P. (2000). Origins of circulating endothelial cells and endothelia outgrowth from blood. *J Clin Invest.* 105:71-77.

Link,G., Pinson,A. and Hershko,C. (1985). Heart cells in culture: a model of myocardial overload and chelation. *J. Lab. Clin. Med.* 106:147-153.

Liu H, Honmou O, Harada , Nakamura K, Houkin K, Hamada H, and Kocsis JD. (2006). Neuroprotection by PIGF gene modified human mesenchymal stem cells after cerebral ischaemia. *Brain* 129:2734-2745.

Locatelli,F., Vanderson,R., Reed,W., Bernaudin,F., Ertem,M., Grafakos,S., Brichard,B., Li,X., Nagler,A., Giorgiani,G., Haut,P.R., Brochestein,J.A., Nugent,D.J., Blatt,J., Woodard,P., Kurtzberg,J., Rubin,C.M., Miniero,R., Rutz,P., Raja,T., Roberts,I., Will,A.M., Yaniv,I., Vermylen,C., Tannoia,N., Garnier,F., Ionescu,I., Walters,M.C., Lubin,B.H., Gluckman,E. (2003). Related umbilical cord blood transplantation in patients with thalassemia and sickle cell disease. *Blood* 101(6):2137-2143.

Long,M.W. (1992). Blood cell cytoadhesion molecules. *Exp Hematol.* 20:288-301.

Long,M.W., Briddell,R., Walter,A.W., Bruno,E., Hoffman,R. (1992). *Journal of Clinical Investigations*. 90:251-255.

Lord,B.I. (1992). The architecture of bone marrow cell populations. In: Murphy,M., Jr (ed.). *Concise Reviews in Clinical and Experimental Hematology*, p. 225, AlphaMed Press, Dayton, OH.

Lukens,J. (2004). Abnormal hemoglobins, general principles. In: Greer,J.P. *et al.*, (eds.) *Wintrobe's Clinical Hematology*, pp1247-1262, Lippincott Williams and Wilkins, Philadelphia, USA.

Lutty,G.A., McLeod,D.S., Pachnis,A., Costantini,F., Fabry,M.E., and Nagel,R.L. (1994). Retinal and choroidal neovascularization in a transgenic mouse model of sickle cell disease. *American Journal of Pathology*. 145:490-497.

Machado,R.F. (2007). Nitric oxide-based therapies in sickle cell disease: the evidence continues to mount. *Crit Care Med* 35(2):654-655.

Matsuzaki,Y., Kinjo,K., Mulligan,R.C., Okano,H. (2004). Unexpectedly efficient homing capacity of purified murine hematopoietic stem cells. *Immunity* 20:87-93.

Mazo,I., von Andrian,U. (1999). Adhesion and homing of blood borne cells in bone marrow microvessels. *J Leukoc Biol* 66:25-32.

Mazurier,F., Doedens,M., Gan,O.I., and Dick,J.E. (2003). Rapid myeloerythroid repopulation after intrafemoral transplantation of NOD-SCID mice reveals a new class of human stem cells. *Nat Med*. 9(7): 959-963.

Modo M, Rezaie P, Heuschling P, Patel S, Male DK, Hodges H. (2002). Transplantation of neural stem cells in a rat model of stroe:assessment of short term graft survival and acute host immunological response. *Brain Research* 958:70-82.

Montero-Huerta,P., Hess,D.R., Head,C.A. (2006). Inhaled nitric oxide for treatment of sickle cell stroke. *Anesthesiology* 105(3):619-621.

Montplaisir,N., Merault,G., Poyart,C., Rhoda,M.D., Craescu,C., Vidaud,M., Galacteros,F., Blouquit,Y., & Rosa,J. (1986). Hemoglobin S Antilles: a variant with lower solubility than hemoglobin S and producing sickle cell disease in heterozygotes. *Proc. Natl. Acad. Sci. USA*. 83:9363-9367.

Morel,F., Galy,A., Chen.B., Szilvassy,S.J. (1998). Equal distribution of competitive long-term repopulating stem cells in the CD34+ and CD34- fractions of Thy-1^{low}Lin$^{-/low}$Sca-1^{+} bone marrow cells. *Exp Hematol* 26:440-448.

Muzyamba,M.C., Campbell,E.H., Gibson,J.S. (2006). Effect of intracellular magnesium and oxygen tension on K+-Cl- cotransport in normal and sickle human red cells. *Cell Physiol Biochem* 17(3-4):121-128.

Nagel,R.L., Fabry,M.E. (2001). The panoply of animal models for sickle cell disease. *Br J Hematol* 112(1):19-25.

Nilsson,S.K., Dooner,M.S., Tiarks,C.Y., Weier,H.-U., and Quesenberry, P.J. (1997). Potential and distribution of transplanted hematopoietic stem cells in a nonablated mouse model. *Blood* 89(11):4013-4020.

Nilsson,S.K., Johnston,H.M., Coverdale,J.A. (2001). Spatial localization of transplanted hemopoietic stem cells: inferences for the localization of stem cell niches. *Blood* 97(8):2293-2299.

Nystedt J, makinen S, Lain J, Jolkkonen J. (2006). Human cord blood CD34+ cells and behavioral recovery following focal cerebral ischemia in rats. *Acta neurobiol Exp* (Wars) 66:293-300.

obinson S, Von Os R, Sheridon T, Mauch P. (2000). Reduction of marrow hematopoietic progenitor and stem cell content is not sufficient for enhanced syngeneic engraftment. *Stem Cells* 18:93-101.

Okuno,Y., Huettner,C.S., Radomska,H.S., Petkova,V., Iwasaki,H., Akashi,K., Tene,D.G. (2002). Distal elements are critical for human CD34 expression in vivo. *Blood* 100:4420-4426.

Oliveri,N.F. and Brittenham,G.M. (1997). Iron chelating therapy and the treatment of thalassemia. *Blood* 89:739-761.

Oliveri,N.F. and Brittenham,G.M. (1997). Iron chelating therapy and the treatment of thalassemia. *Blood* 89:739-761.

Osawa,M., Hanada,K., Hamada,H., Nakauchi,H. (1996). Long-term lympho-hematopoietic reconstitution by a single CD34- low/negative hematopoietic stem cells. *Science* 273:242-245.

Osawa, M., Hanada,K., Hamada,H., Nakauchi,H. (1996). Long-term lympho-hematopoietic reconstitution by a single CD34- low/negative hematopoietic stem cells. *Science* 273:242-245.

Paszty, C., Brion, C.M., Manci,E., Witkowska,H.E., Stevens,M.E., Mohandas,N., and Rubin,E.M. (1997). Transgenic knock-out mice with exclusively human sickle hemoglobin and sickle cell disease. *Science*. 278:876.

Peled,A., Kollet,O., Ponomaryov,T., Petit,I., Franitza,S., Grabovsky,V., Slav,M.M., Nagler,A., Lider,O., Alon,R., Zipori,D., Lapidot,T. (2000). The chemokine SDF-1 activates the integrins LFA-1, VLA-4, and VLA-5 on immature human CD34+ cells: role in transendothelial/stromal migration and engraftment in NOD/SCID mice. *Blood* 95:3289-3296.

Phinney,D.G., Kopen,G., Isaacson,R.L., Prokop,D.J. (1999). Plastic adherent stromal cells from the bone marrow of commonly used strains of inbred mice: variations in yield, growth and differentiation. *J Cell Biochem*. 72:570-585.

Piomelli,S. (1995). The management of patients with Cooley`s anemia: transfusions and splenectomy. *Sem Hematol* 32:262-268.

Pittenger,M.F., Mackay,A.M., Beck,S.C, Jaiswal,R.K., Douglas,R., Mosca,J.D., Moorman,M.A., Simonetti,D.W., Craig,S., Marshak,D.R. (1999). Multilineage potential of adult human mesenchymal stem cells. *Science*. 284:143-147.

Prockop,D.J. (1997). Marrow stromal cells as stem cells for nonhematopoietic tissues. *Science*. 276:71-74.

Quesenberry PJ, Stewart M, Becker P, D'Handt L, Freimberger A, Lambert JF, Miller C, Heyes C, et al. 2001. Stem cell engraftment strategies. *Ann N Y Acad. Sci.* 938:54-61.

Quesenberry,P., Colvin,G., and Abedi,M. (2005). Perspective: fundamental and clinical concepts on stem cell homing and engraftment: a journey to niches and beyond. *Experimental Hematology* 33:9-19.

Quesenberry,P.J. and Becker,P. (1998). Stem cell homing: Rolling, crawling and nesting. *Proc. Natl. Acad. Sci. USA* 95:15155-15157.

Robertson,S.M., Kennedy,M., Shannon,J.M., Keller,G. (2000). A transitional stage in the commitment of mesoderm to hematopoiesis requiring the transcription factor SCL/tal-1. *Development* 127:2447-2459.

Rubin,E.M., Witkowska,H.E., Spangler,E., Curtin,P., Lubin,B.H., Mohandas,N., and Clift,S.M. (1991). Hypoxia-induced in vivo sickling of transgenic mouse red cells. *Journal of Clinical Investigations*. 87:639-647.

Rust,M.B., Alper,S.L., Rudhard,Y., Shmukler,B.E., Vicente,R., Brugnara,C., Trudel,M., Jentsch,T.J., Hubner,C.A. (2007). Disruption of erythroid K-Cl cotransporters alters erythrocyte volume and partially rescues erythrocyte dehydration in SAD mice. *J Clin Invest* 117(6):1708-1717.

Ryan,T.M., Ciavatta,D.J., and Townes,T.M. (1997). Knock-out transgenic mouse model of sickle cell disease. *Science*. 278:873-878.

Ryan,T.M., Townes,T.M., Reilly,M.P., Asakura,T., Palmiter,R.P., and Behringer,R.R. (1990). Human sickle hemoglobin in transgenic mice. *Science*. 247:566-568.

Sabin,F. (1920). Studies on the origin of blood vessels and of red blood corpuscules as seen in the living blastoderm of chicks during the second day of incubation. *Contrib Embryol Carnegie Inst Washington* 9:214-262.

Saleh,A.W., Hillen,H.F. (1997). Pharmacological induction of fetal hemoglobin synthesis in sickle cell disease. *Neth J Med* 51(5):169-178.

Sato,T., Laver,J.H., Ogawa,M. (1998). Reversible expression of CD34 by murine hematopoietic stem cells. *Blood* 94:2548-2554.

Schofield,R. (1978). The relationship between the CFU-S and the hemopoietic stem cell. *Blood Cells* 4:7-25.

Schrier,S.L., Rachmilewitz,E., Mohandas,N. (1989). Cellular and membrane properties of alpha and beta thalassemic erythrocytes are different: implication for differences in clinical manifestations. *Blood* 74:2194-2202.

Shear,H.L., Roth,E.F., Jr, Fabry, M.E., Costantini, F., Pachnis, A., Hood, A., and Nagel, R.L. (1993). Transgenic mice expressing human sickle hemoglobin are partially resistant to rodent malaria. *Blood*. 81:222-226.

Shehee, W.R., Oliver, P., and Smithies, P. (1993). Lethal thalassemia after insertional disruption of the mouse major adult β-globin gene. *Proc. Natl. Acad. Sci. USA*. 90:3177-3181.

Shi, Q., Rafii, S., Wu, M.H., Wijelath, E.S., Yu, C., Ishida, A., Fujita, Y., Kothari, S., Mohle, R., Sauvage, L.R., Moore, M.A., Storb, R.F., Hammond, W.P. (1998). Evidence for circulating bone marrow-derived endothelial cells. *Blood*. 92:362-367.

Shinar, E., Rachmilewitz,E.A., Lux,S.E. (1989). Differing erythrocyte membrane skeletal protein defects in alpha and beta-thalassemia. *Journal of Clinical Investigations* 83:404.

Skalr,C.A., Lew, L.Q., Yoon,D.J., David,R. (1987). Adrenal function in thalassemia major following long-term treatment with multiple transfusion and chelation therapy: evidence for dissociation of cortisol and adrenal androgen secretion. *Am J Dis Child* 141:327-330.

Skow, L.C, Burkhart, B.A., Johnson, F.M., Popp, R.A., Goldberg, S.Z., Anderson, W.F., Barnett, L.B., and Lewis, S.E. (1983). A Mouse model for β-thalassemia. *Cell*. 34:1043-1052.

Skow, L.C, Burkhart, B.A., Johnson, F.M., Popp, R.A., Goldberg, S.Z., Anderson, W.F., Barnett, L.B., and Lewis, S.E. (1983). A Mouse model for β-thalassemia. *Cell*. 34:1043-1052.

Smith, L.G., Weissman, I.L., Heimfeld, S. (1991). Clonal analysis of hematopoietic stem cell differentiation in vivo. *Proc. Natl. Acad. Sci. USA* 88:2788-2792.

Sonakul, D., Thakerngpol, K. and Pacharee, P. (1988). Cardiac pathology in 76 thalassemic patients. *Birth Defects Orig. Artic. Ser.* 23:177-191.

Sorrentino, B. (2004). Clinical strategies for expansion of hematopoietic stem cells. *Nat Immunol* 4:878-888.

Spangrude, G.J., Brooks, D.M., Tumas, D.B. (1995). Long term repopulation of irradiated mice with limiting numbers of purified hematopoietic stem cells: In vivo expansion of stem cell phenotype but not function. *Blood* 85:1006-1016.

Spangrude, G.J., Heimfeld, S., Weissman, I.L. (1998). Purification and characterization of mouse hematopoietic stem cells. *Science* 241:58-62.

Steinberg,M.H. (1999). Management of sickle cell disease. *N Engl J Med* 340:1021.

Steinberg, M.H. (1999). Management of sickle cell disease. *N Engl J Med* 340:1021.

Steinberg, M.H. (2003). Therapies to increase fetal hemoglobin in sickle cell disease. *Curr Hematol Rep* 2(2):95-101.

Stocker, J.W., Franceschi,L.D., McNaughton-Smith,G.A., Corrocher,R., Beuzard,Y., Brugnara,C. (2003). ICA-17043, a novel Gardos channel blocker, prevents sickled red blood cell dehydration in vitro and in vivo in SAD mice. *Blood* 101(6):2412-2418.

Szilvassy, S., Bass, M.J., Van Zant, G., and Grimes, B. 1999. Organ selective homing defines engraftment kinetics of murine hematopoietic stem cells and is compromised by ex-vivo expansion. *Blood.* 93(5):1557-1566.

Tagushi A, Soma T, Tanaka H, Konda T, Nishimura H, Yoshikawa H, Tsukamoto Y, Iso H et al. 2004. Administration of CD34+ cells after stroke enhances neurogenesis via angiogenesis in a mouse model. *JCI* 114:330-338.

Thein, S.L., Sampietro,M., Rohde,K., Rochette,J., Weatherall,D.J., Lathrop,G.M., Demenais,F. (1994). Detection of a major gene for heterocellular hereditary persistence of fetal hemoglobin after accounting for genetic modifiers. *Am J Hum Genet* 54:514.

Trudel, M., De Paepe,M.E., Chretien,N., Saadane,N., Jacmain,J., Sorette,M., Hoang,T., and Beuzard,Y. (1994). Sickle cell disease of transgenic SAD mice. *Blood.* 84:3189-3197.

Trudel, M., Saadane,N., Garel,M.C., Bardakdjuan-Michau,J., Blouquit,Y., Guerquin-Kern,J.L., Rouyer-Fessard,P., Vidaud,D., Pachniss,A., Romeo,P.H., Beuzard,Y., and Costantini,F.M. (1991). Towards a transgenic mouse model of sickle cell disease: SAD mice. *EMBO journal.*10:3157-3168.

Uchida, N., Fujisaki,T., Eaves,A.C., Eaves,C.J. (2001). Tranplantable hematopoietic stem cells in human fetal liver have a CD34+ side population (SP) phenotype. *J Clin Invest* 108:1071-1077.

Uchisda, N., Jerabek, L., and Weissman, I.L. (1996). Searching for hematopiietic stem cells. II. The heterogeneity of Thy-1.1(lo)Lin(-/lo)Sca1+ mouse hematopoietic stem cells separated by counterflow centrifugal elutriation. *Exp Hematol* 24:649-659.

Ukai R, Honmou O, Harada K, Houkin K, Hamada H, Kocsis JD. 2007. Mesenchymal stem cells derived from peripheral blood protects against ischemia. *J of Neurotrauma* 24:508-520.

Urbinati,F., Madigan,C., and Malik,P. (2006). Pathophysiology and therapy for haemoglobinopathies: Part II: thallassaemias. *Expert Rev Mol Med* 8(10), 9.

Van der Loo, J.C., Ploemacher, R.E. 1995. Marrow and spleen seeding efficiencies of all murine hematopoietic stem cell subsets are decreased by preincubation with hematopoietic growth factors. *Blood.* 85:2598-2606.

Van Hennik, P.B, de Koning, A.E., Ploemacher, R.E. 1999. Seeding efficiency of primitive human hematopoietic cells in nonobese diabetic/severe combined immune deficiency mice: implications for stem cell frequency assessment. *Blood.* 94:3055-3061.

Vellodi,A., Picton,S., Downie,C.J.C., Eltumi,M., Stevens,R., Evans,D.I.K. (1994). Bone marrow transplantation for thalassemia: experience of two british centers. Bone *Marrow Transplantation* 13:559-562.

Verfaillie, C.M., Almeida-Porada,G., Wissink,S., Zanjani,E.D. (2000). Kinetics of engraftment of CD34- and CD34+ cells from mobilized blood differs from that of CD34- and CD34+ cells from bone marrow. *Experimental Hematology* 28:1071-1079.

Vermylen, C. and Cornu, G. (1994). Bone marrow transplantation for sickle cell disease. The European experience. *Am J Pediatr Hematol Oncol* 16(1):18-21.

Verstegen, M.M.A., van Hennik, P.B., Terpestra,W., van den Bos,C., Wielenga, J.J., van Rooijen,N., Ploemacher,R.E., Wagemaker,G., Wognum, A.W. (1998). Transplantation of human umbilical cord blood cellsin macrophage-depleted SCID mice: evidence for accessory cell involvement in expansion of immature CD34+CD38- cells. *Blood* 91:1966-1976.

Vichinsky, E., Onyekwere, O., Porter,J., Swerdlow,P., eckman,J., Lane,P., Files,B., Hassell,K., Kelley,P., Wilson,F., Bernaudin,F., Forni,G.L., Okpala,I., Ressayre-Djaffer,C., Alberti,D., Holland,J., Marks,P., Fung,E., Fisher,R., Mueller,B.U., Coates,T. (2007). A randomized comparison of deferasirox versus deferoxamine for the treatment of transfusional iron overload in sickle cell disease. *Br J Hematol.* 136:501-508.

Wagers,A.J., Sherwood,R.I., Christensen,J.L. (2002). Little evidence for developmental plasticity of adult hematopoietic stem cells. *Science* 297:2256-2259.

Walters,M.C., Sullivan,K.M., O`Reilly,R.J., Boulad,F., Brockstein,J., Blume,K., Amylon,M., Johnson,F.L., Klemperer,M., Graham-Pole,J. (1994). Bone marrow transplantation for thalassemia. The USA experience. *Am J Pediatr Hematol Oncol* 16:11-17.

Wang,W. (2004). Sickle cell anemia and other sickling syndromes. In: Greer,J.P. *et al*, eds. *Wintrobe's Clinical Hematology* (11th ed), pp1263-1296, Lippincott Williams and Wilkins, Philadelphia, USA.

Wang,W.C., Kovnar,E.H., Tonkin,I.L., Mulhem,R.K., Langston,J.W., Day,S.W., Schell,M.J., Willimas,J.A. (1991). High risks of recurrent strokes after discontinuance of five to twelve years of transfusion therapy in patients with sickle cell disease. *J Pediatr* 118:377.

Wei JJ, Zeng LF, Fan XT, Wang Y, Ma WB, Li GL, Dou WC, Zhang ZX, et al. 2007. *treatment of stroke in rats with bone marrow mesenchymal stem cells*. Zhonghua Yi Xue Za Zhi 87:184-189.

Willing AE, Vendrame M, Mallery J, Cassady CJ, Davis CD, Sanchez-Ramos J, Sanberg PR. (2003). Mobilized peripheral blood cells administered intravenously produce functional recovery in stroke. *Cell transplant* 12:449-454.

Wonke,B., Wright,C., Hoffbrand,A.V. (1998). Combined therapy with deferipone and desferrioxamine. *Br J Hematol* 103:361-364.

Wyrick-Glatzel,J. and Hugues,V.C. (2002). Routine Laboratory Methods, In: Harmening,D.M. *Clinical Hematology and Fundamentals of Hemostasis*, 4th Ed. F.A. Davis Company, Philadelphia PA, pp563-593.

Yanagisawa D, Qi M, Kim DH, kitamura Y, Inden M, Tsuchiya D, Takata K et al. (2006). Improvement of focal ischemia-induced rat dopaminergic dysfunction by striatal transplantation of mouse embryonic stem cells. *Neurosci Lett* 407:74-79.

Yang,B., Kirby,S., Lewis,J., Detloff,P.J., Madea,N., and Smithies,O. (1995). A Mouse model for β^0-thalasemia. *Proc. Natl. Acad. Sci. USA*. 92:11608-11612.

Yokoi T, Kobayashi H, Shimata Y, Eto Y, Ishige N, Kitagawa T, Otsu M, Nakauchi H, Ida H, Odashi T. (2011). Minimum requirement of donor cells to reduce the glycolipid storage following bone marrow transplantation in a murine model of Fabry Disease. *J Gen Med* 13:262-268.

Yong, K.L., Watts, M., Thomas, N.S., Sullivan, A., Ings, S., Linch,D.C. (1998). *Blood.* 91: 1196-1205.

Zanjani, E.D., Almaida-Porada,G., Ascensao,J.L., MacKintosh,F.R., Flake,A.W.(1997). Transplantation of hematopiietic stem cells in utero. *Stem Cells* 15:79-92.

Zanjani, E.D., Almeida-Porada,G., Livingston,A.G., Zeng,H., Ogawa,M. (2003). Reversible expression of CD34 by adult human marrow long-term engrafting hematopoietic stem cells. *Experimental Hematology* 31:406-412.

Zeng, Y.-T., Huang,S.-Z., Ren,Z.-R., Lu,Z.-H., Zeng,F.-Y., Schechter, A.N., Rodgers,G.P. (1995). Hydroxyurea therapy in bet-thalassemia intermedia: improvement in hematological parameters due to enhanced beta-globin synthesis. *Br J Hematol* 90:557-563.

Zhang, J., Niu,C., Ye, L., Huang,H., He,X., Tong,W.G., Ross,J., Haug,J., Johnson, T., Feng, J.Q., Harris,S., Wiedemann,L.M., Mishina,Y., Li,Y. (2003). Identification of the hematopoietic stem cell niche and control of the niche size. *Nature* 425:836-841.

Zhao, Y., Lin, Y., Zhan, Y., Yang,G., Louie,J., Harrison,D.E., Anderson, W.F. (2000). Murine hematopoietic stem cell characterization and its regulation in bone marrow transplantation. *Blood*.96:3016-3022.

Zin'kova NN, Gilerovich EG, Sokolova IB, Shvedova EV, Bilibina AA, Krugliakov PV, Polyntsev DG. 2007. Mesenchymal stem cells transplantation influences upon dynamics of morphological changes in rat brain after stroke. *Tsitologila* 49:923-932.

In: Hematopoietic Stem Cells: New Research ISBN 978-1-62257-468-1
Editors: Wesley G. Montgomery and Heather I. Burton

Chapter 3

PSYCHOLOGICAL HEALTH AND ADJUSTMENT OF FAMILIES OF CHILDREN WHO UNDERGO HEMATOPOIETIC STEM CELL TRANSPLANTATION

Marta Tremolada,[1*] Sabrina Bonichini[2] and Marta Pillon[1]
[1]Department of Paediatrics, Oncology Hemathology Division,
University Hospital of Padova, Italy
[2]Department of Developmental and Social Psychology,
University of Padova, Italy

ABSTRACT

Background: Having a child undergoing Hematopoietic Stem Cell Transplantation (HSCT) is a stressful and upsetting experience for parents.

Especially mothers have a key role in children's everyday adaptation to the transplantation experience and for this reason their psychological health has received comparatively large attention in the literature in different phases of medical treatment (pre-HSCT, during the isolation, post HSCT). The presence of a child undergoing HSCT in the family may place also siblings at risk for psychological difficulties.

Aims: This chapter reviews the research published in the last 20 years on the psycho-social health and adaptation of parents and siblings of children who have undergone HSCT.

Method: Articles were found using four electronic databases (PubMed, PsycINFO, Web of Science and SCOPUS) employing various search strategies: the search terms used included MeSH, headings, text words, or keywords relevant to the following terms: ''QoL,'' ''adaptation,'' ''psychology,'' ''HSCT'', "parents" and "siblings". The search was limited to English-language literature published in the last 20 years and to those articles including families of patients who received any type of HSCT as children.

Results: A corpus of 38 empirical studies was selected and will be presented here. From this selection three main topics emerged: psychological health and adaptation of

* Corresponding author: Marta Tremolada, PhD, Haematology-Oncology Division, Department of Paediatrics, University Hospital of Padova, Italy, Via Giustiniani 3 – 35128 Padova, Italy, Tel.+39 3474868835, Fax +39 0498213510, E-mail: marta.tremolada@unipd.it.

parents of children undergoing HSCT (N=24); psychosocial adjustment of siblings of HSCT patients (N=8); psychosocial interventions for families of children undergoing HSCT (N=8, 2 of which also included in the second topic).

The information emerged from the review of the literature will be discussed with special attention to methodological issues and directions for future research will be proposed.

INTRODUCTION

Hematopoietic Stem Cell Transplantation (HSCT) has become an accepted form of therapy for many childhood diseases. Pharmacological and technical improvements in HSCT procedure have lead to a growing number of its applications every year and to an important increase in survival rates (Clarke, Eiser and Skinner, 2008). While the therapeutic success of paediatric HSCT is improving, in the last two decades several studies have outlined the significant risk of aversive consequences on physical health, but also on quality of life, psychological adjustment, cognitive aspects and social functioning (Bonichini et al., 2011).

Parental distress associated with HSCT is often involved not only with the health of the patient, but with the sibling donor/no donor as well: the siblings of HSCT patients are often the best stem cell donor candidates or match for the patient (MacLeod et al., 2003) and they can suffer from both psychosocial and behavioral problems, such as post-traumatic stress reactions, anxiety, low self-esteem, feelings of guilt and school problems (Packman, 1999). Most studies have focused on the mother's psychological well-being (Rodrigue et al., 1997), although the entire family's psychological distress during HSCT needs to be considered. Family cohesion, communication and adaptation to conflicts when encountering stressful situations are part of healthy functioning within the family as the child adjusts to their medical illness (Jobe-Shields et al., 2009)

In this chapter, the psychosocial effects on parents and siblings were reviewed. To this aim, we conducted a literature search using four electronic databases (PubMed, PsycINFO, Web of Science and SCOPUS) employing various search strategies: the search terms used included MeSH, headings, text words, or keywords relevant to the following terms: ''QoL,'' ''adaptation,'' ''psychology,'' ''HSCT'', "parents" and "siblings". The search was limited to English-language literature published in the last 20 years (1991–2011) and to those articles including families of patients who received any type of HSCT as children. We considered the full text of the selected papers to examine all the specific characteristics of each study. One of the eligibility criteria was that the papers dealt with siblings and parents and we excluded the reviews.

The results of this search yielded a total of 38 relevant journal articles. The investigators distilled the most crucial psychological issues related to families of pediatric HSCT and combined that with their knowledge to provide an overview for clinicians and recommendations for future advancements in treating the families of children undergoing HSCT. Studies on these topics have been increasing considerably in recent times, but there is still a gap in the literature in terms of discussion and organization of this information that would allow a clearer idea of the methodologies adopted and formulation of general conclusions from the existing data.

From this selection three main topics linked to family adjustment to pediatric HSCT emerged: psychological health and adaptation of parents of children undergoing HSCT (N=24; Theme 1); psychosocial adjustment of siblings of HSCT patients (N=8; Theme 2); psychosocial interventions for families of children undergoing HSCT (N=8, Theme 3).

Theme 1: Psychological Health and Adaptation of Parents of Children Undergoing BMT

Having a child undergoing HSCT is a universally stressful and upsetting experience for parents and analysing the literature it emerges that in particular maternal psychological health has received comparatively large attention in the literature in different phases of the medical treatment (pre-HSCT, during the isolation, post HSCT), because mothers have a key role in children's everyday adaptation to the transplantation experience.

In general, the studies report various types of stress problems (Rodrigue et al., 1996; Rodrigue et al., 1997; Kronenberger et al., 1998; Streisand et al., 2000) and psychological symptoms in parents, especially mothers, such as anxiety and depression (Barrera et al., 2000; Manne et al., 2001; Manne et al., 2002; Jalmsell et al., 2011; Manne et al., 2004), PTSD and cognitive problems (Duhamel et al., 2004) at various time-points related to HSCT (Phipps et al., 2004).

Other studies show the influences of mothers' symptomathology and life family styles on child's health related quality of life (Barrera, 2009; Vrijmoet-Wiersma et al., 2009; Jobe-Shields et al., 2009). Another group of studies reports the possible coping strategies and family life styles identified as possible factors that dampen stress level and psychological symptoms (Manne et al., 2002; Manne et al., 2003; Rini et al., 2004; Rini et al., 2007; Duhamel et al., 2007). The last group of articles is represented by qualitative studies narrating the parents' experiences of having a child undergoing HSCT by their direct voices (Forinder, 2004; Oppenheim et al., 2002; Wu et al., 2005; Asadi et al., 2011).

At the phase of transplantation, mothers report significant levels of stress in caregiving (Rodrigue et al., 1996; Streisand et al., 2000), in social life (Kronenberger et al., 1998), about family finances (Rodrigue et al., 1997), report high levels of anxiety and depressive symptoms (Barrera et al., 2000; Manne et al., 2002), PTSD and some problems in cognitive processing (Duhamel et al., 2004; Duhamel et al., 2007). Bereaved parents of children undergoing HSCT may be at greater risk of decreased psychological well-being (depression, anxiety, psychological wellbeing, quality of life, physical health) than other bereaved parents of children with cancer (Jalmsell et al., 2011).

For example, Rodrigue et al (1996) evaluated stress, coping resources and family functioning of 36 mothers of children awaiting transplantation, finding that 20% of mothers reported clinically significant stress responses and that parenting stress was higher for mothers of children with solid organ transplantation than in mothers of children with bone marrow transplantation (BMT).

Table 1. Theme 1: Psychological health of parents of children undergoing BMT

authors	sample	type of transplant	type of diagnosis	age range at transplant	Study design	assessment time points	functional area assessed	type of assessment
Sormanti et al. (1994)	N = 73 parents	BMT (allogeneic, autologous)	Malignant haematological disease	BMT time: 1-20 years prior to the study	retrospective study	1-20 years after BMT	psychosocial issues	Profile of Mood States, Cancer Patient Behavior scale
Phipps and Mulhern (1995)	parents	BMT (allogeneic, autologous)	Malignant haematological disease		prospective study	T1: pre-BMT T2/3: 6/12 months after BMT	social competence, self-concept, family cohesion and expressiveness	Questionnaires
Rodrigue et al. (1996)	N = 36 mothers	BMT, liver, kidney or heart transplantation	see type of transplant	Mothers' mean age = 33,6 years (SD=8,1); Children's mean age = 8 years (SD=5,5)	1 time point study	T = awaiting transplantation (12 month period)	stress, coping resources, family functioning	Parenting Stress Index, Coping Health Inventory for Parents, Family Environment Scale, Impact on Family Scale
Rodrigue et al. (1997)	N = 27 mothers	BMT, liver, kidney or heart or transplantation	see type of transplant	Mothers' mean age = 34.6 years (SD = 7.3). Children's mean age = 8.4 years (SD=4.5)	prospective study	T1: pretransplantation (mean of 4.9 weeks pre-transplantation; SD= 6.5) T2: 1 month posttransplantation T3: 6 months posttransplantation	parenting stress, coping resources, and perceptions of family functioning	Parenting Stress Index, Coping Health Inventory for Parents, Family Environment Scale, Impact on Family Scale, Family Inventory of Resources and Management
Kronenberger et al. (1998)	N = 24 mothers	BMT (allogeneic, autologous)	Malignant haematological disease	Mothers' mean age = 36,2 years (SD= 6,6) Children's mean age = 10,3 years (SD = 5,2)	1 time point study	T = 0-4 months pre-BMT	stress, coping and family factors	Demographic and medical measures, Hassles Scale, Life Experiences Survey, Chronic Illness Parental Stress Questionnaire, Coping Strategies Inventory, Family Environment Scale, Symptom Checklist-90-R
Streisand et al. (2000)	N = 22 mothers; N = 11 control mothers	SCT	Non Malignant/Malignant haematological disease	Mothers' mean age = 37,2 (SD = 5,2) Children's ages: 2-6	prospective study (with control group)	T1: BMT preadmission T2: 3 weeks post-BMT	level of stress	Daily Stress Inventory, Parenting Stress Index, Semi-structured Interview, Adherence

authors	sample	type of transplant	type of diagnosis	age range at transplant	Study design	assessment time points	functional area assessed	type of assessment
Manne et al. (2001)	N = 115 mothers	SCT	Non Malignant/Malignant haematological disease	Mothers' mean age = 37,8 years (SD = 7,34) Children's mean age: 9,2 years (SD = 5,56)	retrospective study	Mean time since diagnosis: 1,8 years (SD 25,3 months)	psychological health: maternal distress and coping	Beck Depression Inventory, Beck Anxiety Inventory
Manne et al. (2002)	N = 90 mothers	SCT	Non Malignant/Malignant haematological disease	Mothers' mean age: 37,6 years (SD = 7,35) Children's mean age = 8,75 years (SD = 5,51)	prospective study	T1: BMT infusion T2: 3 months post-BMT T3: 6 months post-BMT	emotional distress, BMT-related fears, family's and friends negative responses	paper-and-pencil structured interview methods (SCID-BP-PTSD, PCL-C), BDI, BAI, Fear Network, Cancer Support Inventory
Oppenheim et al. (2002)	N = 40 parents	SCT autologous/ High dose Chemotherapy	Malignant haematological disease	-	1 time point study	over 9 months	key words to ensure that similar themes were discussed	open-ended psychiatrist-psychoanalyst's interviews
Manne et al. (2003)	N = 207 mothers	BMT	Malignant haematological disease	T1 mothers' mean age = 37,1 years (SD = 6,9); T1 children's mean age = 8,3 years (SD = 5,5)	prospective study	T1 : BMT time T2 : 3 months post-BMT T3 : 6 months post-BMT	maternal coping strategies in depressive symptoms	COPE scale, BDI, Appraisal of Fear/Worry, Medical Risk
Manne et al. (2004)	N = 111 mothers	HSCT	Malignant haematological disease	Mothers' mean age = 34.6 (SD = 7.4) Children's mean age = 8.2 (SD = 5.4)	prospective study	T1 : 2 days before HSCT T2 : 18 months post-HSCT	anxiety, depression and PTSD symptoms, social support, quality of life, previous traumatic events	Beck Anxiety Inventory, Beck Depression Inventory, Impact of Event Scale, Traumatic Stress Schedule, Ways of coping, COPE scale, SCID-NP
DuHamel et al. (2004)	N = 91 mothers	SCT	Malignant haematological disease	T1 mothers' mean age = 37,85 years (SD = 7,30)	prospective study	T1: 3 days before BMT/SCT T2: 3 months post-BMT/SCT	cognitive processing in maternal adjustment	Fear Network, Impact of Events scale, BAI, BDI
Forinder et al. (2004)	N = 20 parents	BMT	Malignant haematological disease		retrospective study	T1 : 4-8 years post-BMT T2 : 4 years post T1	in-depth knowledge of the parents' situation during a critical time	self-report questionnaire for coping, two series of qualitative interviews
Phipps et al. (2004)	N = 151 parents	SCT	Malignant haematological disease		prospective study	T1 : week -1 ; T2 : weekly +6 T3: monthly +6	patterns of distress cf parents and children	parent and child reports

Table 1. (Continued)

authors	sample	type of transplant	type of diagnosis	age range at transplant	age range at transplant	assessment time points	functional area assessed	type of assessment
Rini et al. (2004)	N = 100 mothers	BMT	Malignant haematological disease	T1 mothers' mean age = 37 years (SD = 6,82) T1 children's mean age: 8 (SD = 5,49)	prospective study	T1 : during BMT hospitalization T2 : 1 year post-T1	life stress and basic beliefs about self-worth	Janoff-Bulman's World Assumption Scale, Traumatic Stress Schedule, Life Experiences Survey, SF-36 Health Survey, Mental Health Inventory, Medical and demographic information
Phipps et al. (2005)	N = 151 parents	SCT	Malignant haematological disease (most leukemia)	T1 children's age = 8,9 years	prospective study	T1 : prior BMT admission T2 : weekly +6 post-BMT T3 : monthly +6 post-BMT	psychosocial predictors of distress	Profile of Mood States, Perceived Stress Scale, Caregiving Burden Scale, Prior Illness Experience Scale, Family Environment Scale, Inventory for Socially Supportive Behaviors, Ways of Coping Questionnaire
Wu et al. (2005)	N = 11 parents and grandparents	HSCT	Malignant haematological disease	Children's mean age = 10.5 years; Fathers' mean age = 41.8 years; Mothers' mean age = 37.2 years	1 time point study	within 2 weeks after the children received transplants	life experiences and feelings of parents	semi-structured interviews
DuHamel et al. (2007)	N = 140 mothers	HSCT	Non Malignant/Malignant haematological disease	Mothers' mean age = 37 years (SD = 6.99) and most Caucasian (77.1%). Children's mean age = 8 years (SD = 5.57)	prospective study	T1: during their child's hospitalization for HSCT T2: 3-months post-HSCT; T3: 6-months post HSCT	maternal optimism, recent negative life events, lifetime history of traumatic events	Fear Appraisals scale, Life Orientation Test, Life Experiences Survey, Traumatic Stress Schedule

authors	sample	type of transplant	type of diagnosis	age range at transplant	age range at transplant	assessment time points	functional area assessed	type of assessment
Rini et al. (2008)	N = 163 mothers	HSCT	-	Primary caretaker of a child age 21 or younger undergoing HSCT, English-speaking, and age 18 or older	prospective study	T1: prior to HSCT infusion T2: 3-months post-HSCT T3: 6-months post-HSCT; T4: 12-months post-HSCT	maternal psychological functioning, spouse/friends support	Interviews, SF-36, Cancer Support Inventory
Barrera (2009)	N = 99 mothers	SCT	Malignant haematological disease	Mothers' mean age = 36.40 years (SD = 12.30); Children's mean age at SCT = 8.27 (SD = 4.38)	prospective study	T1: 1-2 weeks pre-SCT; T2: 12-months post-HSCT T3: 24 months post-HSCT	health related quality of life (HRQOL) outcomes, family cohesion, maternal distress	Child Health Questionnaire (CHQ-PF50), Pediatric Oncology Quality of Life Scale (POQOLS) (cancer-specific), Family Adaptability and Cohesion Evaluation Scale (FACES-III), Beck Depression Inventory
Jantien Vrijmoet-Wiersma et al. (2009)	N = 31 parents of 21 children (19 mothers + 12 fathers)	SCT allogeneic	Non Malignant/Malignant haematological disease	Parents' mean age at T1 = 42 (SD = 5.5); Children's average age at T1 = 11 years (SD = 4.8)	prospective study	T1: 2 weeks pre-SCT T2: on average 10 months post-SCT (SD = 4.7)	parenting stress	The Dutch version of the parenting stress index (PSI) , named NOSI
Jobe-Shields et al., 2009	N = 146 parents (82% mothers, 12% fathers, and 6% another caretaker)	HSCT (allogenic, autologous, matched sibling)	Non Malignant/Malignant haematological disease	Children's mean age = 13.2 years (SD = 3.7)	1 time point study	prior to HSCT	parental depressive symptoms and family environment (cohesion, expressiveness, and conflict)	Center for Epidemiologic Studies Depression Scale (CES-D), The Family Environment Scale (FES)
Asadi et al. (2011)	N = 6 parents	BMT	Malignant haematological disease	-	1 time point study	parents of children who undergoing BMT	qualitative study	Semi-structured and in-depth face to face interviews

Table 1. (Continued)

authors	sample	type of transplant	type of diagnosis	age range at transplant	age range at transplant	assessment time points	functional area assessed	type of assessment
Jalmsell et al. (2011)	N = 97 parents	HSCT	Children diagnosed with a malignancy before their 17th birthday and died before the age of 25.	Parents' age at child diagnosis: < 29 years = 14 years = 50 >40= 32	1 time point study		psychological and physiological well-being, anxiety, depression and quality of life	self-reports of their psychological and physiological well-being over the last month at the time of the study, on a visual digital scale (VDS), State-Trait Anxiety Inventory (STAI-T), the Center for Epidemiological Studies Depression Scale (CES-D).

Table 2. Psychosocial adjustment of siblings of BMT patients

authors	sample	type of siblings	type of transplant	age range at assessment	Study design	Functional area assessed	Type of assessment
Packman, Crittenden, Fisher et al. (1997)	N = 44 N = 44 parents	21 donors + 23 nondonors	BMT	6-18 years old	Retrospective study	Views, concerns, struggles	Interviews to siblings and to parents
Packman, Crittenden, Shaffer et al. (1997)	N = 44	21 donors + 3 nondonors	BMT	6-18 years old	Retrospective study	Behaviour, psychological distress, sense of self	Self-report measures, teacher-related scales
MacLeod et al. (2003)	N = 15	8 successful transplant; 7 no successful transplant	HSCT (hematopoietic stem cell transplant)	Assessment mean age = 19,6 years HSCT mean age = 13,3 years	Retrospective study	Psychosocial experience	Interviews
Packman et al. (2003)	N = 42	donors and nondonors	BMT	Ages 6-18 years	Retrospective study	Psychosocial experience	Humane Figure Drawing
Parmar et al. (2003)	N = 1	donors	HSCT		Retrospective study	Psychosocial experience	Reflections on donor's experience
Packman et al. (2004)	N = 44	21 donors + 23 nondonors	HSCT (hematopoietic stem cell transplant)	6-18 years old	Retrospective study	Psychosocial adjustment	Measures of psychosocial development (self-report measure)

authors	sample	type of siblings	type of transplant	age range at assessment	Study design	Functional area assessed	type of assessment
Wilkins and Woodgate (2007)	N = 8	donors and nondonors	BMT	11–24 years old; Mean age = 18 years; All female	6 months period Mean time since BMT = 53 months	Lived experience of the BMT trajectory	semistructured, open-ended interviews; demographic forms; and field notes
Wiener et al. (2008)	N = 14	donors	peripheral blood stem cell (PBSC) transplantation	average age of 18.6 years old (range 9–28).	Retrospective study. ≥4 months post-donation	Experiences of PBSC sibling donors	interviews

In another prospective study, Rodrigue et al. (1997) showed in mothers significant disruption in family planning and activities, as well as strong associations between lower socioeconomic status and higher parental stress. Increased parenting stress, financial strain, caregiver burden, and family stress were reported following transplantation and persisted for several months. The mostly used coping strategies reported by mothers were characterized by attempts to maintain family integration and to understand the child's medical situation.

The study by Streisand et al. (2000) also showed increased levels of stress in 22 mothers during pre-transplant time comparing with the 3 weeks post-transplant. Manne et al. (2001) examined anxiety and depressive symptoms by questionnaires and structured clinical interviews in 115 mothers of children undergoing HSCT a week before the infusion. Again, about 20% of the mothers received at least one of three severe diagnosis: generalized anxiety disorder, panic disorder or major depressive disorder. In another prospective study of Manne et al. (2004) nearly one third of mothers who had 1 of the 4 diagnoses (generalized anxiety disorder, panic disorder, major depressive disorder and Post-Traumatic Stress Disorder) at 18 months after HSCT, were younger and had higher anxiety and depressive symptoms at the time of HSCT.

A prospective study (Phipps et al., 2004) assessed patterns of distress in 151 parents of children undergoing HSCT. The period of most elevated distress of parents seemed to be from admission through week +3, resolving by 4-6 months post-transplant. Parental distress resulted related to parental socioeconomic status and it was predicted by child distress level at the time of admission for HSCT.

Another study of the same research group (Phipps et al., 2005) showed significant changes in parental distress across the course of HSCT. Several significant predictors of parental distress trajectories were identified: prior parent and patient illness-related distress, pre-morbid child internalizing behaviour problems, the family relationship dimensions of the family environment, and parental avoidant coping behaviours. In this way, it was possible to identify the parents at higher risk for increased distress during the acute phase of transplant.

The findings of a retrospective study by Sormanti et al. (1994) were that the majority of parents do not experience long-term psychosocial problems and that the most difficult period is during the child's hospitalization. The most distressed parents were those whose child had received the transplant less than 24 months before the study. However, parents reported several psychosocial concerns about the child's health, insurance, finances and their own physical and mental health.

The PTSD-related cognitive processing was examined in 91 mothers of children undergoing HSCT (Duhamel et al., 2004). The authors used a structured interview about fears, intrusions, avoidance and distress regarding their child's HSCT at two time points: During the child's hospitalization and approximately 3 months later. The main hypothesis was that paediatric HSCT would lead to development of a "Fear Network" (Threat of Life, Potential for Suffering, Magnitude of Fear) that would be associated with mother's distress. The findings of this study showed that mothers' fears played a primary role in their adjustment to their child's transplantation. At both time of assessments, mothers who had a grater Fear Network were more distressed. Mothers' avoidance of thoughts, feelings and reminders of their child's illness during the child's transplantation was associated with their distress 3 months later. The child's risk for an unsuccessful transplantation outcome was not associated with mothers' fears or distress during the child's hospitalization, but it was associated with mothers' distress during the child's post-hospital course of recovery.

Results of the study by Kronenberger et al. (1998) indicated that mothers who had experienced severe major life stresses (in addition to their children's illness) and social stresses reported significantly more symptoms of depression and ruminative worries. Another relevant finding was that mother social stress and avoidant coping negatively predicted the adjustment of children preparing to undergo HSCT.

In this sense, maternal depression was negatively associated with children's physical and psychosocial health related quality of life (HRQoL): Higher maternal education and older age at pre-HSCT predicted improvements in children's physical domains 2 years post-HSCT (Barrera, 2009). Parenting stress was higher post-HSCT than pre-HSCT and high levels of parenting stress were predictive of poor parental ratings of child HRQoL post-HSCT (Vrijmoet-Wiersma et al., 2009). Parental symptoms of depression, family cohesion, and family expressiveness emerged as significant predictors of child-reported distress: When parental depressive symptomatology was high, child distress was high regardless of family environment. However, when parental depressive symptomatology was low, family cohesion and expression served as protective factors against child distress (Jobe-Shields et al., 2009). The effect of perceived family environment as a determinant of adjustment of HSCT children was assessed in a prospective study˙ (Phipps and Mulhern, 1995). Results showed that perceived family cohesion and expressiveness act as protective factors, promoting resilience to the stresses of HSCT, whereas family conflict acts directly as a risk factor.

A longitudinal study by Duhamel et al. (2007) investigated several potential antecedents of 140 mothers' fear appraisals using interviews: lower optimism and a greater number of negative life events were independently associated with greater maternal fear appraisals, but no association was found with lifetime history of trauma. Mothers' fear appraisals during their child's hospitalization were, in turn, associated with their fear appraisals up to 6 months later.

Similarly, Manne et al. (2002) analysed the role of cognitive and social processing in mothers' PTSD symptoms using a battery of questionnaires about emotional distress, HSCT-related fears, and negative responses of family and friends at the time of infusion and 3 and 6 months post- HSCT. It was found that the measures at the time of HSCT hospitalization were predictive of later PTSD symptoms. In another study, Manne et al. (2003) evaluated the role of maternal coping strategies in depressive symptoms experienced by mothers of children undergoing HSCT. A total of 207 mothers completed measures of coping and depressive symptoms at the time of child's HSCT, 3 and 6 months post- HSCT. The results showed that acceptance and humour were associated with reduction in maternal depressive symptoms across the 6 months and that greater planning and alcohol/substance use were associated with increases in maternal depressive symptoms across the 6-month time period. Finally, positive reframing, emotional support and religion were negatively associated with the course of the depressive symptoms, but the magnitude of associations differed depending on the use of the coping strategies at the time of transplantation (e.g., acceptance and humour). Rini et al. (2004) studied the relation between life stress and basic beliefs about self-worth and the benevolence and meaningfulness of the world among 100 mothers of children during HSCT hospitalization and 1 year later. Results showed that prior trauma and recent negative events are associated with basic beliefs during hospitalization and also with changes in basic beliefs in the next year, with distress mediating some of these relations. Findings also demonstrated relations between basic beliefs and physical and mental functioning. Rini et al. (2008) investigated also whether social support from family and friends attenuated adverse effects of having low spouse support among 163 mothers of children undergoing HSCT. Their findings indicated that mothers with low spousal support and low family/friend support showed the worst functioning across all time points, while mothers with low spousal support and high family/friend support demonstrated significantly better functioning. Moreover, mothers with high family/friend support demonstrated trajectories of physical health-related functioning that were more stable than the trajectories of mothers with low family/friend support.

A retrospective study adopting a narrative approach (Forinder, 2004) showed that the child's illness and treatment play an important role in the parents' lives for many years. Those parents who managed to put reason before emotion, rated their coping as better. They also reported that their sense of participation was an useful coping strategy.

From pre-HSCT in-depth interviews (Oppenheim et al., 2002), parents expressed great distress, considerable difficulty in assuming their parental role (with feelings of helplessness and guilt), and had distorted relations with the child whose behavior was unusual and incomprehensible. The relation with care providers, who should be 'all-powerful' and harmless, was ambivalent and the couple went through a crisis. Temporal and social landmarks were disturbed with loss of social and professional relations.

Another qualitative study that used in-depth interviews (Wu et al., 2005) indicated that the experiences of parents of children undergoing HSCT include 4 themes: parental psychological distress, family lifestyle disturbances, parents' coping patterns, and family resources. Other themes that emerged (Asadi et al., 2011) were: pending between dread and hope of transplantation result, exalting spirituality, worry about circumstantial difficulties and life lessons learned.

Discussion and Research Recommendations

The area of investigation about parental psychological health and adaptation related to their child HSCT is well developed. The studies' designs are principally prospective (58.33%), followed by one-time points (29.62%) and by retrospective ones (12,05%). The use of the prospective design is really necessary and useful to investigate parents' mental health during the different HSCT phases. The one-time point studies (Rodrigue et al., 1996; Kronenberger et al., 1998) focused on the pre-transplant phase as a critical period. Pre-transplant phase as a critical period is confirmed also by other prospective (Rini et al., 2004) and retrospective (Manne et al., 2001) studies. Another evidenced critical period for parents of children who undergo HSCT is the acute phase of transplant hospitalization (Manne et al., 2002; Manne et al., 2003; Phipps and Mulhern, 1995). These studies suggest the importance of a good screening of parental mental health to find out the parents more at risk and to adopt an early psychological supportive intervention for them.

Most of the studies in this area of investigation assessed mothers' psychological health (54.16%), while a few studies focused on both parents' experience (45.84%) and none focused specifically on fathers' psychological health. The reason for the absence of specific studies on fathers' experience can be due to the major presence of mothers as caregiver during the child HSCT hospitalization. However it would be useful to have more information also about fathers' mental health and coping styles in order to have global point of view on the entire family, its resources and its needs.

The type of assessment in the different studies is similar, with self-report questionnaires to test parents' mental health, quality of life and coping strategies. Only 6 out of the 24 studies (25%) used qualitative interviews with parents. Future research could focus more on parents' direct words to better understand their point of view and their principal needs in this critical event regarding their child health.

Another methodological consideration is that these studies rarely differentiate between types of transplant, of diagnosis and also do not take into account properly child's age discussing the findings. Future research should address these issues as well.

THEME 2: PSYCHOSOCIAL ADJUSTMENT OF SIBLINGS OF HSCT PATIENTS

In the last 20 years there were only few studies (N=8) that investigated the siblings of pediatric HSCT patients. Table 2 reports the articles retrieved about this issue.

In particular, there were 5 studies of the same research group on the same group of 44 siblings of transplanted patients (Packman, Crittenden, Fischer, et al., 1997; Packman, Crittenden, Schaeffer, et al., 1997; Packman, 1999; Packman et al., 2003; Packman et al., 2004). In the first study (Packman, Crittenden, Fischer, et al., 1997), views, concerns and struggles of 44 siblings (21 donors and 23 nondonors) of surviving pediatric HSCT patients were explored by interviews. It was found that donors had significantly more anxiety, lower self-esteem and more adaptive skills in schools that did nondonors, whereas nondonors exhibited significantly more school problems. In another study (Packman, Crittenden, Schaeffer, et al., 1997) the same siblings were tested also by quantitative measures. One-third of the siblings in each group (donors and nondonors) reported a moderate level of post-traumatic stress reaction. MacLeod et al. (2003) examined the psychosocial experience of 15 hematopoietic stem cell transplant siblings donors (8 successful and 7 unsuccessful) by qualitative interviews. Results showed that siblings in the unsuccessful transplant group reported greater negative impact and feelings of guilt following HSCT and were less likely to experience positive psychological effects. Both groups reported that informed consent involved "no choice" and that psychological aspects of the procedure outweighed physical aspects.

Few reports have been written from the donor's perspective, an example in this sense was the study of Parmar et al. (2003). Another study that used in-depth interviews was that of Wilkins et al. (2007). Interruption in family life emerged as the essence of siblings' experience. Four themes supported this essence: Despite family life being interrupted, life continued on for siblings ("life goes on" theme); the HSCT experience made feeling like a part of a family challenging for siblings ("feeling more or less a part of a family" theme); use of spirituality and religious beliefs for dealing with life events (faith in God that things will be okay); and emotional reactions of siblings to the interruption in family life associated with the HSCT ("feelings around families" theme).

Packman et al. (2003) measured also the siblings' emotional distress among 42 siblings aged 6-18 years. Feelings of isolation, anger, depression, anxiety and low self-esteem emerged as the major results. In another study (Packman et al., 2004) donor siblings reported significantly more anxiety and lower self-esteem than did nondonors. Nondonors showed significantly more school problems. Approximately one third of all siblings reported moderate to severe posttraumatic stress.

In conclusion, these findings indicate the importance of attending to siblings' needs throughout the transplantation process.

Also peripheral blood stem cell (PBSC) donors felt anxious about the procedure and expressed concerns about physical harm to themselves and their sibling recipient (Wiener et al., 2008). Age appears to play a key role, as a larger percentage of older donors reported feeling 'pretty nervous' or 'extremely nervous' about the apheresis procedure compared to younger donors. Donors reported that while the informational session with the transplant team staff provided useful information, additional preparation sessions about transplant outcome and complications would have been helpful.

Discussion and Research Recommendations

Research findings on the psychological adaptation of siblings of a chronically ill children suggest that the presence of a child with a chronic illness in the family may place siblings at risk for psychological difficulties (Packman et al., 2004). A significant difference in psychological health between donor and nondonor siblings is showed (Packman, Crittenden, Fischer, et al., 1997; Packman, Crittenden, Schaeffer, et al., 1997; MacLeod et al., 2003; Packman et al., 2004).

There are really a few studies about siblings' experience (only 8 studies) and future research should fill in this gap.

THEME 3: PSYCHOSOCIAL INTERVENTIONS FOR PARENTS AND SIBLINGS OF THE CHILDREN UNDERGOING HSCT

The HSCT procedure can be divided into several stages, each accompanied by particular emotional tones and psychological issues. The psychological care of the patient, donor and family has to follow these stages, from pre-HSCT consultation, through informed consent, hospitalization and convalescence (Lesko, 1994). We considered here the interventions directed to parents or to siblings of children undergoing HSCT.

Two studies investigated the preparing process and the experience of siblings to be bone marrow donors: Heiney et al. (2002) underlined the efficacy of education and therapeutic interventions consisting in a teaching book to use after transplantation, while Shama (1998) developed an age-appropriate medical play and a discussion of feelings and concerns about their role obtaining a successful rate of 97.5%. Also the above cited studies by Packman, Crittenden, Fisher et al. (1997) and Wilkins et al. (2007), underlined that participation in support groups is helpful for siblings, increasing their understanding of the transplant process and facilitating changes in their mood (eg, less fearful and less anxious). Interviews and opportunities to talk for donor and nondonor siblings are recommended also post-donation and post-HSCT in sibling support groups (Packman, 1999).

Streisand (1999; 2000) measured the efficacy of a new program to reduce mothers' distress while their children were inpatients in a bone marrow transplant unit. The instruments adopted were self-report measures and a semi-structured interview. The intervention strategy consisted mostly in teaching coping styles and it was applied to 11 mothers out 22. Results indicated a limited support for the efficacy of the intervention, with only a few differences between the intervention program-group and the standard treatment-group. Increased levels of parenting distress in pre-transplant phase suggested the need for additional psychological intervention at that time.

Finally, Phipps (2002) reviewed the potential benefits of a number of techniques from the field of complementary medicine (relaxation/imagery; massage; humour therapy, expressive therapy) for reducing transplant-related distress. Based on patient and parent evaluations, massage and humour therapy emerged as the most promising approaches.

Discussion and Research Recommendations

Research findings in this field underline the importance of education and therapeutic interventions and of complementary therapies (like play therapy program, art therapy intervention, relaxation/imagery, music therapy, massage; humour therapy, expressive therapy) during the different stages of pediatric HSCT, for both parents and siblings.

This area of investigation is not enough developed yet and future research should better address this issue.

Conclusion

This chapter reviewed the research published in the last 20 years on parents and siblings of children undergoing hematopoietic stem cell transplantation, identifying three main topics linked to family psychological adjustment to HSCT: psychological health and adaptation of parents of children undergoing HSCT, psychosocial adjustment of siblings of HSCT patients and psychosocial interventions for families of children undergoing HSCT.

Several studies underlined that parents' psychological health and adaptation can influence child's health related quality of life, for this reason it is important to improve family supportive interventions, in order to increase child's quality of life. The studies reported here documented various types of stress problems and psychological symptoms in parents, especially mothers, such as anxiety and depression, PTSD and cognitive problems at various time-points related to HSCT. The use of the prospective design is really necessary and useful to investigate parents' mental health and adaptation processing during the different HSCT phases. The pre-transplant phase and the acute phase of transplant hospitalization result as the most critical periods for parents.

The possible coping strategies and family life styles identified as factors that dampen stress level and psychological symptoms were also underlined, for example prior parent illness-related distress, lower parental socioeconomic status, the family relationship dimensions of the family environment, parental avoidant coping behaviours, acceptance and humour, positive reframing, emotional support (friend/family) and religion.

Future research could be directed to have more information also about fathers' mental health and coping styles, to compare these variables with the mothers' ones and to have a global point of view on the entire family of the children who undergo HSCT. Another research strategy that seems to be promising is the mixed-method that allows collecting data directly from parents' narrations, in order to better understand their own point of views and principal needs in this critical event.

The issues about psychosocial adjustment of siblings of HSCT patients and psychosocial interventions for families of children undergoing HSCT have not been yet well developed. The studies underlined how the presence of a child with a chronic illness in the family may place siblings at risk for psychological difficulties and how donor and nondonor perspectives and experiences were different, but low possible clinical indications were showed, exclusively related to siblings' needs at pre-transplant phase, such as giving them the possibility to have the right information.

Also the area of investigation of psychosocial interventions for families of children undergoing HSCT was not enough developed yet and future research should better address this issue.

References

Asadi, M., Manookian, A., Nasrabadi, A. N. (2011). Parents' experiences of their children bone marrow transplantation: A qualitative study, *International Journal of Hematology Oncology and Stem Cell Research*, Jan.: 1-7.

Barrera, M., Atenafu, E., Hancock, K. (2009). Longitudinal health-related quality of life outcomes and related factors after pediatric SCT, *Bone Marrow Transplantation* 44(4):249-56.

Barrera, M., Boyd Pringle, L. A., Sumbler, K., and Saunders, F. (2000). Quality of life and behavioral adjustment after pediatric bone marrow transplantation, *Bone Marrow Transplantation*, 26:427-435.

Bonichini, S., Tremolada, M., Aloisio, D., Pillon, M., Messina, M., Carli, M. (in press). Quality of life, psychosocial sequelae and medical treatment late effects in pediatric patients undergoing hematopoietic stem cell transplantation. In: Cell Transplantation: New Research, Nova Science Publishers.

Clarke, S. A., Eiser, C., Skinner, R. (2008). Health-related quality of life in survivors of BMT for paediatric malignancy: a systematic review of the literature, *Bone Marrow Transplantation*, 42: 73–82.

Duhamel, K. N., Manne, S., Nereo, N., Ostroff, J,. et al. (2004). Cognitive processing among mothers of children undergoing bone marrow/stem cell transplantation, *Psychosomatic Medicine*, 66:92-103.

DuHamel, K. N., Rini, C., Austin, J., Ostroff, J., Parsons, S., et al. (2007). Optimism and life events as predictors of fear appraisals in mothers of children undergoing hematopoietic stem cell transplantation, *Psycho-Oncology*, 16: 821-833.

Forinder, U. (2004). Bone marrow transplantation from a parental perspective, *Journal of Child Health Care*, 8(2): 134-148.

Heiney, S. P., Bryant, L. H, Godder, K., Michaels, J. (2002). Preparing children to be bone marrow donors, *Oncol. Nurs. Forum*, 29(10):1485-9.

Kronenberger, W. G., Carter, B. D., Edwards, J., Morrow, C., et al. (1998). Psychological adjustment of mothers of children undergoing bone marrow transplantation: The role of stress, coping and family factors, *Children's Health Care*, 27(2): 77-95.

Jalmsell, L., Onelöv, E., Steineck, G., Henter, J. I., Kreicbergs, U. (2011). Hematopoietic stem cell transplantation in children with cancer and the risk of long-term psychological morbidity in the bereaved parents, *Bone Marrow Transplantation*, 46(8):1063-70.

Jobe-Shields, L., Alderfer, M. A., Barrera, M., Vannatta, K., Currier, J. M., Phipps, S. (2009). Parental depression and family environment predict distress in children before stem cell transplantation, *J. Dev. Behav. Pediatr.*, 30(2):140-6.

Lesko, L. M. (1994). Bone marrow transplantation: support of the patient and his/her family, *Support Care Cancer*, 2(1); 35-49.

MacLeod, K. D., Whitsett, S. F., Mash, E. J., and Pelletier, W. (2003). Pediatric siblings donors of successful and unsuccessful hematopoietic stem cell transplants (HSCT): a qualitative study of their psychosocial experience, *Journal of Pediatric Psychology*, 28(4): 223-230.

Manne, S., DuHamel, K., Nereo, N., Ostroff, J., et al. (2002). Predictors of PTSD in mothers of children undergoing bone marrow transplantation: The role of cognitive and social processing, *Journal of Pediatric Psychology*, 27(7): 607-617.

Manne, S., DuHamel, K., Ostroff, J., Parsons, S., et al. (2003). Coping and the course of mother's depressive symptoms during and after pediatric bone marrow transplantation, *J. Am. Acad. Child Adolesc. Psychiatry*, 42(9):1055-1068.

Manne, S., DuHamel, K., Ostroff, J., Parsons, S., Martini, D. R., et al. (2004). Anxiety, depressive, and posttraumatic stress disorders among mothers of pediatric survivors of hematopoietic stem cell transplantation, *Pediatrics,* 113(6): 1700-1708.

Manne, S., Nereo, N., DuHamel, K., Ostroff, J., Parsone, S., et al. (2001). Anxiety and depression in mothers of children undergoing bone marrow transplant: Symptom prevalance and use of the Beck Depression and Beck Anxiety Inventories as screening instruments, *Journal of Consulting and Clinical Psychology*, 69(6): 1037-1047.

Oppenheim, D., Valteau-Couanet, D., Vasselon, S., and Hartmann, O. (2002). Psychosocial considerations. How do parents perceive high-dose chemotherapy and autologous stem cell transplantation for their children, *Bone marrow Transplantation*, 30: 35-39.

Packman, W. L. (1999). Psychosocial impact of pediatric BMT on siblings, *Bone marrow Transplantation*, 24:701-706.

Packman, W. L., Beck, V. L., VanZutphen, K. H., Long, J. K., et al. (2003). The human figure drawing with donor and nondonor siblings of pediatric bone marroe transplant patients, *Art Therapy*, 20(2):83-91.

Packman, W. L., Crittenden, M. R., Fischer, J. B., Schaeffer, E., et al. (1997). Siblings' perceptions of the bone marrow transplantation process, *Journal of Psychosocial Oncology*, 15(3-4):81-105.

Packman, W. L., Crittenden, M. R., Schaeffer, E., Bongar, B., et al. (1997). Psychosocial consequences of bone marrow transplantation in donor and nondonor siblings, *J. Dev. Behav. Pediatr.*, 18(4): 244-53.

Packman, W. L., Gong, K., VanZutphen, K., Shaffer, T., and Crittenden, M. R. (2004). Psychosocial adjustment of adolescent siblings of hematopoietic stem cell transplant patients, *Journal of Pediatric Oncology Nursing*, 21(4): 233-248.

Parmar, G., Wu, J. W., Chan, K. W. (2003). Bone marrow donation in childhood: one donor's perspective, *Psychooncology*, 12(1): 91-94.

Phipps, S. and Mulhern, R. K. (1995). Family cohesion and expressiveness promote resilience to the stress of pediatric bone marrow transplant: a preliminary report, *J. Dev. Behav. Pediatr.*, 16(4):257-63.

Phipps, S. (2002). Reduction of distress associated with paediatric bone marrow transplant: complementary health promotion interventions, *Pediatr. Rehabil.*, 5(4): 223-234.

Phipps, S., Dunavant, M., Lensing, S., and Rai, S. N. (2004). Patterns of distress of children undergoing stem cell transplantation, *Pediatr. Blood Cancer*, 43(3): 267-74.

Phipps, S., Dunavant, M., Lensing, S., and Rai, S. N. (2005). Psychosocial predictors of distress in parents of children undergoing stem cell or bone marrow transplantation, *Journal of Pediatric Psychology*, 30(2):139.153.

Rini, C., Manne, S., DuHamel, K., Austin, J., et al. (2004). Change in mothers' basic beliefs following a child's bone marrow transplantation: the role of prior trauma and negative life events, *Journal of Traumatic Stress*, 17(4): 325-333.

Rini, C., Manne, S., DuHamel, K., Austin, J., Ostroff, J., et al. (2008), Social support from family and friends as a buffer of low spousal support among mothers of critically ill children: A multilevel modeling approach, *Health Psychology*, 27(5):593-603.

Rodrigue, J. R, Hoffmann, R. G., MacNaughton, K., Graham-Pole, J., et al. (1996). Mothers of children evaluated for transplantation: stress, coping resources, and perceptions of family functioning, *Clinical Transplantation*, 10: 447-450.

Rodrigue, J. R., MacNaughton, K., Hoffmann, R. G., Graham-Pole, J., Andres, J. M., Novak, D., Fennel, R. S. (1997). Transplantation in children. A longitudinal assessment of mothers' stress, coping, and perceptions of family functioning, *Psychosomatics*, 38: 478-486.

Shama, W. L. (1998). The experience and preparation of pediatric sibling bone marrow donors, *Soc. Work Health Care*, 27(1): 89-99.

Sormanti, M., Dungan, S., Rieker, P. P. (1994). Pediatric bone marrow transplantation: Psychosocial issues for parents after a child's hospitalization, *Journal of Psychosocial Oncology*, 12(4): 23-42.

Streisand, R. M. (1999). An intervention designed to reduce stress in mothers of children undergoing bone marrow transplantation, *Dissertation-Abstract-International: Section B: The Sciences and Engineering*, 59(5-B):5133.

Streisand, R. M. (2000). Brief report: Parents of children undergoing bone marrow transplantation: Documenting stress and piloting a psychological intervention program, *Journal of Pediatric Psychology*, 25(5):331-337.

Vrijmoet-Wiersma, C. M., Kolk, A. M., Grootenhuis, M. A., Spek, E. M., van Klink, J. M., Egeler, R. M., Bredius, R. G., Koopman, H. M. (2009). Child and parental adaptation to pediatric stem cell transplantation, *Support Care Cancer*, 17(6):707-14.

Wiener, L. S., Steffen-Smith, E., Battles, H. B., Wayne, A., Love, C. P., Fry, T. (2008). Sibling stem cell donor experiences at a single institution, *Psychooncology*, 17(3):304-307.

Wilkins, K. L., Woodgate, R. L. (2007). An interruption in family life: siblings' lived experience as they transition through the pediatric bone marrow transplant trajectory, *Oncol. Nurs. Forum*, 34(2):E28-35.

Wu, J., Mu, P. F., Tsai, S. L., and Chiou, T. J. (2005). Parental experience of family stress during hematopoietic stem cell transplantation of pediatric patients in germ-free isolation in Taiwan, *Cancer Nursing,* 28(5):363-371.

In: Hematopoietic Stem Cells: New Research ISBN 978-1-62257-468-1
Editors: Wesley G. Montgomery and Heather I. Burton ©2012 Nova Science Publishers, Inc.

Chapter 4

NEW INSIGHTS INTO THE IMMUNOGENETICS OF UNRELATED HEMATOPOIETIC STEM CELL TRANSPLANTATION FOR THALASSEMIA

G. Caocci[1]*, R. Littera[2], S. Orrù[2], C. Carcassi[2] and G. La Nasa[1]
[1]Hematology Unit, Bone Marrow Transplant Center, R. Binaghi Hospital, Department of Internal Medicine, University of Cagliari, Italy
[2]Medical Genetics, Department of Internal Medicine, University of Cagliari, Italy

ABSTRACT

Beta-thalassemia major, also known as Cooley's anemia, is designated by the World Health Organization (WHO) as one of the world's most common inherited genetic blood disorders. Although regular transfusions of red blood cells can correct the anemia and effectively suppress the ineffective erythropoiesis, patients will eventually develop some of the typical clinical complications of iron overload such as cardiac dysfunction, liver disease and impairment of the endocrine system. Allogeneic hematopoietic stem cell transplantation (HSCT) is currently the only treatment potentially capable of liberating patients from the weight of chronic lifelong transfusion therapy. The first successful bone marrow transplantation (BMT) for beta thalassemia major was performed in Seattle, Washington in 1981. Since then, enormous progress has been made, and estimates for overall survival (OS) and thalassemia-free survival (TFS) now range from 70%-95% and 65%-90%, respectively, depending upon the patient's age and clinical conditions before HSCT. The parallel availability of an international network of voluntary stem cell donor registries has significantly increased the odds of being able to find a suitable human leukocyte antigen (HLA) matched donor for patients lacking a compatible family donor. Graft versus host disease (GVHD) remains a prominent cause of death and morbidity following HSCT. The complex mechanisms that mediate induction of donor-specific tolerance and facilitate engraftment have tempted many investigators. Scientific studies

* Corresponding author: Dr. Giovanni Caocci, Cattedra di Ematologia, Centro Trapianti di Midollo Osseo, P.O. "R. Binaghi", Via Is Guadazzonis 3, 09126 Cagliari, Italy, Tel:++39 070 6092800; Fax:++39 070 6092936; E-mail: gcaocci@alice.it.

conducted in recent years have uncovered a correlation between certain immunogenetic variables and the occurrence of GVHD which is bound to lead to considerable improvement in donor selection criteria. This review addresses some of the most intriguing new findings within this field.

Keywords: Thalassemia; systematic review; HSCT; immunogenetics

1. Clinical Background of Unrelated Hematopoietic Stem Cell Transplantation for Thalassemia

Beta thalassemia major (Cooley's anemia) is a common hemolytic hemoglobinopathy with a high prevalence in the area known as the "thalassemia belt", a stretch of land extending from the Mediterranean region through Turkey, Iran and India to Southeast Asia and Africa. The typical symptoms of the disorder become apparent within a few months of birth. Affected infants fail to thrive and become progressively pale. Microscopic examination confirms the presence of small and short-lived red blood cells resulting from deficient hemoglobin synthesis [1]. The reduced or absent synthesis of beta globins generates an excess of free alpha globin chains that precipitate and cause an increased rate of intravascular and extravascular red cell destruction.

As a result, large amounts of free iron are deposited in the heart, liver and pancreas, causing dilated myocardiopathy, cirrhosis and diabetes mellitus. Reduced fertility due to hypogonadism and impairment of growth are other common features in thalassemia patients. Regular transfusion regimens are necessary to alleviate anemia and maintain blood oxygen carrying capacity. However, frequent blood transfusions lead to the progressive accumulation of excess iron in body organs and tissues. The most important life-limiting complication of iron overload is myocardial disease, responsible for about 70% of deaths in these patients [1]. For this reason, therapy with iron chelating agents is mandatory [2].

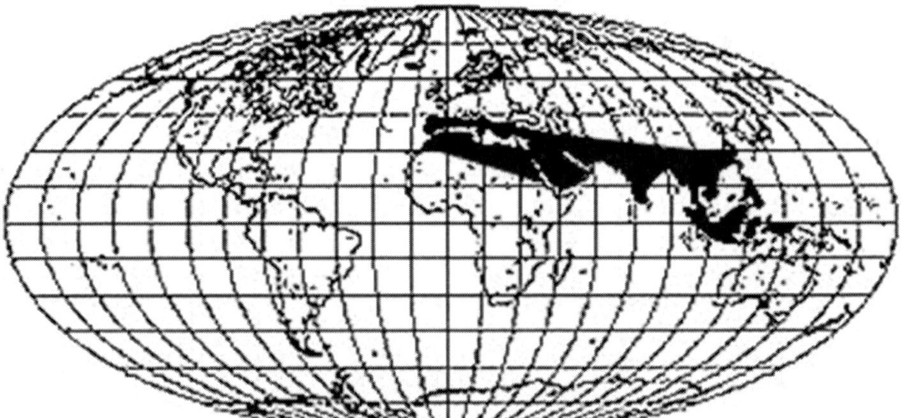

Figure 1. the "thalassemia belt" that extends from the Mediterranean area to the Middle East, India, Southeast Asia and Africa.

Over the last twenty years, progress in the development of iron-chelating therapy for iron overload associated with regular transfusions has substantially changed the prognosis and quality of life of thalassemia patients. Previous reports have shown that almost 70 percent of patients with beta-thalasemia are still alive at the age of 35 years and that survival rates continue to improve for patients born in recent years [3]. Nevertheless, blood transfusions and iron chelation are considered standard supportive but not curative treatments. The only definitive cure for thalassemia is allogeneic hematopoietic stem cell transplantation (HSCT). After successful HSCT, the iron overload in patients with new and sustained hematopoiesis either resolves spontaneously or can be reduced by repeated phlebotomy, thus eliminating any further need for treatment with iron-chelating drugs. Acute and chronic graft-versus-host disease (GVHD) remain the most worrisome complications of HSCT. Contemporarily, it should not be underestimated that growth failure, endocrinopathies, liver and/or heart complications can still occur [4].

A human leukocyte antigen (HLA) identical sibling is the donor of choice for patients requiring allogeneic HSCT. However, the probability of finding a compatible donor within the family ranges from 25 to 30% which means that more then 70% of patients who might benefit from HSCT lack a suitable donor. When an HLA-matched sibling donor is not available, HSCT from an unrelated voluntary donor is a feasible alternative, provided that the donor is selected according to stringent HLA compatibility criteria. Bone marrow registries worldwide now include more than 15 million volunteer donors, thus making it possible for most patients to find an acceptable HLA-matched donor. Experience has shown that by applying highly stringent criteria for donor selection, the outcome of HSCT is not much different from that obtained when using a compatible sibling [5]. Recent reports of the results achieved in Italy are very encouraging, with a 5-year probability of overall survival (OS) of 84% and a thalassemia-free survival (TFS) of 75% [6], but once again confirm that acute and chronic GVHD are the main treatment-related causes of death in thalassemia patients. Undeniably, prevention of GVHD is essential to the optimization of unrelated HSCT in thalassemia.

Historically, several pre-transplantation clinical conditions have played an important role in the outcome of HSCT, particularly the presence of hepatomegaly, the extention of liver fibrosis and the severity of iron accumulation (Pesaro criteria). In adult thalassemia patients with hepatomegaly, portal fibrosis and a history of irregular iron chelation, the procedure is burdened by an elevated risk of transplantation-related mortality (TRM), equal to 29 percent according to the most recently published papers [7, 8].

Over the past decade, research within this field has led to a growing interest in a variety of immunological variables that seem to have a potential role in the outcome of transplantation for thalassemia, capable of predicting engraftment, rejection or the onset of GVHD. Thalassemia patients constitute an ideal cohort for the evaluation of immunogenetic factors and their role in transplantation since the results are not hampered by heterogeneity of the diseases, disease status at transplantation, and the different protocols employed for both conditioning and graft-versus-host disease (GVHD) prophylaxis. Different to patients affected by onco-hematologic diseases, thalassemia patients have a competent immune system that has not been previously compromised by chemotherapy and other aggressive treatment schemes. This review discusses the choice of unrelated hematopoietic stem cell transplantation for thalassemia and the role of immunogenetics in preventing GVHD and TRM.

2. An Important Milestone: Human Leukocyte Antigen (HLA) Matching of Donors and Recipients

Hematopoietic stem cell transplantation is a relatively new medical procedure used to treat diseases once thought to be incurable. Since its first successful application to thalassemia major in 1981, more than 1700 patients have been transplanted around the world [9-13]. Unfortunately, the majority of thalassemia patients lack an HLA-identical donor within the family. For this reason, centers engaged in the cure of thalassemia have become increasingly exposed to pressure and questioning from both patients and their families as to the possibility of transplantation utilizing alternative donors. The first large consecutive series of thalassemia patients transplanted from an unrelated donor was published by La Nasa et al. in 2002 [5] In this preliminary study of 32 patients (median age 14 years, range 2-28 years), donor selection criteria was based on extended haplotype analysis and family segregation studies. Alleles at the HLA-A, -B, -Cw, -DRB1, -DRB3, -DRB4, -DRB5, -DQA1, -DQB1, and -DPB1 loci were identified using the polymerase chain reaction with sequence-specific primers (PCR-SSP).Of the 32 donor/recipient pairs, 24 were identical for HLA-A, B, C, DRB1, DRB3, DRB4, DRB5, DQA1, and DQB1 loci; 7 pairs were identical for 2 extended haplotypes, and 15 pairs shared one extended haplotype. Grade II-IV acute GVHD developed in 41% of cases and chronic GVHD in 25%. Rejection and mortality rates were 12.5% and 19%, respectively. Sixty-nine percent of the patients were alive (OS) with a thalassemia-free survival (TFS) of 66%. The authors concluded that HSCT from unrelated donors, especially when identical for at least one extended haplotype, may offer a probability of success comparable to that observed when using HLA-identical family donors [5].

Since this preliminary study, more than 170 thalassemia patients have been transplanted from an unrelated donor. Further advances of this exciting new approach were released by La Nasa et al in 2005 in a report of 68 thalassemia patients (median age 15 years; range 2-37) transplanted from donors selected according to stringent compatibility criteria [10]. Fourteen patients were classified in risk class I, 16 in risk class II and 38 in risk class III of the Pesaro classification. Overall survival and TFS were 79.3% and 65.8%, respectively.The results improved further when only patients belonging to risk classes I and II were considered, reaching OS and TFS rates of 96.7% and 80%, respectively. Nine patients (13%) developed primary or secondary graft failure. Forty percent of the patients developed grade II to IV acute GVHD and 18% developed chronic GVHD. In 2011, Locatelli and La Nasa published an updated report of the Italian experience of unrelated HSCT for thalassemia. The study was performed on a cohort of 122 thalassemia patients (age range at the time of HSCT 1-35 years, median 10,5) transplanted in one of 4 participating Italian bone marrow transplantation centers [6] Donor and recipient matching was performed using high-resolution molecular typing of class I and II HLA loci and stringent criteria of immune-genetic compatibility. Among pediatric patients, 39 pertained to risk class I, 41 to risk class II and 16 to risk class III of the Pesaro classification. One hundred and five donor/recipient pairs were matched for the HLA-A, -B, -C, -DRB1 loci; 17 donor/recipient pairs had a disparity at the HLA-C locus, but both HLA-C molecules pertained to the same HLA-C ligand group. The patients were prepared for the allograft using a myeloablative conditioning regimen based on the combination of busulfan/treosulfan (BU/TREO), thiotepa (TT) and either cyclophosphamide (CY, 54 patients), or fludarabine (FLU, 68 patients). Graft-versus-host disease (GvHD) prophylaxis was homogeneous in all patients and consisted of cyclosporin-A, short-term methotrexate (15 mg/m2 on day +1 and 10 mg/m2 on days +3, +6 and + 11) and anti-thymocyte globulin (ATG, 2.5 mg/Kg from day –4 to –2). Twenty patients died and 16 patients experienced rejection, the 5-year probability of OS and TFS being 84% and 75%, respectively.

Twenty-eight percent of the patients developed grade II-IV acute GVHD and 13% developed chronic GVHD. The chance of being alive for children belonging to risk classes I, II and III of the Pesaro classification was 97%, 85% and 78%, respectively, while that of adults was 65%. Overall, the results of this study showed that transplantation from well-matched unrelated volunteer donors is able to cure a large proportion of patients with thalassemia major, the results approaching those obtained when the donor is an HLA-compatible sibling. Other authors have reported data obtained on smaller groups of patients. Hongeng et al [12] reported a 2-year thalassemia-free survival of 71% for recipients of unrelated donor stem cells. Three of their patients experienced autologous recovery. Another 3 patients died of sepsis, GVHD or bleeding. The incidence of acute and chronic GVHD was 42% and 14%, respectively.

Table 1. Outcomes of unrelated hematopoietic stem cell transplantation and cord blood transplantation in young adult and pediatric thalassemia patients BM: bone marrow; CB: cord blood; OS: overall Survival; TFS: Thalassemia Free Survival; TRM: Transplant-related mortality; aGVHD: acute graft versus host disease; cGVHD: chronic graft versus host disease

Author	N	Source	Age median years (range)	OS (%)	TFS (%)	TRM (%)	Rejection (%)	aGVHD (%)	cGVHD (%)
La Nasa et al (2002)[5]	32	BM	14 (2-28)	79	66	19	12.5	41	25
La Nasa et al (2005)[10]	68	BM	15 (2-37)	79.3	65.8	20	13	40	18
Hongeng et al (2006)[12]	21	BM	4 (0.7-12)	85.7	71	14.3	14.3	42	14
Locatelli et al (2011)[6]	122	BM	10.5 (1-35)	84	75	16.4	13.1	28	13
Ruggeri et al (2011)[15]	35	CB	4 (0.5-14)	62	21	34	57	23	16
Jaing et al (2012)[14]	35	CB	5.5 (1.2-14)	88.5	88.5	11.4	0	47	35

Some interesting reports have focused on the use of cord blood (CB) as an alternative source of hematopoietic stem cells in unrelated transplantation for thalassemia. Only very recently, the largest single-institution unrelated cord blood transplantation (CBT) series for thalassemia has been published [14] This alternative stem cell source has the advantage of being immediately available when required and is not as difficult to match as stem cells from an adult volunteer donor. Indeed, it should soon be possible to extend this life-saving therapy to a much larger pool of patients. Jaing et al. performed unrelated CBT in 35 thalassemia patients. HLA matching at enrolment according to low-resolution typing of HLA-A, -B, and high-resolution typing of DRB1was 6/6 in 23%, 5/6 in 44.4%, 4/6 in 77.1%, or 3/6 in 3% of patients.

The preparative regimens consisted of oral or i.v. Busulphan, i.v. Cyclophosphamide and equine or rabbit antilymphocyte globulin prophylaxis against seizures during treatment. GVHD prophylaxis, consisted of Cycloporin A(CsA) and a course of methylprednisolone. The CsA dose was tapered starting at least 60 days after confirming engraftment and full-donor chimerism. The 5-year OS and TFS survival rates after the first transplant were 88.3% and 73.9%, respectively. The cumulative incidence of TRM at 2 years was 11.7%. Acute grade III-IV GVHD developed in 47% of patients, while chronic skin GVHD was observed in 40% of patients. Thirty patients (85.7%) were alive and transfusion-free. Based on these promising results, the authors conclude that patients without an available HLA compatible sibling or well-matched unrelated donor should be considered for CBT [14]. Ruggeri et al [15] examined the efficacy of unrelated cord blood (CB) transplantation in 35 children with thalassemia, reporting data from the Eurocord Registry. Overall survival (OS) and disease-free survival (DFS) were 62% and 21%, respectively. Primary graft failure was the predominant cause of treatment failure, occurring in 20 patients with thalassemia. The authors suggested that only CB units containing an expected infused cell dose of $>5x10^7$/kg should be considered for transplantation in hemoglobinopathies. Table 1 illustrates the outcome of unrelated HSCT/CBT performed to cure children and young adults with beta thalassemia major.

3. Why the HLA-DPB1 Locus Is So Special!

Human leukocyte antigen (HLA)-DP was first described in 1980 as a distinct group of HLA class II antigens. Since then, increasing evidence has emerged that HLA-DP molecules can trigger both humoral and cellular alloresponses relevant to clinical transplantation. The HLA-DP antigens are heterodimers encoded by genes at the DPA1 locus, which displays limited polymorphism, and at the highly polymorphic DPB1 locus. Because of the weak linkage disequilibrium with other HLA class II loci, unrelated hematopoietic stem cell transplantation (HSCT) is generally performed across HLA-DPB1allelic mismatches. The major obstacles to successful allogeneic HSCT for the cure of beta-thalassemia are graft rejection and GVHD. A wide range of factors are involved in the onset of these complications which can occur even when the donor is an HLA identical sibling. Both major and minor histocompatibility antigens can be presented by major histompatibility complex molecules to donor T-cells which recognize these antigens as non self and trigger an immune response.

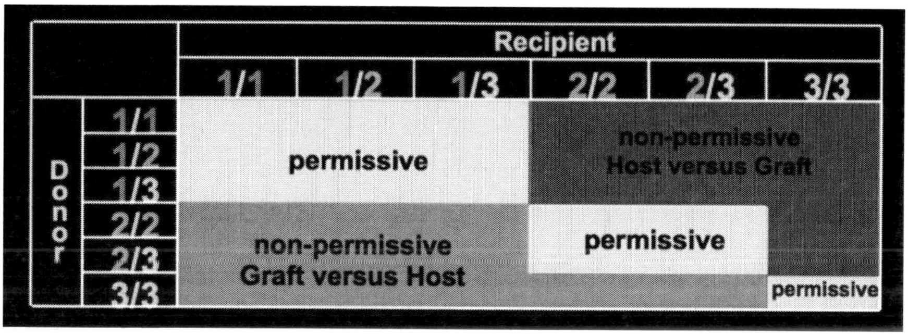

Figure 2. An algorithm for permissiveness of HLA-DPB1 mismatches in HSC donor-recipient pairs. HLA-DPB1 alleles were divided into 3 groups (1-3) according to their in vitro-established immunogenicity. The 3 groups of alleles can be present in 6 different combinations in diploid cells. Numbers indicate the group of the first (before the slash) and the second (after the slash) HLA-DPB1 allele of the donor or recipient. Classification of HLA-DPB1mismatches as permissive or non-permissive in Graft versus Host or in Host versus Graft direction is indicated according to all possible combinations.

To avoid the occurrence of immune-mediated complications in patients with thalassemia, matching of unrelated donor-recipient pairs must be based on high-resolution typing of the HLA-A, -B, -C,-DRB1, and -DQB1 loci. Because of the very weak linkage disequilibria existing between the DR/DQ and DP loci, only 20% of matched unrelated donor-recipient pairs are also compatible for HLA-DPB1. Consequently, more than 80% of unrelated donor transplantations are performed across the HLA-DPB1 transplantation barrier. In 2004, the research team led by Katharina Fleischhauer proposed an algorithm for the determination of non-permissive HLA-DPB1 disparities, which were found to be associated with a significantly increased risk of transplantation-related mortality (TRM) and grade II-IV acute graft-versus-host disease (aGVHD) in patients undergoing transplantation for malignant hematopoietic disorders [16]. The algorithm divided HLA-DPB1 alleles into 3 groups according to in vitro immunogenicity testing.

The 3 groups of alleles could be present in 6 different combinations in diploid cells. Classification of HLA-DPB1 mismatches as permissive or non-permissive in Graft versus Host (GvH) or in Host versus Graft (HvG) direction was indicated according to all possible combinations (Figure 2). A further step ahead was made in 2006 when Fleischhauer and La Nasa showed that the risk of rejection in unrelated donor HSCT for beta-thalassemia was associated with the presence of non-permissive HLA-DPB1 mismatches in the host-versus-graft (HvG) direction, as defined by the previously published algorithm, regardless of the Pesaro patient's class of risk [17]. A retrospective study was performed on 72 beta-thalassemia patients receiving grafts from unrelated donors matched at high resolution for the HLA-A, -B,-C, -DRB1, and -DQB1, loci. In 21 donor-recipient pairs (29%), both HLA-DPB1 alleles were matched. The remaining pairs had one or two HLA-DPB1 disparities, which were classified as permissive (24 pairs, 33%) or non-permissive in HvG (17 pairs, 24%) or GvH (10 pairs, 14%) direction, according to the previously described algorithm. TFS was reduced in patients with non-permissive HLA-DPB1mismatches in HvG (10 of 17; 59%) or GvH (6 of 10; 60%) direction, as compared to the matched or permissive group (35 of 45; 78%). In multivariate analysis, HLA-DP disparity in HvG direction was associated with a statistically significant, lower probability of TFS as compared to patients belonging to the matched or permissive group. These results serve to implement standard criteria for donor selection and highlight the crucial role of immunogenetic factors in the occurrence of complications due to alloreactivity following unrelated donor HSCT for beta-thalassemia. In 2009, Fleischhauer et al. integrated their algorithm with functional data obtained in vitro. Its clinical predictive value was retrospectively evaluated in a study of 621 unrelated HSCT from the Italian Bone Marrow Donor Registry [18]. It was demonstrated that the approach based on T-cell alloreactivity, used to define an algorithm for donor selection, was a powerful strategy for the characterization of non-permissive mismatches in unrelated HSCT. In 2012, the same group of researchers applied the DPB1 algorithm to a large cohort of 8539 transplanted patients: 64% were completely matched for ten HLA alleles (HLA 10/10 matched) and 36% for 9 HLA alleles (HLA 9/10 matched). Only 20% were HLA-DPB1 matched, 31% had non-permissive HLA-DPB1 mismatches, and 49% permissive HLA-DPB1 mismatches [19]. In HLA 10/10-matched transplantations, non-permissive mismatches were associated with a significantly increased risk of overall mortality and severe acute GVHD, compared to permissive mismatches. These findings strongly suggest that HSCT from unrelated donors with a non-permissive T-cell-epitope mismatch at HLA-DPB1 should be avoided and might prove to be a practical clinical strategy for lowering the risks of mortality after unrelated-donor hemopoietic-cell transplantation.

4. An Increasing Interest Surrounds the Role of Killer Immunoglobulin-Like Receptors (KIRs)

HLA class I molecules and killer cell immunoglobulin-like receptors (KIRs) are of pivotal importance for regulating natural killer (NK) cell function [20]. KIRs are encoded within a 100–200 kb region of the leukocyte receptor complex (LRC) on chromosome 19q13.4. The specificity of HLA class I molecules for inhibitory KIRs has only been documented for one activating KIR, namely KIR2DS1 (20, 21). The KIR gene family currently comprises 15 functional genes and 2 pseudogenes organized within the LRC as haplotypes. These haplotypes exhibit extensive variation in the number and type of KIR genes present, producing considerable diversity in the NK cell receptor repertoires. Genetic polymorphism is a primary characteristic of the human major histocompatibility complex HLA class I and class II loci.

Apart from their role in acquired immune response, HLA class I molecules participate in innate immunity as ligands for the killer immunoglobulin-like receptors (KIR). A great complexity of interactions exist between the different types of KIRs and their ligands. KIR haplotypes can be broadly classified as A or B (Figure 3). Group A haplotype has a fixed gene content of seven KIR genes and two pseudogenes and includes a single activating gene (2DS4). Group B haplotype differs for both gene content and allelic polymorphism. In particular, group B haplotypes are distinguished by the presence of a variable number of KIR genes that are not components of group A haplotypes: the inhibitory KIR gene 2DL5 and different combinations of the activating KIR genes 2DS1, 2DS2, 2DS3, 2DS5 and 3DS1.KIRs regulate the activity of NK cells through interaction with HLA class I molecules. HLA-C is the predominant ligand for the 2DL1, 2DL2 and 2DL3 inhibitory KIRs and the 2DS1 activating KIR [20, 21].

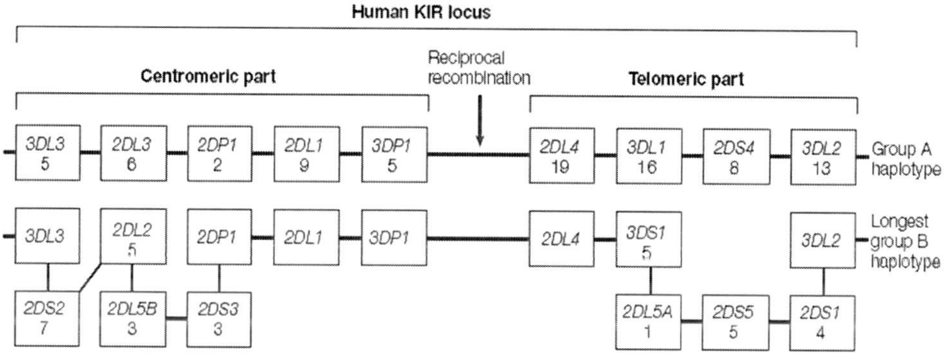

Figure 3. human KIR haplotypes.

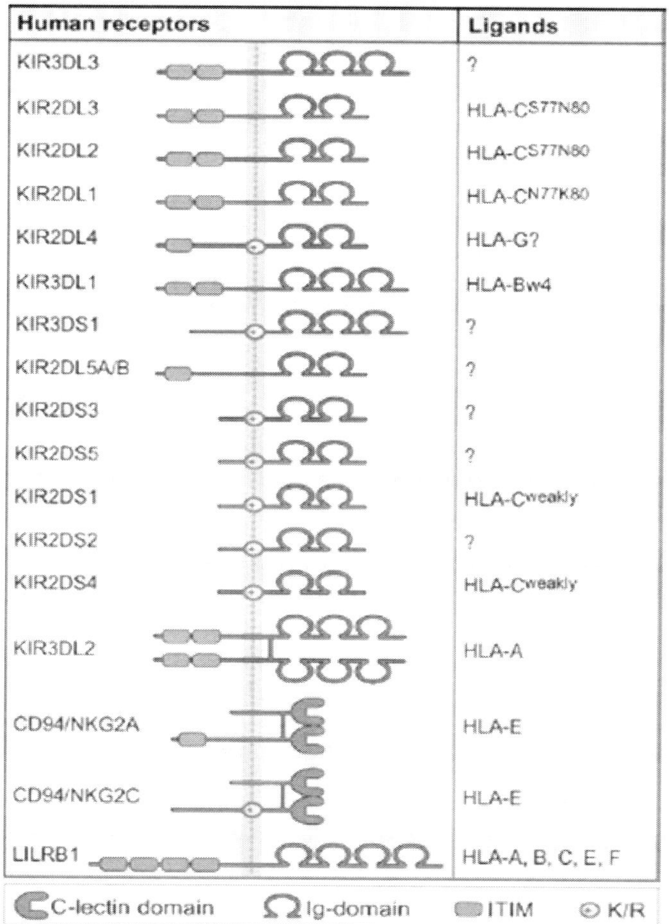

Figure 4. activating/inhibitory KIRs and C1/C2 ligands.

The replacement of an amino acid residue at positions 77 and 80 of the HLA-C alpha-helix makes it possible to divide HLA-C molecules into two groups (C1 and C2), each one selectively recognized by a specific pair of activating/inhibitory KIRs (Figure 4). Several studies have investigated the influence of KIRs on the outcome of both related and unrelated hematopoietic SCT for hematological malignancies, leading to conflicting results. In 2010,

Littera and La Nasa performed a study to follow up on the conclusions drawn from their preliminary report published in 2007 [22, 23]. They retrospectively evaluated 72 consecutive transfusion-dependent beta-thalassemia patients transplanted from an HLA-matched unrelated donor to investigate the impact of KIRs and their ligands on HSCT outcome. The KIR genes 2DL1, 2DL2, 2DL3, 2DL4, 2DL5, 3DL1, 3DL2, 3DL3, 2DS1, 2DS2, 2DS3, 2DS4, 2DS5, 3DS1 were typed in donors and recipients. Combinations of donor 2DS2 and 2DS1 activating KIRs and patient C1 and C2 KIR ligands and combinations of donor 2DL1, 2DL2, 2DL3 and 3DL1 inhibitory KIRs and patient C1, C2 and Bw4 KIR ligands were analysed. The influence on transplantation outcomes of recipient HLA class I KIR ligands (C1, C2, HLA-A11, -A3, -Bw4) was analysed either alone or in combinations with the single activating and inhibitory KIRs of the donors. Donors and recipients were divided into two groups according to combinations of group A and group B KIR haplotypes: those homozygous for KIR haplotype A (AA) and those either heterozygous or homozygous for KIR haplotype B (AB+BB). The authors found that patients transplanted from donors homozygous for KIR haplotype A (AA) had a fourfold risk of developing moderate acute GVHD and a sevenfold risk of developing severe acute GVHD. Considering that the A haplotype only includes one stimulatory KIR (2DS4), which in most cases is not expressed on the NK cell membrane, the authors postulated that NK cells in donors expressing only the A haplotype could display a lower efficiency in killing recipient antigen-presenting cells (APC). It is possible that APCs trigger donor T-lymphocytes into activation of the first step of the pathological cascade leading to acute GVHD occurrence. Another interesting finding of this study was that all nine patients who experienced rejection were either C1 or C2 homozygotes. The strong association observed between C1 or C2 homozygosity and graft failure was confirmed in multivariate analysis.

By interpolating the number of donor activating KIRs with recipient HLA-C KIR ligands, the same authors recently created an algorithm capable of stratifying patients according to the immunogenetic risk of complications following unrelated HSCT [24]. They retrospectively analysed a cohort of 114 thalassemia patients transplanted from an HLA-matched unrelated donor to investigate the effects that combinations of patient HLA-Class I KIR ligands and the number of functional activating KIRs on donor NK cells could have on the outcome of unrelated HSCT for thalassemia, and, more specifically, on the incidence of acute GVHD and rejection. HLA KIR ligand groups C1 and C2 and the number of functional donor activating KIRs had the strongest impact on HSCT outcome. Donors with the AA genotype and only non-functional deletion variants of KIR2DS4 were defined as non-carriers of activating KIRs (aKIR = 0).

By interpolating recipient HLA KIR ligand groups C1/C2, C1/C1 and C2/C2 with the number of donor activating KIRs (0, 1, ≥2), they built two tables each consisting of nine distinct panels. Recipients were then inserted into one of the two tables according to the development of acute GVHD or rejection. The highest risk of acute GvHD was observed for C1/C2 heterozygotes transplanted from donors completely lacking activating KIRs. Conversely, the risk of acute GvHD was totally absent in C2/C2 homozygotes transplanted from donors possessing ≥2 activating KIRs. None of the C1/C2 heterozygotes transplanted from donors totally lacking activating KIRs rejected the graft. 50% of cases of rejection registered in the patient cohort belonged to the group of C2/C2 homozygotes transplanted from donors with ≥2 aKIR. Based on these observations, a transplantation-risk algorithm was developed (Figure 5).

The authors also proposed a possible mechanism for immunological rejection based on a reduction in donor NK cell alloreactivity associated with an increment in recipient NK cell alloreactivity (Figure 6).

Recipient KIR ligands				
C2/C2	Standard risk	Standard risk	Rejection	
C1/C1	aGvHD	Standard risk	Standard risk	
C1/C2	aGvHD	Standard risk	Standard risk	
	0 aKIRs	1 aKIRs	≥ 2 aKIRs	Donor activating KIRs

Figure 5. Unrelated transplantation risk based on recipient KIR ligands and donor activating KIRs.

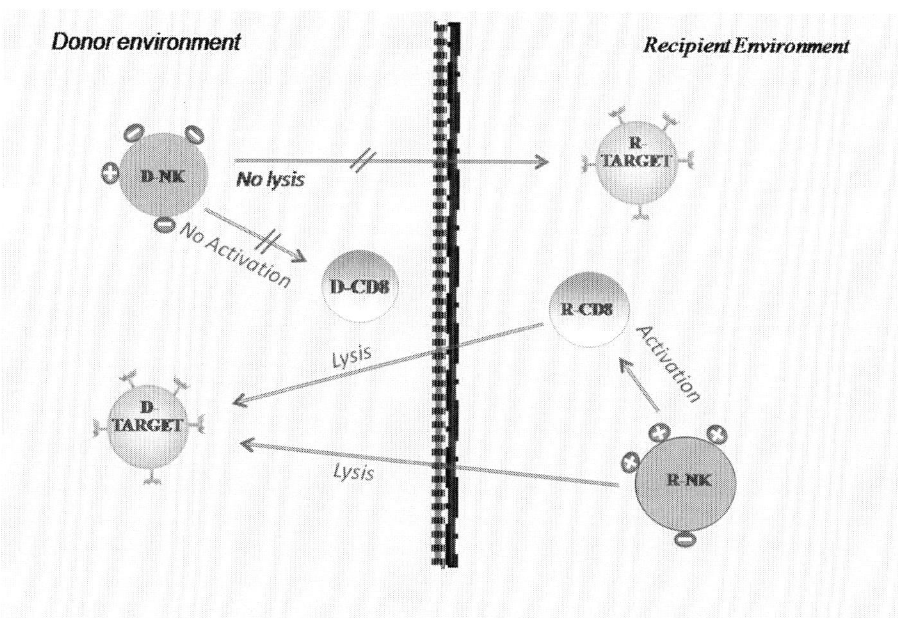

Figure 6. possible immunological interactions between donors and recipients, based on KIR status (see explanation in the text).

Indeed, it would seem that the presence of C2/C2 targets determines a strong inhibitory signal for donor NK cells (KIR2DL1+, KIR2DS1) whereas, on the other hand, activating signals for residual clones of recipient NK-cell subsets (KIR2DS1+) prevail, thus leading to graft failure accompanied by autologous hematopoietic reconstitution. A similar mechanism can be hypothesized for C1/C1 homozygotes (donor NK cells lacking KIR2DS2 versus patient NK cells expressing KIR2DS2).

Also in these cases, it can be hypothesized that recipient NK cell alloreactivity had the upper hand. All considered, it is likely that the proposed algorithm will prove helpful in pre-HSCT risk assessment as well as the delicate process of patient risk counselling when considering the option of unrelated HSCT for a chronic non-malignant disease like thalassemia.

5. The Human Leukocyte Antigen G: From Pregnancy to HSCT

Human Leukocyte Antigen G (HLA-G) represents a "non classic" HLA class I molecule, highly expressed in trophoblast cells [25]. HLA-G plays a key role in embryo implantation and pregnancy by contributing to maternal immune tolerance of the fetus and, more specifically, by protecting trophoblast cells from maternal NK cells through interaction with their inhibitory KIR receptors. It has also been shown that HLA-G expression by tumoral cells can contribute to an "escape" mechanism, inducing NK tolerance toward cancer cells in ovarian and breast carcinomas, melanoma, acute myeloid leukemia, acute lymphoblastic leukemia and B-cell chronic lymphocytic leukemia [26] Additionally it would seem that HLA-G molecules have a role in graft tolerance following HSCT. These molecules exert their immunotolerogenic function towards the main effector cells involved in graft rejection through inhibition of natural killer (NK) and cytotoxic T lymphocyte (CTL)-mediated cytolysis and CD4+T-cell alloproliferation [27]. HLA-G transcript generates 7 alternative mRNAs that encode 4 membrane-bound (HLA-G1, G2, G3, G4) and 3 soluble protein isoforms (HLA-G5, G6, G7).

Moreover, HLA-G allelic variants are characterized by a 14-basepair (bp) deletion-insertion polymorphism located in the 3'-untranslated region (3'UTR) of HLA-G. The presence of the 14-bp insertion is known to generate an additional splice whereby 92 bases are removed from the 3'UTR [28]. HLA-G messenger ribonucleic acids (mRNAs) having the 92-base deletion are more stable than the complete mRNA forms, and thus determine an increment in HLA-G expression. Therefore, the 14-bp polymorphism is involved in the mechanisms controlling post-transcriptional regulation of HLA-G molecules Following these observations, in 2007 La Nasa et al. investigated the influence of the 14-bp deletion/insertion polymorphism on the outcome of HSCT in patients affected by thalassemia major [29]. Fifty-three beta-thalassemia major patients transplanted from an unrelated donor were retrospectively evaluated. The donor/recipient pairs were typed at high resolution level for the HLA-A, -B and -C loci and the HLA-DRB1, -DQB1 and-DPB1 loci. The recipients shared the same HLA-G and HLA-G 14-bp deletion/insertion genotypes with their donors. The presence of the 14-bp deletion/insertion polymorphism in the 3'UTR of HLA-G was determined and the recipients were divided into three groups according to the HLA-G 14-bp genotype: homozygotes for the 14-bp insertion, heterozygotes for the 14-bp deletion/insertion and homozygotes for the 14-bp deletion. The authors found that patients homozygous for the

14-bp deletion had a higher risk of developing acute GVHD compared to patients carrying the 14-bp insertion, while no significant differences were observed for rejection, TFS or OS. They attributed this finding to the increased production of HLA-G1 and -G5 molecules and suggested that incorporation of the HLA-G 14-bp insertion-deletion polymorphism in the pre-transplantation risk-assessment process could assist the hematologist in the HSCT decision-making process and improve the planning of conditioning regimens, immunosuppressive therapy and treatment schedules, all of which translate into a beneficial impact on the outcome of transplantation.

6. Cytotoxic T Lymphocyte Associated Antigen-4: A Key Role in Unrelated Transplantation?

As mentioned in the previous paragraphs, acute GVHD is the result of donor T-cell alloreactivity against disparate major and minor histocompatibility antigens of the recipient. This process is also influenced by several membrane-bound receptors and soluble molecules capable of regulating the duration and severity of the immune response. Among these, the cytotoxic T lymphocyte–associated antigen-4 (CTLA-4) cell surface molecule could play a key role.

CTLA-4 is a member of the immunoglobulin superfamily, encoding a protein that transmits an inhibitory signal to T cells that downregulates their activation. In humans, the CTLA-4 protein is encoded by a gene located on chromosome 2p22 and exists as 2 isoforms: a membrane-bound (flCTLA-4) and a soluble form (sCTLA-4); the alternative splicing that generates these isoforms seems to be regulated by genetic polymorphisms within or in close proximity to the CTLA-4 gene [30]. Polymorphisms of the CTLA-4 gene have been associated with autoimmune diseases and it has recently been reported that donor genotypes correlate with the outcome of allogeneic HSCT in leukemia patients [31]. Given these interesting data, Orrù and La Nasa studied the role of CTLA-4 gene polymorphisms in the development of acute GVHD in 72 thalassemia patients given HSCT from an unrelated donor [32].

The mean age of patients (41males and 31 females) was 13 years. Genotypes for CTLA-4 polymorphisms were determined by direct cycle sequencing and the genotype distribution for each polymorphism was compared versus either the presence or absence of acute GVHD. It was found that genetic variability of CTLA-4 is implicated in the development of acute GVHD following allo-HSCT. Acute GVHD was significantly more frequent in patients homozygous for the CT60-A allele than in patients with the CT60-G allele. These data support the hypothesis that the G-allele determines protection against acute GVHD by reducing the expression of sCTLA-4. The significantly increased expression of sCTLA-4 associated with the CT60-AA genotype seems to determine susceptibility to acute GVHD by impeding or reducing the possibility of binding between B7 and membrane-bound CTLA-4 expressed on activated T lymphocytes.

7. Dealing with Such a Complex Scenery: The Role of Mathematical Tools

Transplantation from unrelated donors is burdened by an increased risk of acute GVHD with a consequent negative impact on overall survival. Therefore, every effort needs to be made to carefully evaluate the risk of GVHD before performing unrelated-HSCT. GVHD remains the major barrier to the successful outcome of HSCT in thalassemia. HLA disparity between the donor and the recipient is clearly the most powerful risk factor, but also older age, gender mismatch, Pesaro risk class, cytomegalovirus (CMV) positivity, as well as higher median infused hematopoietic stem cell doses have been shown to increase the risk for GVHD. As previously discussed, evidence emerging from recent reports indicates a correlation between certain immunogenetic variables and the occurrence of GVHD: donor-recipient HLA-Cw ligand groups for KIR receptors, KIR genotypes, the HLA-G 14-basepair (bp) polymorphism and HLA-DPB1 disparity.

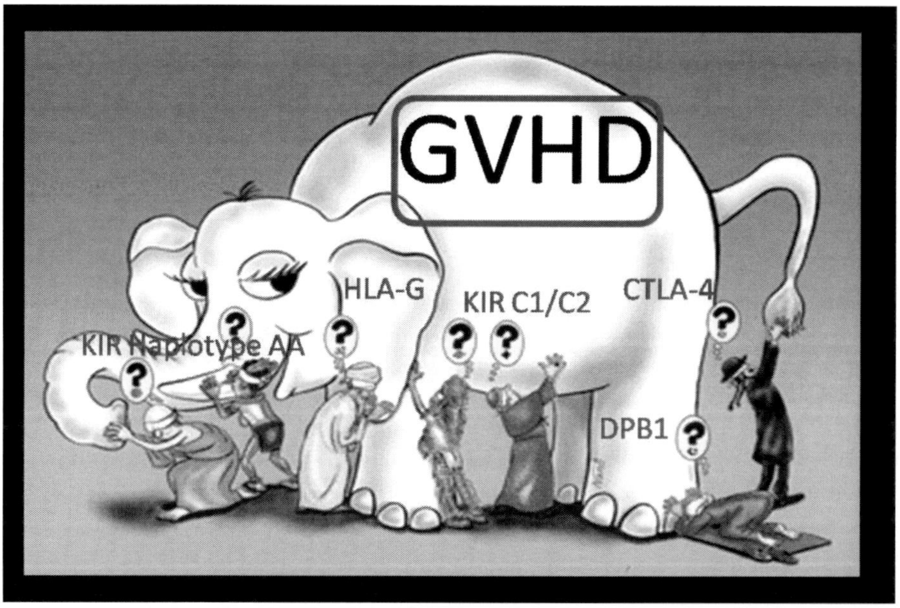

Figure 7. Researchers are currently involved in the study of several variables that seem to have a role in GVHD onset. Unfortunately, a simple prognostic tool that is capable of analyzing the most relevant predictive variables and predicting GVHD is still missing.

Although this information may contribute to our understanding of the pathogenesis of GVHD, it is difficult to apply in clinical practice. We feel like we are groping in the dark for small parts of a big problem (Figure 7). We need a tool capable of analyzing the most relevant predictive variables. In medicine, several tools have been developed for the prediction of outcomes following drug treatment and other medical interventions. The standard approach for a binary outcome is to use logistic regression (LR) but over the past year, artificial neural networks (ANNs) have increasingly been used as an alternative to LR analysis for prognostic and diagnostic classification in clinical medicine [33]. The growing interest in ANNs has mainly been triggered by their ability to mimic the learning processes of the human brain.

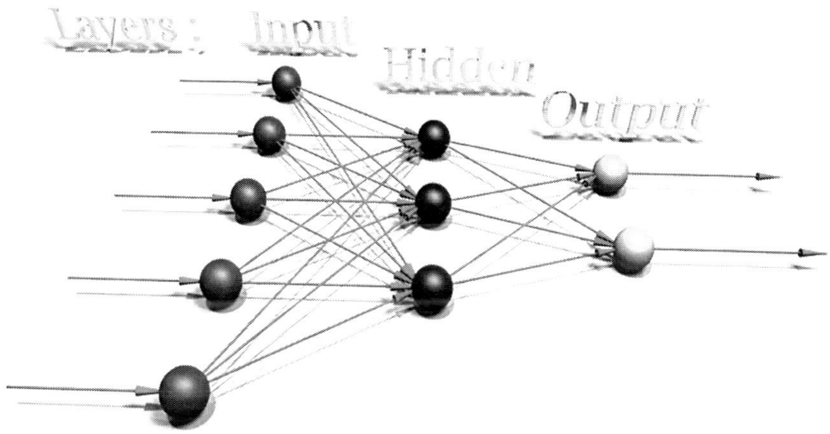

Figure 8. The structure of ANN usually consists of three layers of artificial neurons. The input layer accepts data sets from an external source (input variables). The next layer is called the hidden layer because its neuron values are not visible outside the net. The use of one or more hidden layers increases the net's learning abilities. The final layer is the output layer.

ANNs have been successfully applied in the fields of mathematics, engineering, medicine, economics, meteorology, psychology, neurology, and many others. Indeed, in medicine, they offer a tantalizing alternative to multivariate analysis. However, the issue remains as to how these ANNs actually succeed in recognizing patterns within data that are too complex for the human brain—the so-called "black-box" aspect of ANNs (Figure 8). This all led up to the intriguing challenge of discovering whether ANNs were capable of predicting the outcome of HSCT after analyzing donor and recipient pre-transplantation clinical and immunogenetic variables [34].

Caocci et al [35] set up an ANN to analyze a series of immunogenetic parameters in 72 thalassemia patients who underwent unrelated HSCT: recipient gender, recipient age, donor gender, donor age, the combination male recipient/female donor versus the other possible combinations, recipients and/or donors with positive CMV serology versus donor and recipient pairs with negative CMV serology, the Pesaro risk class at transplantation, HCV-RNA positivity, median infused CD34 cell dose, Treosulfan-containing conditioning regimen versus other regimens, HLA Class I mismatch, presence of HLA-A11, non-permissive HLA-DPB1 disparity in GvH direction, presence of the HLA-G 14-basepair deletion/deletion polymorphism in recipients, presence of the HLA-G 14-basepair deletion/deletion polymorphism in donors, heterozygosity for HLA-Cw ligand groups 1 and 2 in patients, recipient KIR ligand/donor activating KIR (recipient C1 absent/donor KIR2DS2 present versus the other three combinations; recipient C2 absent/donor KIR2DS1 present versus the other 3 combinations), recipient KIR ligand/donor inhibitory KIR (patient C1 absent/donor KIR2DL2 present versus the other three combinations, recipient C1 absent/donor KIR2DL3 present versus the other three combinations, patient C2 absent/donor KIR2DL1 present versus the other three combinations), donor homozygosity for KIR haplotype A.

It was firstly reported the usefulness of ANNs in predicting onset of acute GVHD following HSCT for thalassemia. The decision to perform analyses in this particular clinical setting was motivated by the complexity of clinical decision-making that surrounds the difficult choice of unrelated HSCT donors for thalassemia patients and the relatively large number of immunogenetic and other variables that have been shown to influence the onset of GVHD in this patient cohort. When comparing the prognostic performance of LR to ANN, the ability of predicting acute GVHD was 21.7% for LR versus 83.3% for ANN. The advantage of ANNs over LR can theoretically be explained by their ability to evaluate complex nonlinear relations among variables. By contrast, ANNs have been faulted for functioning as black boxes and for being unable to assess the relative importance of the single variables, while LR determines a relative risk for each variable. In many ways, these two approaches are complementary and their combined use should considerably improve the clinical decision-making process and prognosis of unrelated HSCT in thalassemia.

Conclusion

The immune system of thalassemia patients undergoing allogeneic HSCT is less compromised than that of patients undergoing transplantation for hematologic malignancies. Understanding the role of genetic factors capable of influencing the outcome is fundamental to the increasingly safer application of HSCT. Genetic factors conferring protection or susceptibility to acute GVHD are particularly important, considering that this complication is the main cause of morbidity and mortality following HSCT for thalassemia, but, conversely, can have a beneficial effect on the survival of patients transplanted for leukemias or lymphomas. Within this context, all the immunogenetic variables taken into consideration in this review should be evaluated in thalassemia patients to establish pre-transplantation risk. This approach, combined with the other currently known risk factors, can form the basis for appropriate tailoring of strategies aimed at preventing the onset of acute GVHD and rejection following HSCT for a chronic non-malignant disease.

References

[1] Rund D, Rachmilewitz E. Beta-thalassemia. *N. Engl. J. Med.* 2005; 353: 1135-46.

[2] Borgna-Pignatti C, Vergine G, Lombardo T, Cappellini MD, Cianciulli P, Maggio A, et al. Hepatocellular carcinoma in the thalassaemia syndromes. *Br. J. Haematol.* 2004; 124:114-7.

[3] Borgna Pignatti C. The life of patients with thalassemia major. *Haematologica* 2010; 95:345-347.

[4] Lucarelli G, Giardina C, Baroncini D. Bone marrow transplantation in thalassemia. *Semin. Hematol.* 1995; 32:297-303.

[5] La Nasa G, Giardini C, Argiolu F, Locatelli F, Arras M, De Stefano P, et al. Unrelated donor bone marrow transplantation for thalassemia: the effect of extended haplotypes. *Blood* 2002; 99: 4350-56.

[6] Locatelli F, Littera R, Pagliara D, Contoli B, Giorgiani G, Bernardo ME, et al. Outcome of unrelated donor bone marrow transplantation for thalassemia major patients. *Blood* 2011; 118: Abstract 149.

[7] La Nasa G, Caocci G, Argiolu F, Giardini C, Locatelli F, Vacca A, et al. Unrelated donor bone marrow transplantation in adult patients with thalassemia. *Bone Marrow Transplant.* 2005; 36:971-5.
[8] Cohen A.R, Galanello R, Pennell D.J, Cunningham MJ, Vichinsky E. Thalassemia. *Hematology Am. Soc. Hematol. Educ. Program* 2004: 14-34.
[9] Lucarelli G, Andreani M, Angelucci E. The cure of thalassemia by bone marrow transplantation. *Blood Rev.* 2002; 16: 81–85.
[10] La Nasa G, Argiolu F, Giardini C, Pession A, Fagioli F, Caocci G et al. Unrelated bone marrow transplantation for beta-thalassemia patients: the experience of the Italian Bone Marrow Transplant Group. *Ann. N. Y. Acad. Sci.* 2005; 1054: 186–195.
[11] Locatelli F, Rocha V, Reed W, Bernaudin F, Ertem M, Grafakos S et al. Related umbilical cord blood transplantation in patients with thalassemia and sickle cell disease. *Blood* 2003; 101: 2137–2143.
[12] Hongeng S, Pakakasama S, Chuansumrit A, Sirachainan N, Kitpoka P, Udomsubpayakul U et al. Outcomes of transplantation with related- and unrelated-donor stem cells in children with severe thalassemia. *Biol. Blood Marrow Transplant.* 2006; 12: 683–687.
[13] Gaziev D, Galimberti M, Lucarelli G, Polchi P, Giardini C, Angelucci E et al. Bone marrow transplantation from alternative donors for thalassemia: HLA-phenotypically identical relative and HLA-nonidentical sibling or parent transplants. *Bone Marrow Transplant.* 2000; 25: 815–821.
[14] Jaing TH, Hung IJ, Yang CP, Chen SH, Chung HT, Tsay PK, et al. Unrelated cord blood transplantation for thalassaemia: a single-institution experience of 35 patients. *Bone Marrow Transplant.* 2012; 47:33-9.
[15] Ruggeri A, Eapen M, Scaravadou A, Cairo MS, Bhatia M, Kurtzberg J, et al. Umbelical cord blood transplantation for children with thalassemia and sickle cell disease. *Biol. Blood Marrow Transplant.* 2011; 17:1375-1382.
[16] Zino E, Frumento G, Marktel S, Sormani MP, Ficara F, Di Terlizzi S, et al. A T-cell epitope encoded by a subset of HLA-DPB1 alleles determines nonpermissive mismatches for hematologic stem cell transplantation. *Blood* 2004; 103:1417-24.
[17] Fleischhauer K, Locatelli F, Zecca M, Orofino MG, Giardini C, De Stefano P, et al. Graft rejection after unrelated donor hematopoietic stem cell transplantation for thalassemia is associated with nonpermissive HLA-DPB1 disparity in host-versus-graft direction. *Blood* 2006; 10:2984-92.
[18] Crocchiolo R, Zino E, Vago L, Oneto R, Bruno B, Pollichieni S, Sacchi N, et al. Nonpermissive HLA-DPB1 disparity is a significant independent risk factor for mortality after unrelated hematopoietic stem cell transplantation. *Blood* 2009; 114:1437-44.
[19] Fleischhauer K, Shaw BE, Gooley T, Malkki M, Bardy P, Bignon JD, et al. Effect of T-cell-epitope matching at HLA-DPB1 in recipients of unrelated-donor haemopoietic-cell transplantation: a retrospective study. *Lancet Oncol.* 2012 Feb 14 [Epub ahead of print].
[20] Moretta A, Locatelli F, Moretta L. Human NK cells: from HLA class I-specific killer Ig-like receptors to the therapy of acute leukemias. *Immunol. Rev.* 2008; 224: 58–69.
[21] Trowsdale J. Genetic and functional relationships between MHC and NK receptor genes. *Immunity* 2001; 15: 363–374.

[22] La Nasa G, Littera R, Locatelli F, Giardini C, Ventrella A, Mulargia M, et al. Status of donor-recipient HLA class I ligands and not the KIR genotype is predictive for the outcome of unrelated hematopoietic stem cell transplantation in beta-thalassemia patients. *Biol. Blood Marrow Transplant.* 2007; 13:1358-68.
[23] Littera R, Orrù N, Vacca A, Bertaina A, Caocci G, Mulargia M, et al. The role of killer immunoglobulin-like receptor haplotypes on the outcome of unrelated donor haematopoietic SCT for thalassaemia. *Bone Marrow Transplant.* 2010; 45:1618-24.
[24] Littera R, Orrù N, Caocci G, Sanna M, Mulargia M, Piras E, et al. Interactions between killer immunoglobulin-like receptors and their human leucocyte antigen Class I ligands influence the outcome of unrelated haematopoietic stem cell transplantation for thalassaemia: a novel predictive algorithm. *Br. J. Haematol.* 2012; 156:118-28.
[25] Kovats S, Main EK, Librach C, Dtubblebine M, Fisher SJ, DeMars R. A class I antigen, HLA-G, expressed in human trophoblasts. *Science,* 1990; 248:220-223.
[26] Carosella ED, Favier B, Rouas-Freiss N, Moreau P, LeMaoult P. Beyond the increasing complexity of the immunomodulatory HLA-G molecule. *Blood* 2008; 11:4862-4870.
[27] Le Rond S, Aze´ma C, Krawice-Radanne I, Durrbach A, Guettier C, Carosella ED, Rouas-Freiss N. Evidence to support the role of HLA-G5 in allograft acceptance through induction of immunosuppressive/ regulatory T cells. *Journal of Immunology,* 2006; 176:3266–3276.
[28] Harrison GA, Humphrey KE, Jakobsen IB, Cooper DW. A 14-bp deletion polymorphism in the HLA-G gene. *Human Molecular Genetics,* 1993; 2:2200.
[29] La Nasa G, Littera R, Locatelli F, Lai S, Alba F, Caocci G, et al. The human leucocyte antigen-G 14-basepair polymorphism correlates with graft-versus-host disease in unrelated bone marrow transplantation for thalassaemia. *Br. J. Haematol.* 2007; 139:284-8.
[30] Magistrelli G, Jeannin P, Herbault N, Benoit De Coignac A, Gauchat JF, et al. A soluble form of CTLA-4 generated by alternative splicing is expressed by nonstimulated human T cells. *Eur. J. Immunol.* 1999; 29:3596–602.
[31] Perez-Garcia A, De la Camara R, Roman-Gomez J, Jimenez-Velasco A, Encuentra M, Nieto JB, et al. CTLA-4 polymorphisms and clinical outcome after allogeneic stem cell transplantation from HLA-identical sibling donors. *Blood* 2007; 110:461–467.
[32] Orrù S, Orrù N, Manolakos E, Littera R, Caocci G, Giorgiani G, et al. Recipient CTLA-4*CT60-AA genotype is a prognostic factor for acute graft-versus-host disease in hematopoietic stem cell transplantation for thalassemia. *Human Immunology.* 2012; 73:282-286.
[33] Schwarzer G, Vach W, Schumacher M. On the misuses of artificial neural networks for prognostic and diagnostic classification in oncology. *Stat. Med.* 2000; 19:541-561.
[34] Caocci G, Baccoli R, Vacca A, Mastronuzzi A, Bertaina A, Piras E, et al. Comparison between an artificial neural network and logistic regression in predicting acute graft-vs-host disease after unrelated donor hematopoietic stem cell transplantation in thalassemia patients. *Exp. Hematol.* 2010; 38:426-33.

In: Hematopoietic Stem Cells: New Research ISBN 978-1-62257-468-1
Editors: Wesley G. Montgomery and Heather I. Burton ©2012 Nova Science Publishers, Inc.

Chapter 5

HEMATOPOIETIC STEM CELL THERAPY FOR INFLAMMATORY BOWEL DISEASES

***W. K. van Deen*[1,2], *G. M. Crooks*[3] *and D. W. Hommes*[1]**
[1]Center for Inflammatory Bowel Diseases, UCLA, Los Angeles, CA, US
[2]Department of Gastroenterology and Hepatology, Leiden University Medical Center, Leiden, The Netherlands
[3]Department of Pathology and Laboratory Medicine and Department of Pediatrics, David Geffen School of Medicine, UCLA, Los Angeles, CA, US

ABSTRACT

Inflammatory bowel diseases (IBD) are chronic debilitating inflammatory disorders of potentially any part of the gastrointestinal tract, leading to various intestinal but also extra-intestinal symptoms. It is thought that dysregulation of the normally controlled immune response to commensal bacteria in genetically susceptible patients drives the disease. Although medical therapy for IBD has improved due to an extensive repertoire of immunosuppressive drugs and the introduction of anti tumor necrosis factor-α (TNFα) compounds, the clinical course of the disease cannot be adequately controlled in a substantial group of patients. More than half of the patients require one or more surgical resections during the course of the disease. Therefore, there is an unmet need for more effective therapeutic strategies.

Evidence that hematopoietic stem cell transplantation (HSCT) would be an effective treatment for autoimmune diseases firstly came from several animal models and from incidental case reports on HSCT recipients with coexistent autoimmune disease. Already more than 15 years ago a case report on the positive effect of HSCT on active IBD was published, followed by many others showing improvement of the clinical course of disease after HSCT indicated for other diseases. In the last couple of years, various cases have been reported of successful remission induction of patients with (therapy refractory) Crohn's disease (CD) by means of an autologous HSCT. The most extensive experience on autologous HSCT applied specifically for CD has been reported by the group of Oyama. All treated patients went into remission with a Crohn's Disease Activity Index (CDAI) score of <150. There was no inpatient mortality and neutropenic fever was the most important complication. Recently published long-term follow follow-up data showed a clinical relapse-free survival of 57% at 3 years and 19% at 5 years. The percentage of patients in remission (CDAI<150), steroid free, or medication free at any post-transplant evaluation interval over 5 years post-transplant was 70%, 80% and 60%, respectively.

Although the observed benefit is remarkable, the exact mechanism behind this 'resetting' of the immune system needs to be elucidated. Although the prolonged T cell depletion will probably add to the therapeutic benefit, the thymus most likely plays a dominant role in resetting the T cell repertoire in IBD patients. This chapter will review the evidence for HSCT for IBD and discuss potential mechanisms of HSCT important for clinical benefit.

INTRODUCTION

Inflammatory bowel diseases (IBD) are debilitating disorders characterized by chronic inflammation of the gastrointestinal system and cause a considerable amount of morbidity. Even though treatment options for these patients have improved over the past years, the course of the disease is still hard to control in many patients. Many will require surgery and recurrence is common afterwards. [1, 2] In the past decades hematopoietic stem cell transplantation (HSCT) has been explored as possible therapeutic option for autoimmune disorders (AIDs). Promising results have been published, but the underlying mechanism is still largely unclear. This chapter will review HSCT as a treatment modality for AIDs and for IBD specifically. The possible underlying mechanisms will be discussed as well.

INFLAMMATORY BOWEL DISEASES

Symptoms

Inflammatory bowel diseases are diseases characterized by chronic inflammation of the gastrointestinal tract. Both Crohn's disease (CD) and ulcerative colitis (UC) are part of the IBD spectrum. Patients suffer from relapsing flares, clinically manifesting in bloody diarrhea, abdominal pain and malnutrition. CD and UC can be distinguished by location and type of inflammation. In CD the inflammation can affect the entire gastrointestinal tract and is usually transmural with a discontinuous pattern. In UC the inflammation involves solely mucosa and submucosa and is characterized by a continuous pattern of inflammation starting in the rectum. In UC, the inflammation is confined to the colon and can therefore be cured by colectomy. [1, 3] Next to gastrointestinal complaints, 25 – 40% of IBD patients suffer from extraintestinal manifestations of IBD. The most common extraintestinal manifestations are musculoskeletal manifestations such as ankylosing spondylitis and skin lesions such as pyoderma gangrenosum. [4]

Epidemiology

Incidence rates for IBD differ between regions, with the highest incidence rates reported in the developed world, ranging from 17.4 – 24.3 per 100,000 for UC and 10.6 – 29.3 per

100,000 for CD in Canada, Australia and Northern Europe. Incidence rates for IBD seem to be equally distributed between sexes, with the highest incidence rates between the second and fourth decade of life. [5] Many environmental risk factors have been described to contribute to IBD development, however, many of them remain controversial. Among these risk factors, smoking has most clearly been shown to be positively correlated with CD and negatively with UC. [6]

Pathophysiology

Dysregulation of the intestinal immune system seems to be a leading cause in the development of IBD in a genetically prone individual. The intestinal immune system is exposed to both pathogenic microorganisms and to high concentrations of luminal commensal bacteria. Therefore, a strict immune regulation and immune tolerance is necessary to maintain a healthy bowel. Dysregulation of this balance might contribute to the development of IBD and might be caused by alterations in epithelial barrier function, innate immunity or lymphocyte function. [3] Inflammation in IBD is driven by $CD4^+$ T helper cells. In UC, the response is mainly driven by an atypical T_h2-response, whereas in CD the response is mainly T_h1-driven and also IL-17 producing T_h17 cells are likely to play a role in CD development. [1]

Genetics

Genetic predisposition plays a major role in IBD development, but seems to be more profound in CD than in UC. The concordance rate in monozygotic twins is 10 – 15% in UC and 39 – 35% in CD, suggesting that genetic factors are more important in CD development, while environmental factors are more important in UC development. The first gene identified to be associated with IBD was the *NOD2* gene, a gene that is implicated in modulation of both innate and adaptive immune responses. Since then, many other genes have been found to be associated with IBD development using genome wide association studies. Both protective and predisposing alleles have been described, and single nucleotide polymorphisms (SNPs) in both coding and non-coding regions. By now approximately 100 genetic risk loci have been described, of which 30% overlap between CD and UC. These loci are important in many different pathways involved in IBD pathogenesis. Genes have for example been found to be associated with epithelial barrier function, regulation of reactive oxygen species, innate and adaptive immune regulation, autophagy and metabolic pathways. Interestingly about 50% of the identified genes involved in IBD development overlap with genes involved in the development of other AIDs. [7]

Treatment

IBD treatment consists of induction therapy, to subside the acute phase, and maintenance therapy, to prevent relapse. Depending on the extent and severity of inflammation, maintenance therapy for UC usually consists of orally or rectally administered sulfasalazine,

5-ASA or thiopurines. For induction of remission in UC, glucocorticosteroids, administered orally, rectally or intravenously, can be used in addition to maintenance therapy. Infliximab, an anti tumor necrosis factor-α (TNFα) agent is a good alternative for patients who do not respond sufficiently to intravenous corticosteroids or who continue to be glucocorticosteroid dependent. Because of the relatively mild course of the disease usually a step-up treatment regimen is preferred in UC. Medications with fewer side effects are prescribed as initial therapy and only if remission is not achieved another dosage or drug with possibly more side effects will be prescribed. [1] Conventional therapy for CD also follows a step-up approach, starting with glucocorticosteroids during a flare, then adding thiopurines or methotrexate. In case of refractory disease or intolerance to these drugs, anti TNFα agents are started. However, a top-down approach, where initial treatment is started with aggressive anti TNFα therapy with or without other immunosuppressive agents, might be preferable in certain patients with high risk of developing a severe course of the disease. [8]

Complications

Complications in IBD are the cause of many hospitalizations and surgeries and cause substantial morbidity and disability. Acute complications in UC include severe bleeding, bowel perforation and toxic megacolon. 5 – 20% of UC patients eventually have to undergo colectomy during the course of their disease. [1] For CD most common complications are the formation of strictures, abscesses and fistula, which occurs in 50% of patients in the 20 years following diagnosis. 50% of CD patients need surgery within 10 years after diagnosis, 60% of them need a second surgery within the next 15 years. [9] In the long term UC and CD patients have a 40 – 70% increased risk of developing osteoporotic fractures and have an increased risk of developing intestinal malignancies. A slight decrease in life expectancy has been reported for CD patients. [2]

Hematopoietic Stem Cell Transplantation

History

Hematopoietic stem cells (HSCs) are the source of all blood cells. They have the unique capacities to give rise to more differentiated progenitor cells and to self renew. Theoretically one single stem cell can give rise to an entire immune system. Hematopoietic stem cell transplantation (HSCT) has been used for over 50 years to treat many malignant and non-malignant disorders. Animal experiments were the first to show that HSCT could rescue animals treated with total body irradiation from death by generating a new hematopoietic system. [10] The first patients who underwent experimental HSCT for different indications were reported in 1957 [11], and in 1959 the first successful transplantation for end stage leukemia was reported, resulting in remission of leukemia for 3 months after transplantation of bone marrow from an identical twin. [12] Many patients followed afterwards and up till now HSCT is used as a treatment modality for many diseases. Most common indications for HSCT now are hematologic malignancies such as multiple myeloma, Non-Hodgkin's lymphoma and acute leukemia's. In addition, several inherited disorders such as severe combined immunodeficiency and thalassemia are currently treated by HSCT. The use of HSCT has also been reported as treatment option for a variety of AIDs. [10]

Procedure

The HSCT procedure consists of the harvest of stem cells, a preparative regimen and the actual stem cell transplantation. The hematopoietic stem cells (HSCs) can be isolated from the bone marrow (BM), from peripheral blood after a mobilization procedure, usually using granulocyte colony-stimulating factor (GCSF), or from umbilical cord blood. When cells are isolated from peripheral blood the graft contains relatively fewer HSCs and more T cells. HSCs can be derived either from the patient (autologous transplantation) or from a related or unrelated healthy donor (allogeneic transplantation). A preparative regimen is necessary to facilitate marrow engraftment of HSCs and progenitors, and in the case of allogeneic HSCT, to eradicate the recipient's immune system to prevent rejection of the graft. Various preparative regimens are used that combine high dose chemotherapy, with or without total body irradiation. Originally only myeloablative regimens (i.e. those that completely destroy endogenous HSCs) were used with the thought that the preparative regimen was required to "make space" in the host bone marrow. However, experimental models and subsequent clinical studies, have demonstrated that engraftment can occur with less aggressive preparative regimens (so called "reduced intensity" or "nonmyeloablative" conditioning) leading to reduced toxicity from the procedure. The transplantation itself is performed by intravenous administration of the graft. Before allogeneic HSCT, T cell depletion of the graft is sometimes performed to remove alloreactive donor T cells and reduce the incidence of graft-versus-host disease (GvHD). [10, 13]

Complications

The main complications after autologous HSCT are organ toxicity from the preparative regimens and infections, due to the neutropenia and immune deficient state that persists until full immune reconstitution is achieved. The transplant related mortality (TRM) rate for autologous HSCT varies depending on the preparative regimen and pre-transplant status of patients, but overall TRM has been steadily reduced with better supportive measures, now ranging from 2 – 5%. In allogeneic HSCT acute or chronic GvHD, a condition in which the T cells within the graft induce an alloreactive response against the host, is the other main cause of treatment related morbidity and mortality. The mortality rates for allogeneic HSCT range from 10 – 40% depending on various factors, among others the underlying disease and age. [10]

Mechanism

The objective of the preparative regimen is to induce changes in the bone marrow to allow HSC engraftment and to immune suppress the host to prevent rejection of the graft. In the case of hematologic malignancies, the preparative regimen is also used to eradicate the cancer. Compared to a reduced intensity regimen, a myeloablative regimen eradicates more of the cancer and induces a more profound immune suppression with higher engraftment rates. But, because of the higher complication and infection rates associated with a myeloablative regimen, the risks might exceed the benefits. The transplantation, in both allogeneic and in autologous settings, is performed to prevent death due to the damage caused by the preparative regimen, by replacing the immune system with a new one. Allogeneic HSCT though offers another advantage in cancer patients. Donor T cell reactivity against the tumor can promote eradication of eventual tumor rests that have survived the preparative regimen. This effect is called graft-versus-tumor effect (GvT) and resembles the mechanism of graft-versus-host disease (GvHD), where donor derived T cells react against host tissue. [10]

Acute GvHD is caused by infusion and expansion of donor derived alloreactive T cells, that cause an immune reaction against host tissue. Alloreactive T cells also play a central role in chronic GvHD, but the mechanism and optimal treatment of this complication is less clear. Clinical manifestations of chronic GvHD typically arise beyond 100 days post transplantation and often resemble autoimmune disease. To prevent GvHD the graft can be depleted of T cells, either by positive selection of CD34+ hematopoietic cells or by depletion of lymphocytes. However, with T cell depletion the GvT effect is also diminished, and the risk of infection is markedly increased because of delayed immune reconstitution. The best approach must therefore balance between the need to achieve disease remission through GvT effect, while preventing infection, and the need to prevent GvHD, and thus must be tailored for each patient. [13]

Hematopoietic Stem Cell Transplantation in Autoimmune Diseases

History

The first evidence that HSCT could serve as a potential treatment for autoimmune diseases came from preclinical animal experiments [14] and several case reports of patients who suffered from AIDs, who were treated with HSCT for concominant cancer or aplastic anemia. Most patients who were described initially suffered from rheumatoid arthritis (RA), psoriasis or systemic lupus erythematosus (SLE) and underwent either autologous or allogeneic HSCT for malignancies. In some patients, their AID seemed to run a favorable course after HSCT, with a reported remission of RA up to 13 years post allogeneic HSCT for severe aplastic anemia. [15] In 1996 the European League against Rheumatism (EULAR) and the European Group for Blood and Marrow Transplantation (EBMT) came together to discuss the new possibility of treating AIDs with HSCT. They developed a standardized protocol for HSCT specifically for AID treatment, with the objective to stimulate the structured development of phase I/II trials in this field. Furthermore, a database was developed where these trials were registered. They proposed the use of mainly autologous transplants because of the high mortality rate associated with allogeneic HSCT. [16] The first case report was published 1 month later and described a patient suffering from severe systemic sclerosis (SSc) with pulmonary hypertension and skin manifestations unresponsive to conventional therapy.

She underwent autologous HSCT and 6 months post transplantation a clear improvement of skin manifestations was observed and no pulmonary hypertension was detected. [17] Afterwards hundreds of patients were registered in the EBMT database, most of them suffered from SLE, SSc, RA or multiple sclerosis (MS). [18]

Clinical Trials

In 2009 an analysis of the data registered in the EBMT database between 1996 and 2007 was published. 900 patients who had received an autologous HSCT for various types of AID were analyzed. The overall survival after 5 years was 85%, the progression free survival 43%. A 100 day mortality rate of 5% was reported. Half of the total recorded deaths were related to the transplantation procedure, infection being the leading cause of death. A strong correlation between mortality and experience of transplantation center and between mortality and type of autoimmune disease was shown. Interestingly no significant difference in survival between different conditioning regimens was observed. Depleting the graft of T cells did not affect survival either, nor did it affect the progression free survival. [18]

An analysis of 35 patients in the EBMT database who received allogeneic HSCT for AID was also published in 2009. Treatment related mortality was 20% within the first 3 months post transplantation and 30% after 5 years. Complete remission was achieved in 55%, partial remission in 24%. 13% (3 patients) of the cases in whom complete or partial remission was achieved relapsed after a median of 12.3 months after transplantation. Interestingly in all patients who developed chronic GvHD, improvement of their AID was observed post transplantation. Also in this study no significant correlation between outcome and type of preparative regimen or between outcome and T cell depletion of the graft was observed. [19]

Hematopoietic Stem Cell Transplantation for Inflammatory Bowel Diseases

History

The idea of HSCT as a treatment for IBD came from several reports of CD patients undergoing HSCT for concomitant malignancies. The first published case of a CD patient undergoing BM transplantation dates from 1993 and describes a 41 year old CD patient undergoing autologous BM transplantation for non-Hodgkin lymphoma who stayed in remission from CD up till 6 months after HSCT [20]. Since that date several other reports regarding CD and UC patients undergoing autologous HSCT for other indications, who stayed in prolonged remission have been published [21-26].

Several cases of improvement of CD after allogeneic HSCT have also been reported. In 1998, 6 patients with CD and concomitant malignancies undergoing allogeneic HSCT were described. All patients received an allogeneic bone marrow transplant from a related or unrelated donor after undergoing a myeloablative preparative regimen. One patient died 97 days post transplantation of apparent septic shock, four of the other five patients remained in remission from CD during a follow up ranging from 4.5 – 15 years. Interestingly the only patient who did relapse showed a mixed donor-host chimerism and all patients who stayed in remission suffered from chronic GvHD. [27] Another retrospective study described 7 CD and 4 UC patients receiving allogeneic HSCT for other indications. Ten out of 11 patients had no evidence of chronic inflammation during the follow up of 3 – 117 months. Only one patient experienced mild bowel inflammation in the post transplant course. One patient died 10 months after transplantation of pulmonary fungal infection. [28]

Clinical Trials

After these case reports, several reports regarding CD patients who underwent autologous HSCT specifically for CD have been published. In 2003 a patient with a history of CD for 13 years that was not well controlled by conventional therapy underwent a nonmyeloablative conditioning regimen followed by autologous HSCT. Histologic remission was achieved after HSCT and lasted for 9 months after which conventional therapy was restarted prophylactically. [29] A report published in 2004 described another CD patient refractory to all conventional therapy who underwent autologous HSCT after a nonmyeloablative conditioning regimen. The patient stayed in clinical remission up to at least 5 months post transplantation, and endoscopic and histological improvement was also observed. [30] Recently a case report was presented that described a CD patient that remained disease free (clinical and histological) until at least 26 months after autologous HSCT [31].

Our own experience consists of 3 patients with severe CD who underwent autologous HSCT. All patients were refractory to conventional therapy including anti TNFα therapy and surgery was an unattractive option in all of them. The patients were conditioned with cyclophosphamide (CTX) and anti thymocyte globulin (ATG) followed by infusion of $CD34^+$ enriched GCSF-mobilized peripheral blood stem cells. In 1 patient complete clinical remission was achieved after the GCSF mobilization procedure, and did therefore not proceed to conditioning or HSCT. Clinical remission in this patient was retained up to 1.5 years after mobilization. The other 2 patients improved after HSCT. In one patient medication was restarted 12 months after HSCT, no luminal relapse was observed in the 6 years of follow up. In the third patient medication was restarted 6 months after HSCT and the patient relapsed only after 5 years post HSCT. There was no transplant related mortality and side effects appeared manageable. [32]

In 2008 a phase I/II trial was published that described 4 CD patients with a Crohn's Disease Activity Index (CDAI) >250, all refractory to conventional drugs including anti TNFα. All patients underwent autologous HSCT following a nonmyeloablative conditioning regimen. In this trial no CD34+ enrichment of the graft was performed to decrease infection risk. After HSCT clinical remission was achieved in 3 of the 4 patients within 1 month, the 4th patient went into remission within month 3. After a median follow up of 16.5 months 75% of patients remained in remission without further treatment and in all those patients fistula resolved. 1 patient relapsed in the 4th month, and remained a clinical dilemma. All patients experienced neutropenic fever, but blood cultures were negative and no life-threatening infections were reported. [33] Recently this group reported that a total of 10 patients are included in this trial in total now, with a follow up ranging from 23 – 68 months. Remission was achieved within one month post HSCT in 80% of patients. After 1, 3 and 5 year respectively 80%, 40% and 30% of patients remained in remission. [34]

Table 1. Overview of patients undergoing HSCT specifically for CD

Reference	Number of patients	Mobilization	Response to mobilization procedure	Conditioning regimen	CD34+ enrichment of the graft	Complications (number of patients)	Reported remission	TRM
Kreisel e.a. 2003 [29]	1	CTX + GCSF	Clinical, but not histological remission for 10 months	CTX	yes	Neutropenic fever	Restarted CD drugs 9 months post HSCT, in clinical remission during 12 months of follow up.	0%
Scimè e.a. 2004 [30]	1	CTX + GCSF	Clinical response, no endoscopic improvement	CTX + equine ATG	yes	Infection, transfusion requirement	In clinical remission during 5 months of follow up	0%
Cassinotti e.a. 2007 [33]	4	CTX + GCSF	Deterioration in 3 patients, in 1 improvement. 1 developed perianal abscess	CTX + rabbit ATG	no	Pleural/pericardial effusion (1), culture-negative fever (4), hematuria (1)	75% in clinical and endoscopic remission after median follow up of 16.5 months	0%
Burt e.a. 2010 [35]	24	CTX + GCSF	Unquantified improvement in symptoms	CTX + equine/rabbit ATG	yes	Infection (19), sepsis (1), GI complaints (14), pulmonary edema (2), perirectal abscess (1)	91% at 1 year, 57% at 3 years 19% at 5 years, in remission defined as CD drugs not restarted	0% (1 ac-cidental death during follow up)
Kountouras e.a. 2011 [31]	1	CTX + GCSF	n/a	CTX + rabbit ATG	n/a	No reported complications	Clinical, endoscopic and histological remission during 31 months follow up	0%
Hommes e.a. 2011 [32]	3 (1 did not receive HSCT after mobilization)	CTX + GCSF	1 patient 2 years in remission	CTX + equine ATG	yes	Transfusion required (3), allergic reaction to ATG (1), transient deterioration in kidney function (1), infection (2)	1 patient 6 years in clinical remission, 1 patient relapsed after 5 years	0%
Cassinotti e.a. 2012 [34]	10 (incl. 4 reported in 2007 [33])	CTX + GCSF	No improvement	CTX + rabbit ATG	no	Pleural/pericardial effusion (1), hematuria (1), acute pyelonephritis (1)	80% at 1 year, 40% at 3 years 30% at 5 years in clinical remission	0%

ATG=anti thymocyte globulin, CD=Crohn's disease, CDAI=Crohn's disease activity index, CTX=cyclophosphamide, GCSF= granulocyte colony-stimulating factor, HSCT=hematopoietic stem cell transplantation, TRM=treatment related morbidity.

The most extensive experience on HSCT for IBD was recently published by the Oyama group. [35] They performed a phase I/II study, and describe a cohort of 24 patients with active CD undergoing autologous HSCT, with a follow up of 5 years. All patients had a CDAI >250 or a Crohn's Severity Index (CSI)>16 and failed to respond to conventional therapy including anti TNFα biologicals. All patients underwent autologous HSCT after $CD34^+$ enrichment of the graft. A rapid and significant drop in CDAI and CSI was observed after transplantation. The rate of clinical relapse-free survival (defined as not restarting CD medication) was 91% at 1 year, 57% at 3 years and 19% at 5 years. During the entire period more than 70% of the patients were in remission independent of therapy, over 60% were medication free and around 80% were steroid free. No treatment related mortality was observed, and the main reported complications were neutropenic fever and infections. [35] See table 1 for an overview of the abovementioned reports on HSCT specifically for CD.

MECHANISM

Autologous HSCT

The rationale for using autologous HSCT to treat AID is that depletion of autoreactive T and B cells via lympho-ablative preparative regimen will induce remission and that immune reconstitution post HSCT will result in a naïve and tolerant T cell pool without auto-reactive cells and maintenance of remission. Clearly the likelihood of success depends on whether the particular AID is genetically determined and to what extent the disease is induced by environmental factors.

In the first scenario, as autologous HSCs are given, the underlying genetic susceptibility of the host will not be removed, and theoretically the patient will remain at increased risk for developing AID compared to the general population. In the second scenario, if the environmental factors that initially lead to the AID do not appear again, AID will not recur. Observed relapses of AIDs after HSCT might be explained by newly developed autoreactive clones in a susceptible host or by incomplete removal or reinfusion of autoreactive cells.

To prevent reinfusion of autoreactive cells the graft can be depleted of B- and T-cells. However, this approach increases the risk of infection, due to the prolonged depletion of immune cells. [36] The conditioning regimen itself, and even the GSCF mobilization procedure, might also contribute to the observed improvement of AIDs after HSCT, since it induces extensive immune deficiency due to prolonged lymphopenia. [37] However, the observed improvements of AID after HSCT seem to last longer than the duration of the immunosuppressive state. [38, 39]

Allogeneic HSCT

Allogeneic HSCT offers the theoretical advantage of replacing an immune system genetically prone to AID with a healthy one. Transferring susceptibility for developing AID through HSCT has been described in animals [14] and in human [40,41]. Several reports of patients without previous history of IBD who developed UC [42, 43] or CD [44] after undergoing HSCT support this concept as well.

Allogeneic transplantation followed by immune reconstitution by both host and donor HSCs, inducing a state of mixed donor- host hematopoietic chimerism, may also be advantageous by inducing tolerance, even though the genetic susceptibility of the host is not deleted. If both donor and host HSCs give rise to all hematopoietic cells, thymic dendritic cells will also be derived from both host and donor. Negative selection of T cell clones in the thymus will therefore be mediated by both host and donor cells and autoreactive clones will be deleted, thereby inducing a state of tolerance to autoantigens. [36]

Thymic Immune Reconstitution After Hematopoietic Stem Cell Transplantation

Physiology of the Thymus

Lymphoid commitment starts in the bone marrow, where HSCs divide and give rise to various multipotent progenitors. These progenitors subsequently home to the thymus where they pass through a complex series of stages from T lineage commitment and differentiation ultimately developing into mature naïve T cells. In addition to the hematopoietic cells, or thymocytes, the thymus consists of thymic stroma, consisting of a network of epithelial and mesenchymal cells that, in addition to dendritic cells, orchestrate the process of thymopoiesis. As thymocytes differentiate in the thymus, TCR gene rearrangement occurs, providing a diverse T cell repertoire. The twin programs of positive and negative selection result in the production of MHC-restricted and tolerant T cells respectively. First, only T cells with TCRs that interact with self MHC molecules are positively selected and are able to transition from the immature $CD4^{+}CD8^{+}$ (double positive) stage into either $CD4^{+}$ or $CD8^{+}$ cells; those that cannot interact with self MHC undergo apoptosis. Thereafter, T cells undergo a process of negative selection, where those that adhere too strongly to self MHC-peptide complexes are deleted from the T cell repertoire to prevent the release of autoreactive T cells. Following negative selection, naïve tolerant T cells are released into the peripheral blood and travel to the peripheral lymph nodes and spleen. [45]

Although the thymus is essential in generation of new T cells, enumeration of T cells in peripheral blood is not a reliable measure of thymic function because of the contribution of peripheral expansion. T cell receptor excision circles (TRECs), DNA byproducts produced during the process of TCR gene rearrangements in the thymus, can be used as a marker for recent thymic emigrants (RTEs). These TRECs do not duplicate during cell division and are therefore progressively lost during proliferation of mature T cells in the peripheray. To determine T cell diversity, the variability within the lengths of a highly variable region in the TCR is determined or this region can be sequenced directly. [46]

The function of the thymus declines with age, through a process called thymic involution. Throughout life, the thymus is gradually replaced by fat, and epithelial function wanes. This process results in a decline in T cell production. The dysregulation of thymopoiesis from aged and inadequate thymic microenvironment can also lead to a defect in negative selection and escape from the thymus of auto-reactive T cells. Several different approaches have been shown to reverse the process of thymic involution in mice, at least temporarily. These approaches include sex steroid ablation (SSA) or administration of interleukin-7 (IL-7) or keratinocyte growth factor (KGF). [47]

Thymic Function after HSCT

In the aforementioned process of immune replacement after HSCT the thymus appears to play a crucial role. After HSCT protective T lymphocytes from the host are destroyed by the conditioning regimen, thereby causing severe immune deficiency. This causes a high risk of developing infectious complications, so rapid reconstitution of the immune system is necessary for a favorable outcome of HSCT.

Early protective immunity after HSCT can be obtained from the peripheral expansion of mature T cells that either survive the conditioning regimen, or are contained within the infused graft. These memory T cells can respond to antigen quickly but tend to have a narrow TCR repertoir. For an adequate reaction upon new pathogens, a broad repertoire of naïve T cells generated in the thymus is needed. RTEs can be detected within 3 months of HSCT but complete repopulation of the immune system can be delayed for several more months after HSCT. [48]

A functional thymus is a prerequisite for successful repopulation of T cells. Since thymic function decreases with age and is affected by the underlying disease, these factors might influence the outcome of HSCT. Poor thymic function before transplantation has shown to be associated with poorer survival rates, independent of underlying disease. Thymic damage due to the preparative regimen or in case of allogeneic HSCT due to GvHD might also hinder successful recovery. Theoretically, different approaches might be taken to improve thymic function to support repopulation. Therapies might be aimed to improve BM engraftment, to increase homing of precursors to the thymus or to support regeneration of the thymic epithelium. [47]

Function of the Thymus after HSCT Specifically for AID

Since most AIDs are caused by an underlying defect in T cell function, HSCT offers the advantage of creating a new immune system without this T cell defect. However, it is conceivable that thymic function might be more impaired in patients with AID, thus hampering the induction of tolerance after HSCT. Several groups by now have investigated the immune reconstitution after HSCT in patients with AID. [38, 39]

The development of a new and diverse T cell repertoire (TCR) after HSCT was reported in 2005 in a study of seven MS patients followed prospectively for up to 36 months following autologous HSCT after a myeloablative conditioning regimen. All patients stayed in remission from MS during the period of follow up. Six months after transplantation the absolute lymphocyte number had recovered, suggesting that sustained remission beyond this period could not be solely ascribed to the lymphocytopenia induced by the conditioning regimen. Increased numbers of naïve T cells and decreased numbers of central memory T cells were noted. T cells were shown to be of recent thymic origin by TREC assays. Diversity of the TCR repertoire had recovered 2 years after HSCT, without re-emergence of MS. These results demonstrate that T cells with a diverse TCR repertoire were generated in the thymus after autologous HSCT following a myeloablative regimen in patients with MS.[38] Similar findings were reported for seven SLE patients undergoing autologous HSCT, with a follow up of 8 years. [39]

CONCLUSION

Many promising results have been obtained in small phase I/II trials for HSCT as therapy for AIDs in general and for IBD in particular. However, HSCT is associated with a relatively high mortality rate and infection risk and might therefore not be a treatment of first choice for IBD, in which overall mortality tends to be low. [2] However, in certain subgroups of IBD patients who suffer from multiple complications and in whom remission is hard to retain, the balance between risk and benefit might shift towards transplantation. Because allogeneic HSCT is associated with even higher mortality and morbidity, autologous HSCT has been the most common approach.

As yet, no results of randomized controlled trials have been published to truly determine the effectiveness of HSCT for AID. Currently two prospective randomized controlled trials are being performed and analyzed to investigate the effect of HSCT in SSc patients. The SCOT (Scleroderma Cyclophosphamide or Transplant) trial and ASTIS (Autologous Stem Cell Transplantation International Scleroderma) trial both compare immune suppression alone with autologous HSCT. Both trials have finished recruitment now and results are being analyzed. [49] For CD the ASTIC (Autologous Stem Cell Transplantation) trial is currently being performed. ASTIC is a multicentre, prospective, randomized phase III study conducted by the European Crohn's and Colitis Organization (ECCO). The main objective is to evaluate the potential clinical benefit of HSC mobilization followed by high dose immune ablation and autologous HSCT versus hematopoietic stem cell mobilization alone. Patient recruitment is halted since January 2012 and 45 patients have been randomized. [50] It is expected that these trials and others planned will shed light on the effectiveness of HSCT for IBD and AIDs in general.

The most feared complications after HSCT are infections due to prolonged immunosuppression. Promoting immune reconstitution after HSCT might therefore strongly favor the outcome of HSCT by reducing the infection risk. Infusion of mature T cells with the graft offers the advantage of faster immune reconstitution, but this approach also increases the risk of developing GvHD in allogeneic transplantation and the risk of reinfusion of autoreactive T cells in autologous transplantation. To promote thymic output of naive T cells, and thereby promoting faster immune reconstitution, the effect of SSA, IL7 and KGF treatment is currently being investigated. This approach might be of particular interest for patients undergoing HSCT for AID to promote the development of a new diverse immune system without autoimmunity. New research needs to shed light on the feasibility of this approach and on the underlying mechanisms.

Overall, the mechanisms that facilitate the observed benefit of HSCT for AID remain largely unclear and further research is needed in this area. Promoting immune reconstitution after HSCT for AID needs to be further elaborated as well, both to promote safety and effectiveness of HSCT for treating AID. Ideally this will lead to the development of a HSCT protocol specifically tailored to treat IBD, with minimized side effects and maximized disease control.

REFERENCES

[1] Danese, S; Fiocchi, C. Ulcerative colitis. *N. Engl. J. Med.,* 2011, 365(18), 1713-1725.

[2] Peyrin-Biroulet, L; Loftus, EV, Jr.; Colombel, JF et al. Long-term complications, extraintestinal manifestations, and mortality in adult Crohn's disease in population-based cohorts. *Inflamm. Bowel Dis.,* 2011, 17(1), 471-478.

[3] Cho, JH. The genetics and immunopathogenesis of inflammatory bowel disease. *Nat. Rev. Immunol.*, 2008, 8(6), 458-466.

[4] Levine, JS; Burakoff, R. Extraintestinal manifestations of inflammatory bowel disease. *Gastroenterol. Hepatol.* (N Y), 2011, 7(4), 235-241.

[5] Molodecky, NA; Soon, IS; Rabi, DM et al. Increasing incidence and prevalence of the inflammatory bowel diseases with time, based on systematic review. *Gastroenterology,* 2012, 142(1), 46-54.

[6] Molodecky, NA; Kaplan, GG. Environmental risk factors for inflammatory bowel disease. *Gastroenterol. Hepatol. (N Y),* 2010, 6(5), 339-346.

[7] Khor, B; Gardet, A; Xavier, RJ. Genetics and pathogenesis of inflammatory bowel disease. *Nature,* 2011, 474(7351), 307-317.

[8] Ordas, I; Feagan, BG; Sandborn, WJ. Early use of immunosuppressives or TNF antagonists for the treatment of Crohn's disease: time for a change. *Gut.,* 2011, 60(12), 1754-1763.

[9] Peyrin-Biroulet, L; Loftus, EV, Jr.; Colombel, JF et al. The natural history of adult Crohn's disease in population-based cohorts. *Am. J. Gastroenterol.,* 2010, 105(2), 289-297.

[10] Copelan, EA. Hematopoietic stem-cell transplantation. *N. Engl. J. Med.,* 2006, 354(17), 1813-1826.

[11] Thomas, ED; Lochte, HL Jr.; Lu, WC et al. Intravenous infusion of bone marrow in patients receiving radiation and chemotherapy. *N. Engl. J. Med.,* 1957,257(11),491-496.

[12] Thomas, ED; Lochte, HL Jr.; Cannon, JH et al. Supralethal whole body irradiation and isologous marrow transplantation in man. *J. Clin. Invest.,* 1959, 38, 1709-1716.

[13] Roncarolo, MG; Gregori, S; Lucarelli, B et al. Clinical tolerance in allogeneic hematopoietic stem cell transplantation. *Immunol. Rev.,* 2011, 241(1), 145-163.

[14] van Bekkum, DW. Stem cell transplantation for autoimmune disorders. Preclinical experiments. *Best Pract. Res. Clin. Haematol.,* 2004, 17(2), 201-222.

[15] Snowden, JA; Brooks, PM; Biggs, JC. Haemopoietic stem cell transplantation for autoimmune diseases. *Br. J. Haematol.,* 1997, 99(1), 9-22.

[16] Tyndall, A; Gratwohl, A. Blood and marrow stem cell transplants in autoimmune disease. A consensus report written on behalf of the European League Against Rheumatism (EULAR) and the European Group for Blood and Marrow Transplantation (EBMT). *Br. J. Rheumatol.,* 1997, 36(3), 390-392.

[17] Tyndall, A; Black, C; Finke, J et al. Treatment of systemic sclerosis with autologous haemopoietic stem cell transplantation. *Lancet,* 1997, 349(9047), 254.

[18] Farge, D; Labopin, M; Tyndall, A et al. Autologous hematopoietic stem cell transplantation for autoimmune diseases: an observational study on 12 years' experience from the European Group for Blood and Marrow Transplantation Working Party on Autoimmune Diseases. *Haematologica,* 2010, 95(2), 284-292.

[19] Daikeler, T; Hugle, T; Farge, D et al. Allogeneic hematopoietic SCT for patients with autoimmune diseases. *Bone Marrow Transplant.*, 2009, 44(1), 27-33.

[20] Drakos, PE; Nagler, A; Or, R. Case of Crohn's disease in bone marrow transplantation. *Am. J. Hematol.,* 1993, 43(2), 157-158.

[21] Kashyap, A; Forman, SJ. Autologous bone marrow transplantation for non-Hodgkin's lymphoma resulting in long-term remission of coincidental Crohn's disease. *Br. J. Haematol.,* 1998, 103(3), 651-652.

[22] Musso, M; Porretto, F; Crescimanno, A et al. Crohn's disease complicated by relapsed extranodal Hodgkin's lymphoma: prolonged complete remission after unmanipulated PBPC autotransplant. *Bone Marrow Transplant.,* 2000, 26(8), 921-923.

[23] Marti, JL; Mayordomo, JI; Isla, MD et al. PBSC autotransplant for inflammatory bowel disease (IBD): a case of ulcerative colitis. *Bone Marrow Transplant.,* 2001, 28(1), 109-110.

[24] Soderholm, JD; Malm, C; Juliusson, G et al. Long-term endoscopic remission of crohn disease after autologous stem cell transplantation for acute myeloid leukaemia. *Scand. J. Gastroenterol.,* 2002, 37(5),613-616.

[25] Hawkey, CJ. Stem cell transplantation for Crohn's disease. *Best Pract. Res. Clin. Haematol.*, 2004, 17(2), 317-325.

[26] Anumakonda, V; Hayee, B; Chung-Faye, G. Remission and relapse of Crohn's disease following autologous haematopoietic stem cell transplantation for non-Hodgkin's lymphoma. *Gut.,* 2007, 56(9), 1325.

[27] Lopez-Cubero, SO; Sullivan, KM; McDonald, GB. Course of Crohn's disease after allogeneic marrow transplantation. *Gastroenterology,* 1998, 114(3), 433-440.

[28] Ditschkowski, M; Einsele, H; Schwerdtfeger, R et al. Improvement of inflammatory bowel disease after allogeneic stem-cell transplantation. *Transplantation,* 2003, 75(10), 1745-1747.

[29] Kreisel, W; Potthoff, K; Bertz, H et al. Complete remission of Crohn's disease after high-dose cyclophosphamide and autologous stem cell transplantation. *Bone Marrow Transplant.*, 2003, 32(3), 337-340.

[30] Scime, R; Cavallaro, AM; Tringali, S et al. Complete clinical remission after high-dose immune suppression and autologous hematopoietic stem cell transplantation in severe Crohn's disease refractory to immunouppressive and immunomodulator therapy. *Inflamm. Bowel Dis.,* 2004, 10(6), 892-894.

[31] Kountouras, J; Sakellari, I; Tsarouchas, G et al. Autologous haematopoietic stem cell transplantation in a patient with refractory Crohn's disease. *J. Crohns Colitis*, 2011, 5(3), 275-276.

[32] Hommes, DW; Duijvestein, M; Zelinkova, Z et al. Long-term follow-up of autologous hematopoietic stem cell transplantation for severe refractory Crohn's disease. *J. Crohns Colitis*, 2011, 5(6), 543-549.

[33] Cassinotti, A; Annaloro, C; Ardizzone, S et al. Autologous haematopoietic stem cell transplantation without CD34+ cell selection in refractory Crohn's disease. *Gut.,* 2008, 57(2), 211-217.

[34] Cassinotti, A; Onida, F; Annaloro, C et al. P362 Autologous haematopoietic stem cell transplantation without CD34+ cell selection for refractory Crohn's disease: The Milan experience after 5 years. J. Crohns Colitis, 2012, 6(Supp 1), S153-S154.

[35] Burt, RK; Craig, RM; Milanetti, F et al. Autologous nonmyeloablative hematopoietic stem cell transplantation in patients with severe anti-TNF refractory Crohn disease: long-term follow-up. *Blood,* 2010, 116(26), 6123-6132.

[36] Sykes, M; Nikolic, B. Treatment of severe autoimmune disease by stem-cell transplantation. *Nature,* 2005, 435(7042), 620-627.

[37] Gosselin, D; Rivest, S. Immune mechanisms underlying the beneficial effects of autologous hematopoietic stem cell transplantation in multiple sclerosis. *Neurotherapeutics,* 2011, 8(4), 643-649.

[38] Muraro, PA; Douek, DC; Packer, A et al. Thymic output generates a new and diverse TCR repertoire after autologous stem cell transplantation in multiple sclerosis patients. *J. Exp. Med.,* 2005, 201(5), 805-816.

[39] Alexander, T; Thiel, A; Rosen, O et al. Depletion of autoreactive immunologic memory followed by autologous hematopoietic stem cell transplantation in patients with refractory SLE induces long-term remission through de novo generation of a juvenile and tolerant immune system. *Blood,* 2009, 113(1), 214-223.

[40] Daikeler, T; Labopin, M; Di, GM et al. Secondary autoimmune diseases occurring after HSCT for an autoimmune disease: a retrospective study of the EBMT Autoimmune Disease Working Party. *Blood,* 2011, 118(6), 1693-1698.

[41] Daikeler, T; Tyndall, A. Autoimmunity following haematopoietic stem-cell transplantation. *Best Pract. Res. Clin. Haematol.,* 2007, 20(2), 349-360.

[42] Spiers, AS. Ulcerative colitis after bone-marrow transplantation for acute leukemia. *N. Engl. J. Med.,* 1984, 311(19), 1259.

[43] Baron, FA; Hermanne, JP; Dowlati, A et al. Bronchiolitis obliterans organizing pneumonia and ulcerative colitis after allogeneic bone marrow transplantation. *Bone Marrow Transplant.,* 1998, 21(9),951-954.

[44] Sonwalkar, SA; James, RM; Ahmad, T et al. Fulminant Crohn's colitis after allogeneic stem cell transplantation. *Gut.,* 2003, 52(10), 1518-1521.

[45] Parham, P. The Immune System. Second edition. New York, NY: Garland Science. 2005.

[46] Hudson, LL; Louise, MM; Devlin, BH et al. Human T cell reconstitution in DiGeorge syndrome and HIV-1 infection. *Semin. Immunol.,* 2007, 19(5), 297-309.

[47] Lynch, HE; Goldberg, GL; Chidgey, A et al. Thymic involution and immune reconstitution. *Trends Immunol.,* 2009, 30(7), 366-373.

[48] Toubert, A; Glauzy, S; Douay, C et al. Thymus and immune reconstitution after allogeneic hematopoietic stem cell transplantation in humans: never say never again. *Tissue Antigens,* 2012, 79(2), 83-89.

[49] Tyndall, A. Successes and failures of stem cell transplantation in autoimmune diseases. *Hematology Am. Soc. Hematol. Educ. Program,* 2011, 2011, 280-284.

[50] www.nottingham.ac.uk/icr/astic.

In: Hematopoietic Stem Cells: New Research ISBN 978-1-62257-468-1
Editors: Wesley G. Montgomery and Heather I. Burton ©2012 Nova Science Publishers, Inc.

Chapter 6

CONCISE REVIEW: EXTRAMEDULLARY HEMATOPOIESIS LEADING TO THE PRODUCTION OF A NOVEL ANTIGEN-PRESENTING CELL TYPE IN MURINE SPLEEN

Rebecca A. Hinton and Helen C. O'Neill*
Research School of Biology, The Australian National University, Canberra, Australia

ABSTRACT

The concept of extramedullary hematopoiesis for production of organ-specific antigen presenting cells has importance in immunity in terms of the compartmentalisation of the immune response in different tissue sites. A new and distinct dendritic-like antigen presenting cell subtype is described which is dependent on the spleen microenvironment for development. Cells arise by a unique developmental pathway distinct from other dendritic cells (DC). In particular, a self-renewing progenitor of these cells has been identified in spleen upstream of the earliest DC progenitor currently identified in bone marrow. This progenitor depends on the splenic microenvironment for maintenance and proliferation, adding further support for spleen as a site for hematopoiesis.

Keywords: Dendritic cells, development, progenitors, spleen

INTRODUCTION

Dendritic cells (DC) play a specific role in antigen presentation and stimulation of naïve T-cells and are central to the maintenance of peripheral tolerance and the regulation of T-cell responses [1]. Although they develop from bone marrow-derived precursors, *in vivo* studies in both humans and mice have shown that DC reside in various locations throughout the body

* Correspondence: Professor HC O'Neill, Research School of Biology, The Australian National University, Canberra ACT 0200, Australia. Email: Helen.ONeill@anu.edu.au.

including bone marrow, lymphoid tissues like thymus and spleen, as well as blood and peripheral tissues [2]. Populations within these tissues represent specialised subsets which differ in lineage origin and state of maturation and activation, and therefore possess different effector functions for regulation of T-cells [3].

Conventional DC are the most common DC subset in spleen and are relatively small cells with low granularity [4]. They are phenotypically distinct by high expression of the surface markers CD11c and MHC-II [4], and can be divided further by expression of CD8α, such that CD8α$^+$ DC are CD11b$^-$CD11c^{hi}CD8α$^+$CD205$^+$MHC-II$^+$ cells, and are the major population of cells in the thymus and T cell regions of the spleen [3]. CD8α$^-$ DC are CD11b$^+$CD11c^{hi}CD8α$^-$CD205$^-$MHC-II$^+$CD4$^{+/-}$ cells in the splenic marginal zones, which migrate into T-cell areas upon microbial stimulation [3]. They also represent minor populations in thymus and lymph nodes. Another common DC subset is the plasmacytoid (p)DC, found mainly in blood and bone marrow and representing a smaller population within spleen [5]. Plasmacytoid DC are characterised as CD11c^{lo}CD11b$^-$B220$^+$CD8$^{+/-}$MHC-II^{lo} cells, so named for their small plasma cell-like appearance and B220 expression. They have also been termed plasmacytoid pre-DC (p-preDC) based on the fact that they represent the precursors of mature subtypes under inflammatory conditions [6].

Discovery of a Novel Dendritic-Like Cell Type in Spleen

Spleen long-term cultures (LTC) that exclusively support hematopoiesis of dendritic-like cells were first reported more than a decade ago [7, 8]. Cells produced were termed 'LTC-DC' and found to be large cells expressing the common DC surface markers CD11c and CD11b [8]. However, LTC-DC do not express markers like CD8α or B220 which identify murine splenic cDC and pDC, respectively. While they express MHC-I they do not express cell surface MHC-II, and in this way are more like immature DC [8, 9], with high capacity for antigen uptake and processing, but low capacity to activate T cells [10]. LTC-DC were found to be unusual as DC in that they stimulate antigen-specific CD8$^+$ T cell responses, but not CD4$^+$ T cells [8, 11]. These properties distinguish them from common immature and mature DC subsets in spleen, including CD8α$^+$ cDC, CD8α$^-$ cDC and pDC, which are strong activators of both CD4$^+$ and CD8$^+$ T cells. These combined properties potentially differentiate LTC-DC as a novel antigen presenting subset produced within spleen.

Dendritic-like cells reflecting the same phenotype and function as LTC-DC can also be generated from bone marrow and spleen progenitors overlaid in co-cultures above STX3, a stromal cell line derived from an established spleen LTC [12, 13]. These cells, termed 'L-DC', developed within two to three weeks of co-culture, and were identified as progeny of overlaid cells rather than cells arising from progenitors of the stromal cell monolayer [13]. The lineage-depleted (Lin$^-$) fraction of bone marrow is an efficient producer of L-DC characterised by CD11c and CD11b expression, and absence of other DC markers like B220, CD8α and MHC-II (Figure 1). Cells produced are highly endocytic for soluble antigen, but do not resemble macrophages/granulocytes in that they do not express the Gr-1 marker of these cells. Co-cultures established in this way also support L-DC production for up to 12 months (Figure 1).

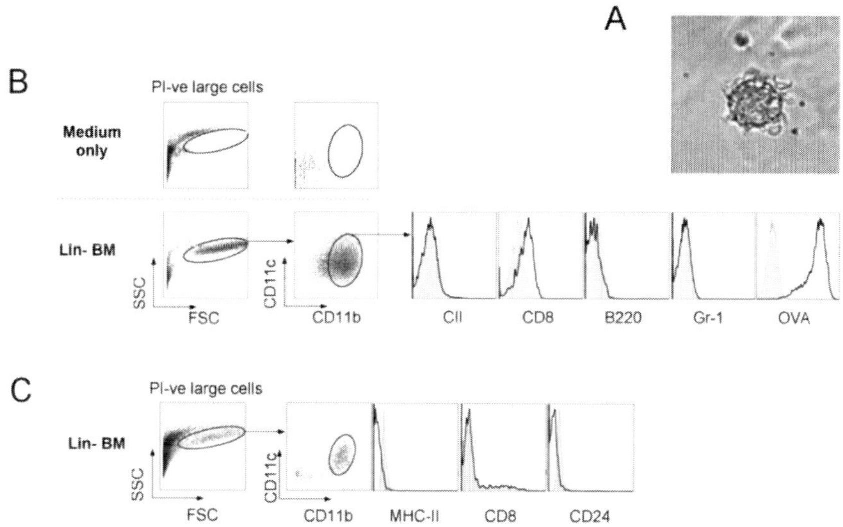

Figure 1. L-DC production in cocultures of BM over stroma. Lineage depleted (Lin⁻) bone marrow was prepared using magnetic MACS® bead technology and cells overlaid in co-cultures over the STX3 splenic stroma. Control stromal cultures contained medium only. A). Photomicroscopy at 14 days under phase contrast reveals dendritic-like cells. (Cell diameter ~50μm). Non-adherent cells were collected and stained B) at 27 days and C) at 12 months using fluorochrome-conjugated antibodies specific for CD11b, CD11c, MHC-II, CD8α, CD24, B220 and Gr-1. Cells were also incubated at 37°C for 40 minutes with OVA-FITC to assess endocytosis. Prior to flow cytometry, cells were stained with propidium iodide for gating of live (PI⁻) cells. For analysis, large cells were gated based on SSC vs. FSC. Numbers in gates reflect % positive cells as set by isotype control antibodies.

Recently *in vivo* splenic counterparts to LTC-DC and L-DC were identified [11]. Cells display the cell surface phenotype of LTC-DC, together with high endocytic capacity and cross-presenting function [8, 13]. Progenitors of this population were found to lie within the $Lin^{-}cKit^{hi}$ population of hematopoietic progenitors in spleen [14]. Their status as L-DC progenitors was identified both after *in vivo* transfer and development in irradiated recipient mice, and after co-culture of isolated progenitors over STX3 stroma for extended periods [14]. This *in vivo* subset has also been tentatively named 'L-DC' and continues to be investigated for its functional potential [11].

L-DC represent steady-state, spleen-resident dendritic-like cells [11], clearly distinct from the currently identified DC populations of spleen, including cDC, pDC, and the lesser known monocyte-derived (mo) DC [15], or regulatory DC described to have regulatory or inhibitory function for T cells (DCreg) [16, 17]. However, their characterisation within the category of classical DC has been difficult. The first identified DC were characterised as a novel subset on the basis of their unique branching morphology and unusual intracellular features [18]. Later, it was found that in addition to their distinct morphology, DC had distinct functions including capacity for antigen-specific activation of naïve T cells [19]. Since immature DC do not consistently display stellate morphology, and since some DC can suppress T cell responses [16, 17], these original described properties are not definitive. Conventional cell surface markers of murine DC like CD11c and MHC-II are also not definitive markers for cells of the dendritic lineage. For example, steady-state pDC are $CD11c^{-/lo}$, and several DC subsets express only low levels of MHC-II [3]. In this way, the definition of cells as 'dendritic' can be difficult and often contentious. Hence the description of LTC-DC and L-DC as dendritic cells is tentative, and used to describe a subset of myeloid, dendritic-like cells which form within the spleen.

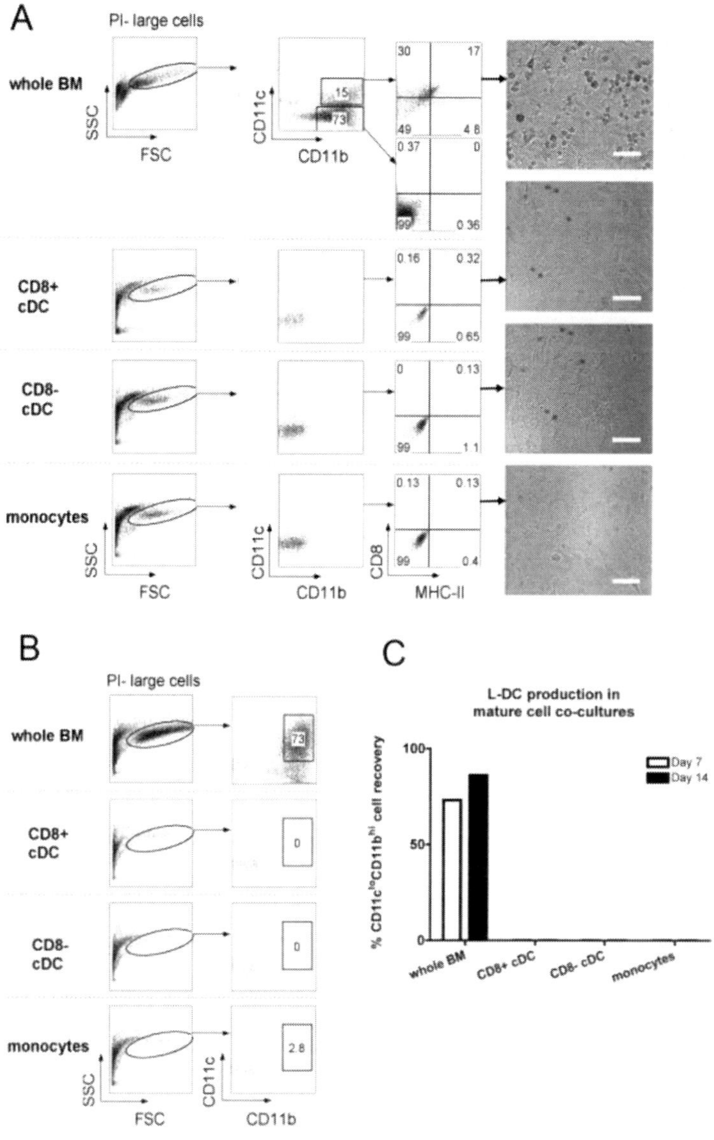

Figure 2. Co-cultures can be established with whole bone marrow cells, but not with sorted CD8α$^+$ cDC, CD8α$^-$ cDC or monocytes. Duplicate flasks were prepared with overlay cells for later detection of cell proliferation. Non-adherent cells were collected at A) 7, and B) 14 days, and stained with fluorochrome-conjugated antibodies specific for CD11b, CD11c, CD8α and MHC-II to detect myeloid and DC subsets. Prior to flow cytometry, cells were stained with propidium iodide (PI) for gating live (PI$^-$) cells. Large cells were gated on SSC vs. FSC plots. Gates were set using isotype controls, and numbers in gates reflect % positive cells. Absence of cell production in cDC and monocyte co-cultures was photographed using phase-contrast microscopy at 23 days (scale bar = 100μm) (A). L-DC recovery from co-cultures established over STX3 with whole BM, CD8α$^+$ cDC, CD8α$^-$ cDC and monocytes is graphed in C) as % viable, CD11b^{hi}CD11c^{lo} cells produced relative to input cell number.

L-DC are clearly distinct from both cDC and pDC in terms of morphology, phenotype and function. Typically, they are $SSC^{hi}FSC^{hi}$ cells (40-50μm in size), with extensive membrane protrusions (Figure 1), and a $CD11b^{hi}CD11c^{lo}CD8^{-}MHC\text{-}II^{-/lo}$ surface marker phenotype [13, 14]. Absence, of MHC-II expression, differentiates L-DC particularly from cDC and mo-DC, and reflects the characteristic of an immature DC type. Whilst L-DC do demonstrate expression of co-stimulators like CD80 and CD86, thus far they have not demonstrated expression of any additional DC subset specific marker and do not express CD24 expressed by some cDC (Figure 1) [8, 11, 14]. Since both L-DC and their *in vitro* correlate (LTC-DC) demonstrate distinct myeloid characteristics including low expression of CD11c, high expression of CD11b with some expression of F4/80 [8, 11], one question to address is whether L-DC represent a monocyte- or macrophage-like cell. It has now been shown that purified subsets of $CD11b^{hi}CD11c^{-}MHC\text{-}II^{-}$ splenic monocytes cannot proliferate or differentiate above STX3 stroma to produce L-DC over 14 days of co-culture, so it is unlikely that L-DC represent monocytes or mo-DC (Figure 2). Control bone marrow however produces a clear population of L-DC by 14 days of co-culture over STX3. Indeed, whilst $CD11b^{+}CD11c^{-}$ myelomonocytic cells have been transiently produced in co-cultures established from heterogeneous populations of spleen and bone marrow cultured over STX3 splenic stroma, these are distinct from L-DC and are only transiently produced within the first 14 days of co-culture [13] (Figure 2B). They are thought to arise from myelomonocytic precursors which respond to soluble stromal factors, while L-DC require stromal cell contact for growth [13]. Altogether, these findings provide strong evidence that L-DC are more representative of a dendritic-like cell than a monocyte/macrophage, although the jury is still out over their lineage origin with respect to macrophages and cDC.

L-DC Have Distinct Functional Potential

Another important question is whether phenotypically distinct L-DC display unique immune functional potential compared with other APC. Recently it was shown that L-DC can activate $CD8^{+}$ T cell responses in a mixed lymphocyte reaction, and in antigen-specific T cell activation assays [11, 14]. When activated with LPS, LTC-DC and L-DC can take up exogenous antigen and 'cross-present' it to $CD8^{+}$ T cells [11]. Cross-presentation, or processing of exogenous antigen via the MHC class I pathway for presentation to $CD8^{+}$ T cells, has previously been identified as an important function of $CD8\alpha^{+}$ cDC [20]. However, cDC have also been shown to stimulate $CD4^{+}$ T cells, whilst L-DC and LTC-DC show activation restricted to $CD8^{+}$ T cells, and not to $CD4^{+}$ T cells [8, 11]. Indeed, LPS treatment *in vitro* upregulates MHC-I and CD86 expression on L-DC produced in co-cultures but fails to upregulate MHC-II expression on these cells (Figure 3). The T cell stimulatory capacity of L-DC (and LTC-DC) is therefore distinct from that of cDC. L-DC are also both functionally and phenotypically distinct from pDC which have low efficiency for endocytosis of antigen and demonstrate poor capacity for antigen-presentation and T activation [6]. Currently it is thought that under steady-state conditions, the primary function of pDC is tolerance induction [21, 22], although the exact mechanism remains unknown. When tested for capacity to suppress or inhibit T cell activation in a mixed lymphocyte reaction, L-DC had no inhibitory capacity but were found instead to enhance T cell proliferation, reflecting uptake of allogeneic APC for presentation to T cells [23]. The failure to inhibit T cell activation suggests that L-DC are also distinct from DCreg. In summary, a novel immune functional capacity for activation of $CD8^+$ T cells and a distinct surface marker phenotype distinguish L-DC as a novel dendritic-like subset developing within spleen.

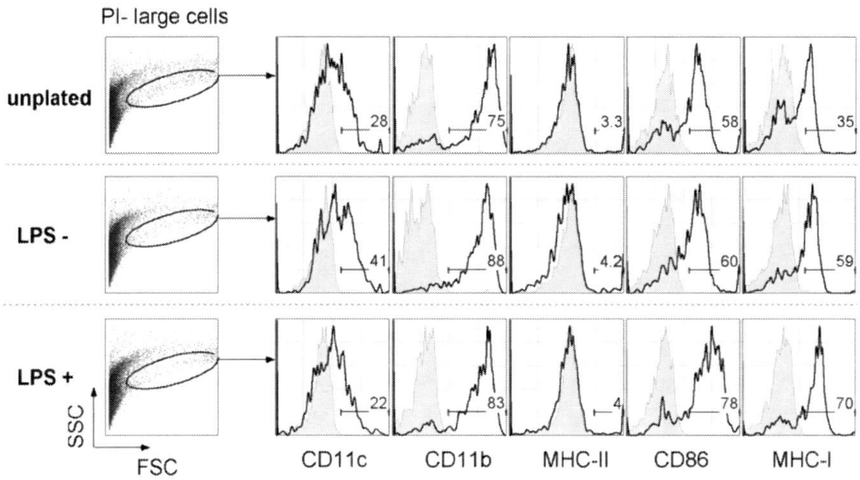

Figure 3. LPS responsiveness of L-DC produced in co-cultures. Co-cultures were established with lineage depleted (Lin^-) bone marrow and maintained for 55 days. Non-adherent cells were collected and then replated for 20 hours ± LPS (10μg/ml) in the absence of stroma to assess activation in terms of marker expression change. After this time, cells were stained with fluorochrome-conjugated antibodies specific for CD11b, CD11c, CD86, MHC-I and MHC-II. Prior to flow cytometry, cells were stained with propidium iodide for gating of live (PI^-) cells. Large cells were gated based on SSC vs. FSC. Numbers in gates reflect % positive cells as set by isotype control antibodies. Isotype controls are shown as an overlay on histograms. Cells stained fresh from cultures (unplated) were controls.

THE DEVELOPMENTAL ORIGIN OF L-DC

The immediate precursors of cDC, known as 'pre-cDC', can be identified in bone marrow and spleen [24], while the precursors of pDC, the 'p-preDC' exist in bone marrow and blood [25]. Since L-DC can be generated by co-culture of spleen or bone marrow in co-cultures over STX3 splenic stroma, one question is whether L-DC derive from mature cDC through a differentiative process induced by the stromal microenvironment. There is evidence that cDC and pDC can differentiate further under certain conditions and act themselves as precursors of different DC subsets [26, 27]. When pure populations of $CD8\alpha^-$ cDC and $CD8\alpha^+$ cDC were isolated from spleen by sorting and overlay over STX3 stroma, neither subset survived the STX3 co-cultures, and did not differentiate to produce progeny resembling L-DC or any other DC subsets (Figure 2). Monocytes can also act as precursors for DC under inflammatory conditions [28], with development of moDC dependent upon cytokines such as GM-CSF and TNF-α. When splenic monocytes were overlaid on to STX3 stroma, they were not maintained and did not differentiate to produce progeny resembling DC (Figure 2). This result is consistent with evidence that STX3 does not produce GM-CSF and TNF-α [29], and confirms that cells of the monocyte/macrophage lineage do not act as precursors of L-DC.

The major DC subsets identified within spleen develop from the $Flt3^+$ bone marrow subsets of common lymphoid progenitors and common myeloid progenitors [30, 31]. More recently, a myeloid dendritic progenitor and a common dendritic progenitor/pro-DC were defined, which are identifiable as $cKit^{lo/+}Sca1^-$ [32] and $CD11c^-cKit^+Sca1^{lo}$ subsets [33, 34], respectively. These progenitors are not present in spleen [35], which immediately distinguishes them from L-DC progenitors. The progenitors of cDC and pDC in bone marrow respond to Flt3L *in vitro* with production of mature DC [32, 33]. Flt3L is, however, not produced by STX3 stroma and so does not drive L-DC differentiation in co-cultures [29, 36]. The L-DC progenitor also appears to be self-renewing since L-DC production *in vitro* in cocultures or in LTC is continuous, as opposed to production of cDC from precursors in Flt3L supplemented bone marrow cultures which is transient [13]. A parallel exists between the development of L-DC with Langerhans cells which both develop from self-renewing progenitors. In the case of Langerhans cells, differentiation occurs in the steady-state from skin-resident progenitors that are self-renewing [37].

In order to directly test whether L-DC derive from self-renewing progenitors in bone marrow, a broad subset of hematopoietic stem cells (HSC) was sorted as the $Lin^-ckit^+Sca1^+$ subset of bone marrow and co-cultured above STX3 stroma [23]. Cells generated within co-cultures morphologically and phenotypically resembled L-DC [11, 13]. The antigen presenting capacity of cells produced in HSC co-cultures was also confirmed, and developing cells had high endocytic capacity, and high ability to activate T cells [23]. Since HSC co-cultures continuously produced a pure population of L-DC, it was reasoned that the $Lin^-ckit^+Sca1^+$ population of bone marrow must also contain an L-DC progenitor. However further characterisation of cells within this population will be needed in order to determine the relationship between the L-DC progenitor and HSC. It is notable that HSC co-cultures can be maintained for >12 months with production of only L-DC[23]. Others have reported the production of $CD45RB^+$ DCreg from HSC co-cultured over spleen endothelial cells [17], but this was not found in our studies using HSC. L-DC appear to develop from a progenitor closely aligned with the HSC subset and by a pathway which distinguishes it from cDC and pDC. STX3 stroma appears to have limited or restricted capacity to support differentiation of L-DC only.

The Ontogeny of L-DC Development

While DC subsets have been well characterised in the adult, limited studies have investigated DC hematopoiesis during embryonic and neonatal development [38, 39]. In this lab we have investigated L-DC prevalence in fetal liver and perinatal spleen. Murine E14.5 fetal liver contains cells expressing high levels of the myeloid marker CD11b but not CD11c, indicating that the known subsets of DC are not present in the early embryo [40]. STX3 co-cultures established using E12.5 fetal liver are not productive, although co-cultures seeded with E14.5 fetal liver generate both L-DC and other cDC-like cells indicating that progenitors for both subsets are present in fetal liver at this stage of development despite an absence of mature DC [40]. Others have also reported that cells with characteristic DC morphology and function can be generated *in vitro* from progenitor cells present in E13.5 fetal liver [41].

Overall, these studies align the L-DC progenitor with primitive hematopoietic cells present in fetal liver, spleen and bone marrow.

In order to test whether L-DC development occurred directly from HSC, L-DC generation in co-cultures was investigated using *Ikaros Plastic* mutant mice developed through an ENU mutagenesis screen [42]. While the Ikaros transcription factor is essential for lymphopoiesis, *Ikaros Plastic* mice contain a point mutation in the zinc finger domain of Ikaros which inhibits HSC self-renewal [42]. The *Ikzf1 plstc* mutant allele shows embryonic lethality at ~E15.5, due to the absence of self-renewing HSC. At E12.5, *plstc/plstc* mice show normal numbers of HSC in fetal liver, whilst at E14.5 they contain no HSC, but an expanded myeloid progenitor population [42]. When *plstc/plstc* fetal liver was tested at E14.5 for capacity to produce L-DC in co-cultures, very low numbers of L-DC were produced after 14 days, and these were completely lost by 21 days. In contrast, fetal liver from wild type littermates showed long-term production of L-DC. Results were consistent with the presence of a progenitor in wild type E14.5 fetal liver, which is self-renewing and can produce L-DC production in STX3 co-cultures. HSC present in E14.5 fetal liver of *plstc/plstc* mice gave only transient L-DC due to loss of self-renewal potential in HSC.

Hematopoietic stem cells which develop in fetal liver migrate to bone marrow, although bone marrow does not become a functioning hematopoietic site until after birth. They also migrate into fetal spleen, which shows hematopoietic development from ~E11.5 [43, 44]. Myelomonocytic cells expressing CD11b but not CD11c have also been identified in spleen before birth, representing the majority of non-lymphoid cells. Cells in spleen expressing the CD11c marker of DC are not detected before birth, but can be detected perinatally, likely representing DC precursors [45]. By day 4, neonatal spleen shows clear subsets of $CD8\alpha^+$ cDC, $CD8\alpha^-$ cDC, pDC and L-DC. However even by day 6, subset size is far less than adult levels, consistent with previous data showing that the DC compartment is not fully competent before 4 weeks of age [46]. While L-DC progenitors exist within the embryo, the splenic microenvironment required for development of L-DC may not form or become competent until the neonatal period. This is consistent with evidence that productive LTC of spleen can only be generated from neonatal mice after day 6 [7]. The presence of L-DC progenitors within spleen during the perinatal period has since been confirmed by establishment of co-cultures over STX3 [45]. The hematopoietic competence of splenic stroma in perinatal mice was also tested in terms of capacity to support productive LTC. LTC established from perinatal spleen before day 6 produced mostly myelomonocytic $CD11c^-CD11b^+$ cells despite evidence that L-DC progenitors are present in spleen as early as day 2 [45]. Indeed, the stromal environment required for L-DC production in spleen may not mature in mice until ~day 6. This timepoint is also consistent with the appearance of L-DC subsets in spleen between day 4 and day 6.

Conclusion: Spleen as a Site for Hematopoiesis of an Endogenous Antigen Presenting Cell

While hematopoiesis in spleen was once thought to be limited to extramedullary production of erythrocytes, we now know that it plays an important role in the development of cDC and pDC from bone marrow-derived precursors entering spleen from blood [47]. In addition, prior to formation of bone marrow in the neonate, spleen acts as a reservoir for progenitors homing from fetal liver [44]. Spleen also acts as a reservoir for bone marrow-derived progenitors in adults under hematological stress [48]. The spleen is largely redundant as a hematopoietic organ, and its loss does not result in significant hematopoietic impairment. Still, it remains a unique hematopoietic organ, comparable only with bone marrow or fetal liver in terms of capacity to fully reconstitute irradiated recipients [49]. We now know that it can be a competent niche for lodgement and maintenance of HSC [49-51], and here we show its role in the extramedullary hematopoiesis of a novel dendritic-like cell type.

In this report we have described a novel dendritic-like subset L-DC, dependent upon the splenic stromal cell microenvironment for development. L-DC can be detected within murine spleen from day 4 after birth, co-incident with the appearance of other known splenic DC subsets [45]. While newborn spleen does not contain these cells, it does contain their progenitors, although the splenic niche is not competent to support L-DC development until neonatal day 4. L-DC can be continuously generated *in vitro* above endothelial splenic stroma when seeded with a source of progenitors [13]. These progenitors have been aligned with self-renewing hematopoietic stem/progenitor cells, and stromal co-cultures can maintain long-term production of L-DC from overlaid hematopoietic progenitors from bone marrow [13], spleen [13, 14], or fetal liver [40]. Whilst *in vitro* studies can misrepresent true physiological development, L-DC produced *in vitro* do have a counterpart cell *in vivo* in spleen [11]. It would appear that the STX3 splenic stroma has specific capacity to maintain self-renewing hematopoietic stem/progenitor cells *in vitro*. These findings reflect on the production of tissue-specific, functionally distinct antigen presenting cells, as well as the *in vitro* maintenance of self-renewing hematopoietic progenitors. The latter has not previously been achieved, and would appear to have clinical importance for amplification of hematopoietic stem cells ahead of transplantation.

ACKNOWLEDGMENTS

This work was supported by project grants to HO from the Australian Stem Cell Centre, and the National Health and Medical Research Council of Australia (Project Grant No. 585443).

Author Disclosure Statement

No competing financial interests exist.

REFERENCES

[1] Liu YJ, H Kanzler, V Soumelis and M Gilliet. (2001). Dendritic cell lineage, plasticity and cross-regulation. *Nat Immunol* 2:585-589.

[2] Wan H and M Dupasquier. (2005). Dendritic cells in vivo and in vitro. *Cell Mol Immunol* 2:28-35.

[3] Shortman K and YJ Liu. (2002). Mouse and human dendritic cell subtypes. *Nat Rev Immunol* 2:151-161.

[4] Xu Y, Y Zhan, AM Lew, SH Naik and MH Kershaw. (2007). Differential development of murine dendritic cells by GM-CSF versus Flt3 ligand has implications for inflammation and trafficking. *J Immunol* 179:7577-7584.

[5] Grouard G, MC Rissoan, L Filgueira, I Durand, J Banchereau and YJ Liu. (1997). The enigmatic plasmacytoid T cells develop into dendritic cells with interleukin (IL)-3 and CD40-ligand. *J Exp Med* 185:1101-1111.

[6] Salio M, MJ Palmowski, A Atzberger, IF Hermans and V Cerundolo. (2004). CpG-matured murine plasmacytoid dendritic cells are capable of in vivo priming of functional CD8 T cell responses to endogenous but not exogenous antigens. *J Exp Med* 199:567-579.

[7] Ni K and HC O'Neill. (1997). Long-term stromal cultures produce dendritic-like cells. *Br J Hematol* 97:710-725.

[8] Quah B, K Ni and HC O'Neill. (2004). In vitro hematopoiesis produces a distinct class of immature dendritic cells from spleen progenitors with limited T cell stimulation capacity. *Int Immunol* 16:567-577.

[9] Pierre P, SJ Turley, E Gatti, M Hull, J Meltzer, A Mirza, K Inaba, RM Steinman and I Mellman. (1997). Developmental regulation of MHC class II transport in mouse dendritic cells. *Nature* 388:787-792.

[10] Tan JK and HC O'Neill. (2005). Maturation requirements for dendritic cells in T cell stimulation leading to tolerance versus immunity. *J Leukoc Biol* 78:319-324.

[11] Tan JK, BJ Quah, KL Griffiths, P Periasamy, YY Hey and HC O'Neill. (2011). Identification of a novel antigen cross-presenting cell type in spleen. *J Cell Mol Med* 15:1189-1199.

[12] Ni K and HC O'Neill. (1998). Hemopoiesis in long-term stroma-dependent cultures from lymphoid tissue: production of cells with myeloid/dendritic characteristics. *In Vitro Cell Dev Biol Anim* 34:298-307.

[13] Periasamy P, JK Tan, KL Griffiths and HC O'Neill. (2009). Splenic stromal niches support hematopoiesis of dendritic-like cells from precursors in bone marrow and spleen. *Exp Hematol* 37:1060-1071.

[14] Tan JK, P Periasamy and HC O'Neill. (2010). Delineation of precursors in murine spleen that develop in contact with splenic endothelium to give novel dendritic-like cells. *Blood* 115:3678-3685.

[15] Cheong C, I Matos, JH Choi, DB Dandamudi, E Shrestha, MP Longhi, KL Jeffrey, RM Anthony, C Kluger, G Nchinda, H Koh, A Rodriguez, J Idoyaga, M Pack, K Velinzon, CG Park and RM Steinman. (2010). Microbial stimulation fully differentiates monocytes to DC-SIGN/CD209(+) dendritic cells for immune T cell areas. *Cell* 143:416-429.

[16] Svensson M, A Maroof, M Ato and PM Kaye. (2004). Stromal cells direct local differentiation of regulatory dendritic cells. *Immunity* 21:805-816.

[17] Zhang M, H Tang, Z Guo, H An, X Zhu, W Song, J Guo, X Huang, T Chen, J Wang and X Cao. (2004). Splenic stroma drives mature dendritic cells to differentiate into regulatory dendritic cells. *Nat Immunol* 5:1124-1133.

[18] Steinman RM and ZA Cohn. (1973). Identification of a novel cell type in peripheral lymphoid organs of mice. I. Morphology, quantitation, tissue distribution. *J Exp Med* 137:1142-1162.
[19] Steinman RM and MD Witmer. (1978). Lymphoid dendritic cells are potent stimulators of the primary mixed leukocyte reaction in mice. *Proc Natl Acad Sci U S A* 75:5132-5136.
[20] Belz GT, FR Carbone and WR Heath. (2002). Cross-presentation of antigens by dendritic cells. *Crit Rev Immunol* 22:439-448.
[21] Bilsborough J, TC George, A Norment and JL Viney. (2003). Mucosal CD8alpha+ DC, with a plasmacytoid phenotype, induce differentiation and support function of T cells with regulatory properties. *Immunology* 108:481-492.
[22] de Heer HJ, H Hammad, T Soullie, D Hijdra, N Vos, MA Willart, HC Hoogsteden and BN Lambrecht. (2004). Essential role of lung plasmacytoid dendritic cells in preventing asthmatic reactions to harmless inhaled antigen. *J Exp Med* 200:89-98.
[23] Hinton RA and HC O'Neill. (2011). In vitro production of distinct dendritic-like antigen presenting cells from self-renewing hematopoietic stem cells. *J Leukoc Biol* Nov 15. [Epub ahead of print].
[24] Naik SH, D Metcalf, A van Nieuwenhuijze, I Wicks, L Wu, M O'Keeffe and K Shortman. (2006). Intrasplenic steady-state dendritic cell precursors that are distinct from monocytes. *Nat Immunol* 7:663-671.
[25] O'Keeffe M, H Hochrein, D Vremec, B Scott, P Hertzog, L Tatarczuch and K Shortman. (2003). Dendritic cell precursor populations of mouse blood: identification of the murine homologues of human blood plasmacytoid pre-DC2 and CD11c+ DC1 precursors. *Blood* 101:1453-1459.
[26] Liu YJ. (2005). IPC: professional type 1 interferon-producing cells and plasmacytoid dendritic cell precursors. *Annu Rev Immunol* 23:275-306.
[27] Martinez del Hoyo G, P Martin, CF Arias, AR Marin and C Ardavin. (2002). CD8alpha+ dendritic cells originate from the CD8alpha- dendritic cell subset by a maturation process involving CD8alpha, DEC-205, and CD24 up-regulation. *Blood* 99:999-1004.
[28] Randolph GJ, K Inaba, DF Robbiani, RM Steinman and WA Muller. (1999). Differentiation of phagocytic monocytes into lymph node dendritic cells in vivo. *Immunity* 11:753-761.
[29] Despars G, K Ni, A Bouchard, TJ O'Neill and HC O'Neill. (2004). Molecular definition of an in vitro niche for dendritic cell development. *Exp Hematol* 32:1182-1193.
[30] D'Amico A and L Wu. (2003). The early progenitors of mouse dendritic cells and plasmacytoid predendritic cells are within the bone marrow hemopoietic precursors expressing Flt3. *J Exp Med* 198:293-303.
[31] Karsunky H, M Merad, A Cozzio, IL Weissman and MG Manz. (2003). Flt3 ligand regulates dendritic cell development from Flt3+ lymphoid and myeloid-committed progenitors to Flt3+ dendritic cells in vivo. *J Exp Med* 198:305-313.
[32] Fogg DK, C Sibon, C Miled, S Jung, P Aucouturier, DR Littman, A Cumano and F Geissmann. (2006). A clonogenic bone marrow progenitor specific for macrophages and dendritic cells. *Science* 311:83-87.
[33] Naik SH, P Sathe, HY Park, D Metcalf, AI Proietto, A Dakic, S Carotta, M O'Keeffe, M Bahlo, A Papenfuss, JY Kwak, L Wu and K Shortman. (2007). Development of

plasmacytoid and conventional dendritic cell subtypes from single precursor cells derived in vitro and in vivo. *Nat Immunol* 8:1217-1226.

[34] Onai N, A Obata-Onai, MA Schmid, T Ohteki, D Jarrossay and MG Manz. (2007). Identification of clonogenic common Flt3+M-CSFR+ plasmacytoid and conventional dendritic cell progenitors in mouse bone marrow. *Nat Immunol* 8:1207-1216.

[35] Liu K, GD Victora, TA Schwickert, P Guermonprez, MM Meredith, K Yao, FF Chu, GJ Randolph, AY Rudensky and M Nussenzweig. (2009). In vivo analysis of dendritic cell development and homeostasis. *Science* 324:392-397.

[36] Wilson HL, K Ni and HC O'Neill. (2000). Proliferation of dendritic cell progenitors in long term culture is not dependent on granulocyte macrophage-colony stimulating factor. *Exp Hematol* 28:193-202.

[37] Merad M, MG Manz, H Karsunky, A Wagers, W Peters, I Charo, IL Weissman, JG Cyster and EG Engleman. (2002). Langerhans cells renew in the skin throughout life under steady-state conditions. *Nat Immunol* 3:1135-1141.

[38] Dakic A, QX Shao, A D'Amico, M O'Keeffe, WF Chen, K Shortman and L Wu. (2004). Development of the dendritic cell system during mouse ontogeny. *J Immunol* 172:1018-1027.

[39] Sun CM, L Fiette, M Tanguy, C Leclerc and R Lo-Man. (2003). Ontogeny and innate properties of neonatal dendritic cells. *Blood* 102:585-591.

[40] Hinton RA, P Papathanasiou and HC O'Neill. (2011). Distinct in vitro myelopoiesis is dependent on the self-renewal of hematopoietic progenitors. *Scand J Immunol* Sep 29. doi: 10.1111/j.1365-3083.2011.02643.x. [Epub ahead of print].

[41] Zhang Y, Y Wang, M Ogata, S Hashimoto, N Onai and K Matsushima. (2000). Development of dendritic cells in vitro from murine fetal liver-derived lineage phenotype-negative c-kit(+) hematopoietic progenitor cells. *Blood* 95:138-146.

[42] Papathanasiou P, JL Attema, H Karsunky, J Xu, ST Smale and IL Weissman. (2009). Evaluation of the long-term reconstituting subset of hematopoietic stem cells with CD150. *Stem Cells* 27:2498-2508.

[43] Bertrand JY, GE Desanti, R Lo-Man, C Leclerc, A Cumano and R Golub. (2006). Fetal spleen stroma drives macrophage commitment. *Development* 133:3619-3628.

[44] Desanti GE, A Cumano and R Golub. (2008). Identification of CD4int progenitors in mouse fetal spleen, a source of resident lymphoid cells. *J Leukoc Biol* 83:1145-1154.

[45] Hinton R, S Petvises and HC O'Neill. (2010). Myelopoiesis related to perinatal spleen. *Immunol Cell Biol* 89:689-695.

[46] Muthukkumar S, J Goldstein and KE Stein. (2000). The ability of B cells and dendritic cells to present antigen increases during ontogeny. *J Immunol* 165:4803-4813.

[47] Tan JK and HC O'Neill. (2007). Concise review: Dendritic cell development in the context of the spleen microenvironment. *Stem Cells* 25:2139-2145.

[48] Litam PP, HD Friedman and TP Loughran, Jr. (1993). Splenic extramedullary hematopoiesis in a patient receiving intermittently administered granulocyte colony-stimulating factor. *Ann Intern Med* 118:954-955.

[49] Tan JK and HC O'Neill. (2010). Investigation of murine spleen as a niche for hematopoiesis. *Transplantation* 89:140-145.

[50] Dor FJ, ML Ramirez, K Parmar, EL Altman, CA Huang, JD Down and DK Cooper. (2006). Primitive hematopoietic cell populations reside in the spleen: Studies in the pig, baboon, and human. *Exp Hematol* 34:1573-1582.

[51] Wolber FM, E Leonard, S Michael, CM Orschell-Traycoff, MC Yoder and EF Srour. (2002). Roles of spleen and liver in development of the murine hematopoietic system. *Exp Hematol* 30:1010-1019.

INDEX

A

accounting, 94
acid, 12, 19, 28, 42, 56, 86
acute leukemia, 31, 32, 34, 35, 133, 139, 150
acute lung injury, 18, 20
acute lymphoblastic leukemia, 128
acute myelogenous leukemia, 35, 36
acute myeloid leukemia, 35, 49, 128
adaptation, viii, ix, 97, 98, 99, 108, 110, 111, 114
adenovirus, 14, 16, 41
adhesion, 54, 86, 90
adjunctive therapy, 42
adjustment, vii, ix, 98, 99, 101, 104, 106, 107, 111, 112, 113
adulthood, 60, 68
adults, 15, 29, 39, 40, 121, 159
advancements, 98
adverse effects, 107
AFO, 20, 21, 22, 24
Africa, 118
age, ix, 3, 13, 14, 15, 18, 19, 21, 24, 35, 56, 62, 100, 101, 102, 103, 104, 105, 107, 109, 110, 117, 119, 120, 129, 130, 131, 139, 145, 146, 158, 159
agonist, 23
AIDS, 12, 38
airflow obstruction, 22, 25, 43, 47
airways, 4, 7, 21, 25, 43, 44, 46
algorithm, 123, 126, 128, 134
allele, 60, 123, 129, 158
allergic reaction, 143
allergic rhinitis, 27
alopecia, 44
alters, 93
alveolar proteinosis, 28, 49
alveoli, 25
amino, 125
amino acid, 125
anchoring, 54
androgen, 93
anemia, ix, 55, 56, 59, 60, 61, 63, 67, 68, 89, 92, 95, 117, 118, 140
anger, 109
angiogenesis, 94
anisocytosis, 55, 60, 61
ankylosing spondylitis, 136
antibiotic, 6, 57
antibody, 15, 28
antigen, vii, x, 5, 13, 33, 34, 88, 122, 126, 129, 134, 146, 151, 152, 153, 155, 157, 159, 160, 161, 162
antigen-presenting cell, vii, 126
antimicrobial therapy, 29, 32
antiviral agents, 16
antiviral therapy, 14, 15, 40, 41
anxiety, 98, 99, 101, 104, 106, 109, 111
anxiety disorder, 106
APC, 126, 155
APCs, 126
aplastic anemia, 43, 140
apoptosis, 23, 89, 145
appraisals, 107, 112
ARDS, 4
arginine, 87
arterial hypertension, 26
arteries, 73
artery, 26, 73, 77
artificial emboli, 73
aspergillosis, 7, 9, 10, 30, 31, 32, 33, 34, 35, 36
Aspergillus terreus, 31, 32, 33
aspirate, 6, 22
aspiration, 4, 10, 27
assessment, 29, 65, 91, 95, 100, 101, 102, 103, 104, 105, 109, 114, 129
asthma, 27, 49
astrocytes, 75
asymmetry, 75
asymptomatic, 16, 21

atmosphere, 74
atopy, 27, 43
atrophy, 75
attractant, 82, 83
autoantigens, 145
autoimmune disease, ix, 129, 135, 140, 141, 148, 149, 150
autoimmune diseases, ix, 129, 135, 140, 148, 149, 150
autoimmunity, 147
autologous bone marrow transplant, 42, 43
autopsy, 31, 45
avoidance, 106

B

bacteremia, 4
bacteria, ix, 4, 14, 16, 135, 137
bacterial infection, 29
bacterial pathogens, 19
base, 128
BBB, 58, 73, 74, 82, 83
BD, 36, 46
Beck Depression Inventory, 101, 103
behavioral problems, 98
beneficial effect, 79, 132, 150
benefits, 23, 140
bioavailability, 14
biopsy, 10, 13, 18, 19, 22, 25, 26
blastoderm, 93
blastomycosis, 12
bleeding, 9, 121, 138
blood clot, 73
blood cultures, 11, 142
blood flow, 57, 76
blood plasma, 39, 161
blood supply, 57
blood transfusion, 55, 56, 118, 119
blood transfusions, 55, 56, 118, 119
blood vessels, 10, 11, 54, 93
blood-brain barrier, 74, 83
bloodstream, 82
body fluid, 9, 12
body weight, 17, 63, 65, 77
bone marrow transplant, ix, 20, 28, 29, 30, 31, 32, 36, 38, 39, 40, 41, 42, 43, 44, 45, 46, 47, 48, 49, 96, 99, 110, 112, 113, 114, 117, 120, 132, 133, 134, 141, 149, 150
BOS, 48
bowel, ix, 135, 136, 137, 138, 142
bowel perforation, 138
brain, vii, 8, 51, 52, 57, 58, 73, 74, 75, 76, 79, 81, 82, 83, 84, 87, 88, 89, 96
branching, 8, 11, 153
breast cancer, 40
breast carcinoma, 128
breeding, 67
bronchiectasis, 21, 25, 27
bronchioles, 21, 25
bronchiolitis, vii, 1, 3, 14, 22, 24, 25, 43, 44, 45, 46, 47, 48
bronchitis, 27
bronchopneumonia, 8
bronchoscopy, 12, 29, 32, 39
Butcher, 90

C

Cairo, 133
CAM, 90
cancer, 11, 28, 31, 33, 34, 36, 37, 40, 47, 84, 99, 103, 113, 128, 140
cancer cells, 128
candida, 12
candidates, 98
candidiasis, 9, 12
capillary, 26
carcinoma, 132
CARD15, 21, 44
caregiving, 99
CD8+, 145, 152, 155
cell death, 73, 79, 83, 84
cell division, 145
cell line, 62, 89, 152, 159
cell surface, 52, 53, 59, 79, 129, 152, 153
cellular immunity, 39
central nervous system, 34, 52
cephalosporin, 6
cerebral cortex, 89
challenges, vii, 1, 74
channel blocker, 94
chemokines, 27
chemotherapeutic agent, 26
chemotherapy, vii, 1, 2, 13, 18, 51, 52, 59, 65, 113, 119, 139, 148
CHF, 3
childhood, 98, 114
children, vii, viii, ix, 16, 43, 45, 49, 85, 88, 97, 98, 99, 100, 101, 102, 103, 106, 107, 108, 110, 111, 112, 113, 114, 121, 122, 133
chromosome, 124, 129
chronic granulomatous disease, 34
chronic illness, 110, 112
chronic lymphocytic leukemia, 128
cirrhosis, 118
classes, 54, 120, 121

classification, 45, 86, 120, 121, 130, 134
clinical application, 60, 84
clinical diagnosis, 18
clinical presentation, 25, 37
clinical trials, 22, 46
coding, 137
codon, 55
cognitive process, 99, 101, 106
cognitive processing, 99, 101, 106
Cold War, 40
colectomy, 136, 138
colitis, 148, 150
collagen, 73
colon, 136
colonization, 4, 9, 21
color, 10, 78
combination therapy, 10, 40
common findings, 13
communication, 98
community, 14, 15, 16, 29, 45
compatibility, 119, 120
compensation, 63
competition, 59
Competitive Repopulation Assay (CRA), viii, 51, 58
complexity, 124, 131, 134
complications, vii, ix, 1, 2, 3, 27, 28, 29, 43, 44, 45, 46, 48, 110, 117, 119, 122, 123, 124, 126, 138, 139, 143, 144, 146, 147, 148
compounds, ix, 135
computed tomography, 32
Concise, v, 91, 151, 162
concordance, 137
condensation, 55
conditioning, vii, 1, 2, 3, 4, 18, 19, 21, 28, 30, 42, 43, 119, 120, 129, 131, 139, 141, 142, 144, 146
conflict, 103
congestive heart failure, 3
conjunctivitis, 15
consensus, 22, 34, 46, 148
consolidation, 4, 8, 10, 13, 25
construction, 3, 11
contamination, 4
control group, 100
controlled trials, 147
controversial, 13, 15, 16, 53, 137
coping strategies, 99, 101, 106, 107, 109, 111
correlation, ix, 43, 46, 88, 118, 130, 141
cortex, 65
corticosteroid therapy, 4, 5, 7, 19, 26, 42
corticosteroids, 8, 11, 12, 18, 20, 22, 23, 24, 26, 27, 47, 138
cortisol, 93
cough, 8, 10, 12, 13, 15, 16, 18, 19, 21, 22, 25, 27
covering, 71
craniotomy, 73, 74
creatinine, 19
critical period, 108, 111
CSF, 13, 17, 20, 28, 36, 42, 156, 160
CT, 6, 8, 10, 27, 28, 31, 32, 38, 40, 43, 46
culture, 6, 7, 8, 9, 10, 11, 12, 13, 38, 40, 89, 90, 143, 152, 153, 155, 156, 162
cure, 52, 56, 57, 119, 120, 121, 122, 133
cures, viii, 52
CV, 36
cycling, 53
cyclophosphamide, 120, 142, 143, 149
cyclosporine, 8, 23, 24
cystic fibrosis, 23
cystitis, 16
cytokines, 17, 20, 21, 23, 82, 83, 86, 156
cytomegalovirus, 3, 28, 31, 38, 39, 40, 130
cytometry, 64, 153, 154, 156
cytoplasm, 55

D

damages, 72
data set, 131
database, 140, 141
DC progenitor currently, x, 151
deaths, 118, 141
decision-making process, 129, 132
defects, viii, 7, 52, 88, 93
defense mechanisms, 21
deficiency, 28, 60, 95, 144, 146
deficit, 79, 80
degradation, 56
dehydration, 57, 86, 93, 94
dendritic cell, x, 145, 151, 154, 160, 161, 162
deposition, 61
deposits, 63, 65, 69, 71
depression, 99, 101, 104, 107, 109, 111, 113
depressive symptomatology, 107
depressive symptoms, 99, 101, 103, 106, 107, 113
depth, 101, 103, 108, 109
derivatives, 10
destruction, 55, 59, 118
detection, 9, 12, 28, 33, 34, 38, 39, 40, 48, 59, 80, 154
developed countries, 58
diabetes, 118
diagnostic criteria, 7, 18, 19, 22, 42
diarrhea, 136
diploid, 123
disability, 138
disease activity, 143

diseases, vii, ix, 13, 30, 35, 51, 52, 55, 72, 84, 98, 119, 120, 135, 136, 138
disequilibrium, 122
disorder, 3, 26, 27, 48, 88, 106, 118
dissociation, 93
distress, 98, 101, 102, 103, 106, 107, 108, 110, 111, 113, 114
distribution, 7, 12, 15, 25, 91, 129, 161
diversity, 124, 145
DNA, 9, 13, 14, 23, 26, 34, 39, 48, 145
donors, 21, 26, 27, 31, 36, 44, 49, 104, 105, 109, 110, 112, 113, 114, 119, 120, 121, 123, 126, 127, 128, 130, 131, 133, 134
dopaminergic, 95
dosage, 138
drawing, 113
drug toxicity, 27
drug treatment, 130
drugs, 119, 138, 142, 143
dyspnea, 8, 10, 12, 13, 15, 18, 19, 21, 22, 25, 26, 27

E

economics, 131
edema, 2
education, 107, 110, 111
effusion, 13
electrolyte, 9
electrophoresis, 59
eligibility criteria, 98
ELISA, 9
emboli, 4, 73
embolization, 4
embryonic stem cells, 58, 60, 76, 86, 95
emotion, 108
emotional distress, 101, 107, 109
emotional reactions, 109
empirical studies, ix, 97
encephalitis, 12
encephalopathy, 17
encoding, 129
endocrine, ix, 117
endocrine system, ix, 117
endothelial cells, 54, 75, 89, 90, 93, 157
endothelium, 26, 54, 160
engineering, 131
England, 32
enlargement, 60, 63
environment, 3, 27, 73, 107, 158
environmental factors, 137, 144
enzyme, 33
enzyme immunoassay, 33
epidemiology, 13, 30, 38
epidural abscess, 8
epithelial cells, 13, 21
epithelium, 146
Epstein Barr, 17
Epstein-Barr virus, 48
erythrocytes, 54, 93, 158
erythroid cells, 59, 72
erythropoietin, 54, 56
ESCs, 54
esophagus, 8
etanercept, 43
etiology, 4, 17, 19, 21, 27, 42
Europe, 137
evidence, x, 10, 16, 22, 27, 28, 31, 35, 62, 91, 93, 95, 122, 130, 136, 140, 142, 155, 156, 158
evolution, 9
excision, 145
exercise, 56
exertion, 26, 27
exposure, 7, 15, 23, 73, 74, 87
expressiveness, 100, 103, 107, 114
extramedullary hematopoiesis, vii, x, 151, 159, 162

F

faith, 109
false positive, 9, 13
families, vii, viii, ix, 97, 98, 99, 109, 111, 112, 120
family conflict, 107
family environment, 103, 106, 107, 111, 113
family factors, 100, 113
family functioning, 99, 100, 114
family life, 99, 108, 109, 111, 114
family planning, 106
family support, 111
fat, 145
fear, 107, 112
fears, 101, 106, 107
feelings, 98, 102, 106, 108, 109, 110
fertility, 118
fetus, 128
fever, x, 4, 8, 12, 13, 16, 18, 19, 25, 27, 135, 142, 143, 144
fibrosis, 25, 26, 27, 71, 119
filament, 73
filtration, 3, 11, 36
financial, 106, 159
fluid, 9, 11, 13, 18, 25, 33, 38, 39
fluorescence, 88
fluoroquinolones, 6
Food and Drug Administration, 9
formation, 13, 55, 63, 67, 68, 73, 138, 159
fractures, 138

fragments, 62
friend support, 108
fungal infection, 9, 11, 22, 30, 31, 32, 34, 35, 36, 37, 142
fungi, 14, 16, 23, 24, 36, 37

G

gastroenteritis, 12, 16
gastrointestinal tract, ix, 135, 136
gene expression, 85
gene therapy, 87, 90
generalized anxiety disorder, 106
genes, 60, 61, 68, 86, 87, 122, 124, 126, 133, 137
genetic factors, 21, 132, 137
genetics, 148
genome, 137
genotype, 126, 128, 129, 134
glia, 83
glial cells, 83
glucose, 59
glutamic acid, 55
God, 109
grades, 77
grading, 77
graft versus host disease (GVHD), vii, 1
grants, 159
growth, viii, 9, 52, 54, 82, 83, 92, 94, 118, 119, 146, 155
growth factor, viii, 52, 54, 82, 83, 94, 146
guanine, 38
guidelines, 6, 7, 31, 32, 35
guilt, 98, 108, 109

H

half-life, 55, 56, 59, 62, 68, 70
haplotypes, 120, 124, 125, 126, 132, 134
HE, 48, 150
headache, 15, 16
health, viii, 97, 98, 99, 100, 103, 106, 107, 108, 109, 111, 112, 114
health promotion, 114
heart transplantation, 100
helplessness, 108
hematologist, 129
hematology, 31
hematopoiesis, x, 60, 86, 92, 119, 151, 152, 157, 158, 160, 162
hematopoietic development, 158
hematopoietic stem cells, vii, 2, 58, 77, 85, 86, 87, 88, 91, 92, 93, 94, 95, 96, 122, 139, 157, 159, 161, 162
hematopoietic stem-cell transplant, 43
hematopoietic system, 138, 163
hematuria, 143
hemisphere, viii, 52, 74, 75, 78, 81, 83
hemochromatosis, 56, 57
hemoglobin, 55, 56, 61, 62, 67, 68, 69, 85, 86, 87, 88, 89, 91, 92, 93, 94, 118
hemoglobinopathies, 122
hemoglobinopathy, 118
hemoptysis, 8, 10, 18, 31
hemorrhage, vii, 1, 2, 3, 8, 18, 30, 42, 75
hepatitis, 12, 16
hepatomegaly, 119
herpes, 3, 17
herpes simplex, 3, 17
herpes virus, 17
herpes zoster, 3
herpesviruses, 38
heterogeneity, 94, 119
heterozygote, 68
high risk patients, 13, 36
histocompatibility antigens, 122, 129
histogram, 78, 156
histology, viii, 51
histoplasmosis, 12
history, 24, 27, 102, 107, 119, 142, 145, 148
HIV, 150
HIV-1, 150
HLA, ix, 26, 117, 119, 120, 121, 122, 123, 124, 125, 126, 128, 130, 131, 133, 134
home oxygen therapy, 21
homeostasis, 162
hospitalization, 11, 102, 106, 107, 108, 110, 111, 114
host, vii, ix, 1, 2, 8, 9, 27, 28, 36, 43, 44, 45, 46, 47, 53, 57, 84, 91, 117, 119, 120, 121, 123, 133, 134, 139, 140, 142, 144, 145, 146
human, ix, 14, 28, 35, 36, 39, 40, 41, 53, 56, 57, 60, 61, 67, 68, 74, 76, 85, 86, 87, 89, 90, 91, 92, 93, 94, 95, 96, 113, 117, 119, 124, 125, 130, 131, 134, 144, 160, 161, 162
human brain, 130, 131
human leukocyte antigen, ix, 117, 119
hyaline, 13
hyperactivity, 75
hyperinflation, 21, 22, 25
hyperplasia, 55, 63
hypersensitivity, 9
hypertension, 87, 141
hypertrophy, 69
hypogonadism, 118
hypothesis, 54, 106, 129
hypoxemia, 12, 13, 15
hypoxia, 17, 75, 86, 87

I

IBD, ix, x, 135, 136, 137, 138, 141, 144, 145, 147, 148, 149
ID, 42
ideal, 73, 119
identification, 161
idiopathic, vii, 1, 3, 17, 22, 43, 44
IL-17, 137
IL-8, 17, 21, 27
imagery, 111
images, 8
immune function, 36, 155
immune reaction, 140
immune regulation, 137
immune response, ix, x, 25, 122, 124, 129, 135, 137, 151
immune system, x, 4, 13, 119, 132, 136, 137, 138, 139, 140, 144, 146, 147, 150
immunity, x, 26, 38, 41, 146, 151, 160
immunocompromised, 9, 32, 34, 35, 38, 40, 41
immunodeficiency, 139
immunogenetics, vii, 118, 119
immunogenicity, 123
immunoglobulin, 46, 124, 129, 134
immunoglobulin superfamily, 129
immunoglobulins, 14, 21, 23, 40
immunomodulator, 149
immunomodulatory, 134
immunoreactivity, 76
immunosuppression, 2, 10, 47, 147
immunosuppressive agent, 11, 23, 26, 138
immunosuppressive drugs, ix, 135
improvements, 64, 76, 98, 107, 144
in utero, 60, 96
in vitro, 94, 123, 124, 155, 157, 159, 161, 162
in vivo, 53, 88, 90, 92, 93, 94, 151, 153, 159, 160, 161, 162
incidence, vii, 1, 2, 4, 6, 7, 8, 11, 12, 13, 14, 15, 17, 18, 19, 20, 21, 24, 26, 29, 38, 39, 41, 42, 43, 121, 122, 126, 136, 139, 148
India, 118
indirect effect, 31
individuals, 56
induction, ix, 36, 56, 81, 85, 86, 89, 93, 117, 134, 135, 137, 146, 155
induction chemotherapy, 36
induration, 7
infants, 118
infection, 3, 4, 6, 7, 8, 9, 10, 11, 12, 13, 14, 15, 16, 17, 18, 28, 30, 31, 36, 37, 38, 39, 40, 41, 46, 140, 141, 142, 143, 144, 147, 150
inferences, 91
inflammation, 8, 13, 25, 136, 137, 142, 160
inflammatory bowel disease, vii, 148, 149
inflammatory cells, 79
infliximab, 23, 31
influenza, 14, 15, 16, 23
influenza a, 14, 23
informed consent, 109, 110
inherited disorder, 139
inhibition, 47, 128
initiation, 14, 23
injections, viii, 51, 57, 58, 64, 65, 66, 71, 72, 79, 82, 84
injury, vii, 1, 18, 19, 21, 26, 43, 73, 82, 89
innate immunity, 124, 137
insertion, 128
integration, 106
integrins, 92
interferon, 10, 35, 36, 161
interferon-γ, 10
interleukin-8, 46
internalizing, 106
interstitial pneumonitis, 13, 19
intervention, 108, 111, 114
intoxication, 56
intracerebral hemorrhage, 90
intravenous immunoglobulins, 6, 15, 24
intravenously, 5, 10, 15, 82, 83, 95, 138
intrusions, 106
involution, 145, 150
ipsilateral, 78, 81
Iran, 118
iron, ix, 36, 55, 56, 57, 60, 61, 63, 65, 69, 71, 90, 95, 117, 118, 119
irradiation, vii, 2, 3, 7, 13, 18, 19, 44, 51, 52, 53, 59, 60, 64, 65, 66, 71, 72, 84, 138, 139, 148
ischemia, 56, 73, 82, 83, 89, 91, 94, 95
isolation, viii, 7, 12, 32, 97, 99, 109, 115
issues, ix, 73, 98, 100, 109, 110, 112, 114
Italy, 97, 117, 119

J

Jordan, 38, 88, 89

K

K^+, 91
keratinocyte, 146
kidney, 63, 65, 69, 100, 143
kidneys, 8, 55, 60, 61, 69, 71
kinetics, 94

L

labeling, 79
laminar, 11
Langerhans cells, 157, 162
lead, ix, 14, 16, 17, 21, 59, 98, 106, 118, 144, 145, 147
learning, 130, 131
learning process, 130
legionella, 4
lesions, 8, 10, 25, 73, 74, 136
leucocyte, 134
leukemia, 14, 19, 24, 43, 44, 45, 102, 129, 138
leukocytes, 12, 39
leukopenia, 28
LFA, 92
life expectancy, 138
life experiences, 102
lifetime, 102, 107
ligand, 120, 124, 126, 130, 131, 160, 161
light, 23, 147
liver, ix, 8, 26, 37, 55, 60, 61, 63, 69, 94, 100, 117, 118, 119, 157, 158, 159, 162, 163
liver disease, ix, 117
liver transplant, 37
liver transplantation, 37
localization, 54, 91
loci, 120, 122, 123, 124, 128, 137
locus, 120, 122
longitudinal study, 39, 107
lower respiratory tract infection, 14, 15, 16, 17, 19
LTC, 152, 153, 154, 155, 157, 158
lung disease, 7, 41, 45, 48
lung function, 19, 22, 24
lung transplantation, 23, 24, 39, 46, 47
lymph, 26, 86, 145, 152, 161
lymph node, 26, 145, 152, 161
lymphocytes, 21, 25, 26, 85, 126, 140
lymphocytosis, 25
lymphoid, 152, 157, 158, 160, 161, 162
lymphoid organs, 161
lymphoid tissue, 152, 160
lymphoma, 5, 139, 141, 149

M

macrophages, 18, 35, 152, 155, 161
magnesium, 57, 87, 91
magnitude, 107
major depressive disorder, 106
major histocompatibility complex, 124
majority, 12, 21, 24, 53, 71, 81, 106, 120, 158
malaria, 93
malignancy, 9, 19, 36, 104, 112
malnutrition, 136
man, 148
management, vii, 1, 10, 11, 14, 18, 22, 23, 29, 31, 32, 35, 36, 92
marrow, 19, 27, 28, 30, 36, 37, 38, 39, 40, 41, 43, 44, 45, 46, 47, 54, 55, 57, 59, 63, 67, 84, 85, 86, 87, 88, 89, 92, 95, 96, 112, 113, 114, 119, 132, 133, 139, 148, 149, 150, 152, 155, 156, 157, 158, 159
Mars, 92
materials, 73
mathematics, 131
maturation process, 161
MB, 40
MCP, 27
MCP-1, 27
measurement, 34
mechanical ventilation, 12, 15, 18, 19
median, 6, 7, 12, 13, 16, 18, 19, 25, 27, 120, 121, 130, 131, 141, 142, 143
medical, viii, ix, 7, 37, 97, 98, 99, 100, 106, 110, 112, 120, 130, 135
medication, x, 15, 17, 23, 136, 142, 144
medicine, 111, 130, 131
Mediterranean, 118
melanoma, 128
memory, 75, 76, 80, 146, 150
meningitis, 8
mental health, 106, 108, 109, 111
mesenchymal stem cells, 58, 74, 76, 83, 89, 90, 92, 95
mesoderm, 92
messenger ribonucleic acid, 128
meta-analysis, 33
metabolic pathways, 137
methylprednisolone, 18, 122
MHC, 133, 145, 152, 153, 154, 155, 156, 160
mice, viii, 36, 51, 53, 60, 61, 62, 63, 64, 65, 66, 67, 68, 69, 70, 71, 72, 74, 75, 76, 77, 78, 79, 80, 81, 82, 83, 84, 85, 86, 87, 88, 89, 90, 91, 92, 93, 94, 95, 146, 151, 153, 158, 161
microorganism, 4
microorganisms, 137
microscopy, 10, 154
microspheres, 73
Middle Cerebral Artery Occlusion (MCAO), viii, 52
Middle East, 118
migration, 92
mitochondria, 55
models, viii, ix, 34, 51, 52, 57, 60, 64, 67, 68, 73, 74, 87, 91, 135, 139
mold, 30, 33
molds, 11

molecules, 56, 86, 90, 120, 122, 124, 125, 128, 129, 145
monoclonal antibody, 8, 15, 48
monolayer, 152
monozygotic twins, 137
morbidity, vii, ix, 1, 2, 16, 21, 55, 58, 113, 117, 132, 136, 138, 139, 143, 147
morphological abnormalities, 55
morphology, 61, 62, 81, 153, 155, 157
mortality, vii, x, 1, 2, 4, 7, 9, 13, 14, 15, 16, 17, 19, 21, 24, 25, 26, 28, 29, 38, 41, 55, 57, 58, 119, 120, 121, 123, 124, 132, 133, 135, 139, 140, 141, 142, 144, 147, 148
mortality rate, 4, 9, 19, 120, 139, 140, 141, 147
mosaic, 22
motor skills, 80
MR, 33, 34, 42, 43, 45, 46, 48
MRI, 89
mRNA, 128
mRNAs, 128
mucormycosis, 31
mucosa, 136
multiple myeloma, 138
multiple sclerosis, 141, 150
multipotent, vii, 51, 52, 145
multivariate, 123, 126, 131
musculoskeletal, 136
music, 111
music therapy, 111
mutagenesis, 158
mutant, 61, 158
mutation, 61, 67, 89, 90
mutations, 67
mycobacteria, 7, 30
mycobacterial infection, 7, 30
myelosuppression, viii, 51, 57, 59, 60, 64, 71, 72
myocardium, 89

N

National Institutes of Health, 19, 22, 46
necrosis, 8, 11
neovascularization, 85, 91
Netherlands, 135
neural network, 130, 134
neural networks, 130, 134
neurogenesis, 75, 89, 94
neurological disease, 52
neurons, viii, 52, 75, 76, 83, 131
neutropenia, 3, 4, 5, 6, 7, 10, 11, 13, 14, 29, 35, 42, 139
neutrophils, 13, 25
nitric oxide, 57, 91
NK cells, 124, 126, 127, 128, 133
nocardiosis, 6, 29
nodules, 6, 8, 11, 13, 14, 15, 32
nucleic acid, 12
nucleus, 55
null, 90

O

obstacles, 58, 122
obstruction, 20, 23, 26, 44, 89
obstructive lung disease, 43, 45
occlusion, 26, 56, 73, 74, 77, 78, 81, 83
OH, 91
opacification, 12, 13
open lung biopsy, 6, 8, 11, 13
opportunities, 110
optimism, 102, 107
optimization, 58, 64, 119
organ, x, 9, 20, 26, 28, 30, 36, 37, 39, 45, 55, 56, 59, 60, 61, 63, 67, 68, 87, 99, 139, 151, 159
organism, 6
organs, 8, 11, 12, 52, 55, 58, 61, 63, 69, 71, 84, 118
outpatient, 23, 24
overall survival (OS), ix, 117, 119
overlap, 137
overlay, 154, 156
overtime, 57, 74, 81, 84
oxidation, 88
oxidative damage, 88
oxidative stress, 87
oxygen, 19, 23, 24, 27, 54, 56, 67, 91, 118

P

paediatric patients, 47
pain, 10, 27, 136
pancreas, 88, 118
panic disorder, 106
parallel, ix, 66, 70, 117, 157
paralysis, 78
parenting, 99, 100, 103, 106, 107, 111
parents, viii, ix, 97, 98, 99, 100, 101, 102, 103, 104, 106, 108, 109, 110, 111, 112, 113, 114
pathogenesis, vii, 1, 17, 18, 21, 22, 25, 27, 36, 130, 137, 148
pathogens, 4, 14, 32, 36, 146
pathology, 22, 57, 61, 67, 68, 94
pathophysiology, 52, 86, 89
pathways, 137
PCR, 9, 12, 13, 26, 33, 39, 120
PCT, 48
penicillin, 88

peptide, 145
perianal abscess, 143
pericardial effusion, 143
pericardium, 10
perinatal, 157, 158, 162
peripheral blood, 2, 17, 20, 23, 29, 38, 39, 44, 52, 58, 59, 61, 62, 63, 64, 66, 68, 69, 70, 71, 72, 76, 94, 95, 105, 110, 139, 142, 145
peripheral blood mononuclear cell, 23
permeability, 17, 58, 67, 72, 83
phenotype, 54, 56, 57, 58, 59, 60, 61, 64, 68, 73, 84, 94, 152, 153, 155, 156, 161, 162
phenotypes, viii, 51
Philadelphia, 88, 89, 91, 95
phlebotomy, 119
phosphate, 59
photophobia, 10
physical health, 98, 99, 108
physiology, 18, 64
pilot study, 46
placebo, 35, 47
plasticity, 95, 159
platelets, 52, 53
pleura, 8
pleural effusion, 8, 10, 15
pleural rub, 10
pleuritic chest pain, 8
PM, 28, 33, 48, 148, 160
pneumococcus, 23
pneumocystis pneumonia, 12
pneumonia, vii, 1, 2, 3, 4, 6, 12, 13, 14, 15, 16, 17, 18, 19, 22, 24, 25, 27, 28, 29, 31, 34, 36, 37, 38, 39, 40, 42, 43, 44, 46, 47, 48, 150
pneumonitis, 12, 13, 38, 39, 48
pneumothorax, 45
point mutation, 55, 158
polar, 56
polymer, 68
polymerase, 34, 40, 120
polymerase chain reaction, 34, 40, 120
polymerization, 56, 67
polymorphism, 21, 122, 124, 128, 129, 130, 131, 134
polymorphisms, 129, 134, 137
polyphenols, 88
polysaccharide, 9, 28
population, 6, 15, 27, 53, 59, 69, 79, 94, 144, 148, 152, 153, 155, 157, 158
Portugal, 42
post-transcriptional regulation, 128
post-transplant, x, 4, 6, 7, 13, 16, 20, 26, 48, 69, 106, 136
posttraumatic stress, 110, 113
potential benefits, 111
precursor cells, 162
prednisone, 23, 26
pregnancy, 128
premature death, 63
preparation, 110, 114
prevention, 14, 26, 29, 30, 38, 39, 40, 48, 57, 86, 119
primary function, 155
priming, 160
principles, 87, 88, 91
probability, 7, 119, 120, 121, 123
progenitor cells, 54, 79, 85, 86, 88, 90, 138, 157, 159, 162
prognosis, 16, 17, 20, 24, 27, 119, 132
pro-inflammatory, 23
project, 22, 46, 67, 159
proliferation, x, 26, 53, 66, 75, 145, 151, 154, 155
promoter, 60
propagation, 58, 74, 82
prophylactic, 5, 6, 12, 14, 23, 37
prophylactic agents, 12
prophylaxis, vii, 1, 4, 6, 11, 12, 13, 14, 17, 19, 24, 36, 37, 39, 41, 43, 119, 121, 122
protection, viii, 52, 79, 81, 83, 84, 129, 132
protective factors, 107
proteins, 12, 85
Pseudomonas aeruginosa, 29
psoriasis, 140
psychiatrist, 101
psychological distress, 98, 104, 108
psychological health, vii, viii, ix, 97, 99, 101, 108, 110, 111
psychological well-being, 98, 99
psychology, viii, 97, 98, 131
psychosocial development, 104
psychosocial interventions, ix, 98, 99, 111, 112
PTSD, 99, 101, 106, 107, 111, 113
pulmonary alveolar proteinosis, 28, 49
pulmonary edema, 17, 26, 143
pulmonary function test, 19, 21, 46
pulmonary hypertension, 140
pulmonary rehabilitation, 23, 24
pulp, 63
purification, 52, 53
purity, 53
pyelonephritis, 143
pyoderma gangrenosum, 136
pyridoxine, 5

Q

quality of life, 98, 99, 101, 103, 104, 107, 109, 111, 112, 119
questioning, 120

questionnaire, 101

R

radiation, 18, 24, 148
rash, 15, 17
RE, 29, 31, 33, 34, 38, 40, 41, 46, 47, 48
reactions, 10, 21, 161
reactive oxygen, 137
reactivity, 140
receptors, 54, 124, 128, 129, 130, 133, 134
recognition, 85
recombination, 60
recommendations, 35, 98
recovery, 8, 16, 18, 28, 31, 42, 46, 75, 76, 79, 80, 82, 83, 84, 90, 91, 95, 106, 121, 146, 154
rectum, 136
recurrence, 29, 136
red blood cells, viii, ix, 51, 52, 55, 62, 69, 71, 72, 88, 117, 118
reduction division, 55
regenerate, 53
regeneration, 90, 146
registries, ix, 117, 119
Registry, 122, 124
regression, 81, 130, 134
rejection, 119, 121, 122, 123, 126, 127, 128, 129, 132, 133, 139
relapses, 144
relaxation, 111
relevance, 41
relief, 57
religion, 107, 111
religious beliefs, 109
remission, ix, 135, 138, 140, 141, 142, 143, 144, 146, 147, 149, 150
repair, viii, 52, 84
requirements, 19, 72, 84, 88, 160
researchers, 124
resection, 10, 35
resilience, 107, 114
resistance, 14, 26, 29
resolution, 8, 27, 40, 43, 46, 120, 122, 123, 128
resources, 99, 100, 108, 114
respiratory distress syndrome, 42
respiratory failure, 13, 14, 15, 19, 20, 21, 24, 26, 28, 42, 49
respiratory syncytial virus, 3, 14, 40, 41
Respiratory syncytial virus, 40
response, 4, 11, 14, 18, 20, 25, 26, 27, 38, 40, 47, 54, 91, 137, 139, 143
responsiveness, 67, 156
restrictive lung disease, 19
RH, 37, 44
rheumatoid arthritis, 140
rhinorrhea, 15, 16
rhinovirus infection, 17
Rhizopus, 11
ribonucleic acid, 55
righting, 77
risk, vii, viii, 1, 4, 6, 7, 8, 9, 10, 11, 13, 14, 15, 16, 20, 21, 23, 26, 29, 30, 31, 32, 36, 37, 40, 41, 44, 45, 46, 97, 98, 99, 106, 107, 108, 110, 112, 113, 119, 120, 121, 123, 126, 127, 128, 129, 130, 131, 132, 133, 137, 138, 140, 142, 144, 146, 147, 148
risk assessment, 128
risk factors, vii, 1, 6, 8, 11, 13, 21, 26, 29, 30, 32, 37, 40, 41, 45, 46, 132, 137, 148
risks, 43, 95, 124, 140
rituximab, 23
RNA, 55, 131
rodents, 74
rods, 6
RSV infection, 15

S

safety, 36, 147
sarcoidosis, 27, 48
school, 98, 109, 110
scleroderma, 27
SCT, 100, 101, 102, 103, 112, 125, 134, 149
search terms, viii, 97, 98
secrete, 82, 83
secretion, viii, 52, 93
seeding, 66, 86, 94
segregation, 120
self-concept, 100
self-esteem, 98, 109
self-reports, 104
self-worth, 102, 107
semi-structured interviews, 102
sensitivity, 9, 12, 13, 15, 22, 33
sepsis, 14, 19, 20, 121, 143
septic shock, 4, 141
sequencing, 129
serology, 131
serum, 9, 14, 19, 21, 33, 34, 44
sex, 59, 146
sex steroid, 146
shape, 56, 86
showing, ix, 7, 10, 18, 22, 58, 62, 64, 78, 135, 158
sibling, 43, 98, 103, 105, 110, 114, 119, 121, 122, 133, 134
sibling support, 110

siblings, viii, ix, 97, 98, 99, 104, 105, 109, 110, 111, 112, 113, 114
sickle cell, viii, 51, 52, 55, 56, 67, 85, 86, 87, 88, 89, 90, 91, 92, 93, 94, 95, 133
sickle cell anemia, 85, 87, 88, 89
sickle cell disease (SCD), viii, 51, 52, 55, 85
side effects, 9, 10, 52, 138, 142, 148
signals, 128
signs, 4, 7, 8, 9, 12, 18, 19, 21, 26, 61, 77, 78
silver, 73
sinusitis, 21
skin, 7, 8, 10, 15, 17, 122, 136, 140, 157, 162
smoking, 137
social competence, 100
social life, 99
social stress, 107
social support, 101, 107
socioeconomic status, 106, 111
sodium, 87
solid tumors, 18
solubility, 91
Southeast Asia, 118
SP, 43, 46, 53, 94
Spain, 37
species, 8, 11, 12, 21, 32, 34, 88, 137
spirituality, 108, 109
spleen, vii, x, 26, 52, 59, 60, 61, 63, 64, 65, 69, 71, 90, 94, 145, 151, 152, 153, 155, 156, 157, 158, 159, 160, 162, 163
splenomegaly, 61, 63, 69
spousal support, 108, 114
sprouting, 75
sputum, 6, 8, 10, 13, 22
sputum culture, 22
SS, 31, 32, 43
SSA, 146, 147
stabilization, 21, 22
standard deviation, 63
staphylococci, 6
state, 53, 139, 144, 145, 152, 153, 155, 157, 161, 162
stem cell differentiation, 93
stem cells, vii, 1, 2, 13, 14, 24, 26, 27, 51, 52, 53, 54, 57, 58, 59, 72, 73, 74, 76, 79, 83, 84, 86, 87, 88, 89, 90, 91, 92, 94, 96, 121, 122, 133, 138, 139, 142, 158
sterile, 10
steroids, 19
stimulation, 151, 152, 160
storage, 96
strategy use, 71
stress, 63, 98, 99, 100, 102, 103, 106, 107, 109, 111, 113, 114, 115, 159
stress reactions, 98
stress response, 99
strictures, 138
stroke, viii, 52, 57, 58, 73, 74, 75, 78, 79, 80, 81, 82, 83, 84, 85, 88, 89, 90, 91, 94, 95, 96
stroma, 145, 153, 155, 156, 157, 158, 159, 160, 162
stromal cells, 54, 92
structure, 131
style, 108
subacute, 20, 25, 34
subgroups, 147
submucosa, 136
substance use, 107
substitution, 55
sulfate, 86
Sun, 89, 162
supplementation, viii, 52, 83
suppression, 36, 86, 140, 147, 149
surface area, 17, 65
surfactant, 21, 28, 44
surfactant proteins, 28
surgical debridement, 11
surgical resection, ix, 35, 135
surveillance, 30, 39
survival, viii, ix, x, 5, 6, 14, 19, 35, 41, 42, 44, 47, 51, 58, 59, 61, 74, 75, 79, 80, 84, 91, 98, 117, 119, 120, 121, 122, 130, 132, 135, 141, 144, 146
survival rate, 19, 98, 119, 122, 146
survivors, 19, 27, 47, 112, 113
susceptibility, 129, 132, 144, 145
swelling, 73
symptoms, ix, 4, 7, 8, 12, 13, 15, 18, 19, 21, 22, 23, 56, 57, 99, 101, 106, 107, 111, 118, 135, 143
syndrome, vii, 1, 2, 3, 12, 17, 18, 19, 20, 22, 36, 41, 42, 43, 44, 46, 48, 150
synthesis, 55, 56, 90, 93, 96, 118
systemic lupus erythematosus, 140
systemic sclerosis, 140, 148

T

T cell, x, 12, 13, 23, 26, 48, 129, 134, 136, 139, 140, 141, 144, 145, 146, 147, 150, 152, 153, 155, 157, 160, 161
lymphocytes, 8, 129, 146
Taiwan, 115
target, 21
TCR, 145, 146, 150
techniques, 12, 111
technology, 153
temperature, 17
temporary protection, 84
tension, 91
testing, 15, 33, 60, 123

TGF, 47
thalassemia, vii, viii, ix, 36, 51, 52, 55, 56, 57, 59, 60, 61, 63, 64, 68, 71, 72, 85, 86, 87, 88, 89, 90, 92, 93, 95, 96, 117, 118, 119, 120, 121, 122, 123, 126, 128, 129, 130, 131, 132, 133, 134, 139
thalassemia-free survival (TFS), ix, 117, 119, 120
T-helper cell, 7
therapeutic interventions, 110, 111
thoracoscopy, 13, 22, 25
thoughts, 106
threats, 36
thrombosis, 11
thymus, x, 136, 145, 146, 147, 152
tissue, viii, x, 8, 10, 11, 12, 18, 25, 52, 53, 54, 56, 74, 78, 79, 81, 82, 83, 84, 140, 151, 159, 161
TNF, 8, 17, 19, 20, 21, 23, 148, 150, 156
TNF-α, 17, 21, 23, 156
tones, 110
top-down, 138
toxic megacolon, 138
toxicity, 2, 34, 86, 139
trafficking, 87, 160
trajectory, 105, 114
transcription, 92, 158
transfusion, ix, 10, 39, 57, 85, 86, 93, 95, 117, 118, 122, 126, 143
transgene, 57, 67, 85
transmission, 3, 27, 48
transplant, x, 2, 3, 7, 9, 14, 19, 21, 26, 29, 30, 33, 36, 37, 38, 39, 40, 41, 42, 44, 45, 46, 47, 64, 66, 79, 80, 81, 95, 100, 101, 102, 103, 104, 105, 106, 108, 109, 110, 111, 112, 113, 122, 136, 139, 142
transplant recipients, 9, 26, 29, 30, 33, 36, 37, 38, 39, 40, 41, 42, 46, 47
transport, 160
trauma, 52, 107, 114
traumatic events, 101, 102
trial, 10, 33, 36, 37, 39, 41, 44, 46, 47, 87, 88, 90, 142, 147
triggers, 27
tuberculosis, 6, 30
tumor, ix, 36, 43, 44, 47, 135, 138, 140
tumor necrosis factor, ix, 36, 43, 44, 47, 135, 138
tumors, 75
Turkey, 118
turnover, 67, 88

U

ulcerative colitis, 136, 149, 150
ultrasonography, 85
umbilical cord, 2, 20, 43, 49, 76, 90, 95, 133, 139
underlying mechanisms, 136, 147
upper airways, 4
upper respiratory tract, 14, 15, 21, 22, 41
urine, 13, 34
USA, 85, 86, 87, 89, 91, 92, 93, 95, 96

V

vaccinations, 23
vaccine, 4, 5, 14, 29
validation, 87
valine, 55
valuation, 136
vancomycin, 6
variables, ix, 33, 111, 118, 119, 130, 131, 132
variations, 92
vaso-occlusion, 57, 67
ventilation, 11, 19
venules, 26
vessels, 27, 54, 76
viral infection, vii, 1, 14, 15, 16, 17, 21, 22, 24, 40, 41
virus infection, 15, 16, 39, 40, 41
viruses, 2, 13, 14, 17, 40, 41, 45
VLA, 92

W

walking, 77
Washington, ix, 93, 117
weight gain, 17
well-being, 104
wheezing, 22, 25
white blood cells, 52, 59, 62, 70, 71, 72
white matter, 89
wild type, 158
World Health Organization (WHO), ix, 117
worldwide, 119
worry, 108

Y

Y chromosome, 59
yield, 9, 32, 58, 72, 92
young adults, 122

Z

zinc, 158
zygomycosis, 37